# GREEN NANOMATERIALS

*Sustainable Technologies and Applications*

# GREEN NANOMATERIALS

*Sustainable Technologies and Applications*

*Edited by*
**Kaushik Pal, PhD.; DSc**

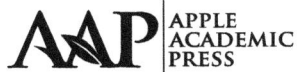

**A∧P** | APPLE
ACADEMIC
PRESS

First edition published 2022

**Apple Academic Press Inc.**
1265 Goldenrod Circle, NE,
Palm Bay, FL 32905 USA
4164 Lakeshore Road, Burlington,
ON, L7L 1A4 Canada

**CRC Press**
6000 Broken Sound Parkway NW,
Suite 300, Boca Raton, FL 33487-2742 USA
4 Park Square, Milton Park,
Abingdon, Oxon, OX14 4RN UK

© 2022 by Apple Academic Press, Inc.

*Apple Academic Press exclusively co-publishes with CRC Press, an imprint of Taylor & Francis Group, LLC*

**Library and Archives Canada Cataloguing in Publication**

Title: Green nanomaterials : sustainable technologies and applications / edited by Kaushik Pal, PhD.
Names: Pal, Kaushik, editor.
Description: First edition. | Includes bibliographical references and index.
Identifiers: Canadiana (print) 20210280352 | Canadiana (ebook) 20210280425 | ISBN 9781771889650 (hardcover) | ISBN 9781774639665 (softcover) | ISBN 9781003130314 (ebook)
Subjects: LCSH: Nanostructured materials—Environmental aspects. | LCSH: Nanotechnology—Environmental aspects.
Classification: LCC TA418.9.N35 G74 2022 | DDC 620.1/15—dc23

**Library of Congress Cataloging-in-Publication Data**

Names: Pal, Kaushik, editor.
Title: Green nanomaterials : sustainable technologies and applications / edited by Kaushik Pal.
Description: First edition. | Palm Bay, FL : Apple Academic Press, 2022. | Includes bibliographical references and index. | Summary: "Recent technological advancements in green nanotechnology have opened a brand new avenue for research and development in the field of medicinal plants-mediated nanoparticles, biopolymer, biotechnology, and antimicrobial and biomedical research. This new volume, Green Nanomaterials: Sustainable Technologies and Applications, explores a number of eco-friendly technologies in green materials synthesis, which are of considerable importance. It takes an inter- and cross-multidisciplinary approach to the green chemistry of nanoengineering and green nanotechnology application in materials research. It provides informative coverage of this exciting and dynamic new field as well as relates the fundamentals of soft-nanomaterials fabrication and brand new spectroscopic integration. The book explores bio-inspired self-assembly green nanomaterials for multifunctional applications as well as the design and synthesis of green polymeric nanomaterials for a number of pharmaceutical and biomedical applications, including biosensors, drug delivery, antimicrobial applications, etc. Also discussed is the fabrication of green polymer nanocomposites from waste and natural fibers, such as chitin fiber, chitin whisker fiber, cellulose fiber, nano cellulose fiber, eggshells, and cotton waste. The book is a unique mixture of exclusive ideas from peer-reviewed papers, reports from the latest research newsletters, mini reviews, and invited papers on key developments in the field. It will be a helpful resource for scientists and researchers, industry professionals, and faculty and advanced students in this area"-- Provided by publisher.
Identifiers: LCCN 2021036350 (print) | LCCN 2021036351 (ebook) | ISBN 9781771889650 (hardcover) | ISBN 9781774639665 (paperback) | ISBN 9781003130314 (ebook)
Subjects: MESH: Nanostructures | Nanotechnology | Biocompatible Materials
Classification: LCC R857.N34 (print) | LCC R857.N34 (ebook) | NLM QT 36.5 | DDC 610.285--dc23
LC record available at https://lccn.loc.gov/2021036350
LC ebook record available at https://lccn.loc.gov/2021036351

ISBN: 978-1-77188-965-0 (hbk)
ISBN: 978-1-77463-966-5 (pbk)
ISBN: 978-1-00313-031-4 (ebk)

# About the Editor

**Kaushik Pal, PhD.; DSc**

*Laboratório de Biopolímeros e Sensores, Instituto de Macromoléculas, Universidade do Rio de Janeiro, Rio de Janeiro – RJ, 21941-901, Brazil.*

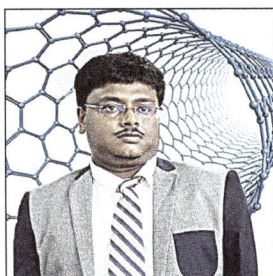

Kaushik Pal, PhD, is a Distinuished Professor at Laboratório de Biopolímeros e Sensores, Instituto de Macromoléculas, Universidade do Rio de Janeiro, Brazil, as well as former fellow Scientist at Wuhan University, Republic of China. Prior to that, he was a Visiting Professor at the International and Inter University Centre for Nanoscience and Nanotechnology (IIUCNN) School of Energy Materials, Mahatma Gandhi University, Kottayam, Kerala, India, as well as Chief-Scientist and Faculty (CAS) Fellow at the Chinese Academy of Science. In the year 2020, he received the Honoris Causa Doctor of Science (DSc) award from the Ministry of Education, Govt. of Malaysia, Institut Kemahiran Tinggi Belia Negara, Sepang, Selangor, Malaysia.

Dr. Pal supervises a significant number of students pursuing their bachelor, master, PhD, and postdoctoral degrees. He has published more than 110 significant research articles in several international top-tier journals, including those published by IOP Nanotechnology, Royal Chemical Society, Elsevier, Springer, IEEE publications, CRC Press Taylor and Francis, etc. He has also edited and published book chapters and review articles. Dr. Pal is an editorial member of the *World Journal of Nanoscience and Nanotechnology, Current Graphene Science, Journal of Chemical Reviews,* and others. Professor Pal is an expert group leader as well as the associate member of various scientific societies, organizations, and professional bodies. He was the chairperson of 35 national or international events, symposia, conferences, workshops, summer internships and has contributed many plenary, keynote, and invited lectures worldwide. He has also been a reviewer of over 150 journal articles.

Dr. Pal's awards include the Marie-Curie Experienced Researcher (Postdoctoral Fellow), offered by the European Commission in Greece and the Brain Korea (BK-21), National Research Foundation Visiting Scientist Fellowship in South Korea. He also served as Research Professor (Group Leader & Independent Scientist) at Bharath University (BIHER), Research and Development, Chennai, India.

Dr. Pal's research interests include nanofabrication, functional materials, condensed matter physics, CNTs/graphene, liquid crystal, polymeric nanocomposite, switchable devices, electron microscopy and spectroscopy, bio-inspired materials, drug delivery, tissue engineering, cell culture and integration, switchable device modulation, flexible and transparent electrodes, supercapacitor, optoelectronics, green chemistry, and biosensor applications.

# Contents

# Contributors

**Khalid M. Al-Batanyeh**
Department of Biological Sciences, Yarmouk University, Irbid, Jordan

**Alaa A. A. Aljabali**
Department of Pharmaceutical Science, Faculty of Pharmacy, Yarmouk University, Irbid, Jordan,
E-mail: alaaj@yu.edu.jo

**Alaa Alqudah**
Department of Pharmaceutical Science, Faculty of Pharmacy, Yarmouk University, Irbid, Jordan

**S. I. Asiya**
Bharath Institute of Higher Education and Research, Bharath University, 173 Agharam Road,
Selaiyur, Chennai – 600073, Tamil Nadu, India, E-mail: asiya_najeeb@yahoo.com

**Kesana Surendra Babu**
Department of Chemistry (PG Studies), Shree Velagapudi Rama Krishna Memorial College,
Nagaram – 522268, Guntur District, Andhra Pradesh, India

**Stephen Boakye-Ansah**
Department of Chemical Engineering, Henry M. Rowan College of Engineering, Rowan University,
201 Mullica Hill Road, Glassboro, NJ – 08028, United States

**Murthy Chavali**
NTRC-MCETRC and Aarshanano Composite Technologies Pvt. Ltd., Guntur District – 522201
Andhra Pradesh, India, Tel.: +91-8309337736; +91-9642878182,
E-mails: ChavaliM@gmail.com; ChavaliM@outlook.com

**Dinesh Kumar Chellappan**
Department of Life Sciences, School of Pharmacy, International Medical University, Bukit Jalil,
Kuala Lumpur – 57000, Malaysia

**Michael K. Danquah**
Chemical Engineering Department, University of Tennessee, Chattanooga, TN – 37403, USA

**Kamal Dua**
The discipline of Pharmacy, Graduate School of Health, University of Technology, Sydney,
NSW – 2007, Australia

**Harish Dureja**
Department of Pharmaceutical Sciences, Maharshi Dayanand University, Rohtak – 124001, India

**Amal Elhussieny**
Center of Nanoscience and Technology (CNT), Nile University, Nile Avenue, Giza, Egypt

**Kareem M. Abd El-Rahman**
Department of Materials Science, Institute of Graduate Studies and Research, Alexandria University,
Alexandria, Egypt

**Nicola. M. Everitt**
Bioengineering Research Group, Faculty of Engineering, University of Nottingham,
University Park, Nottingham NG7 2RD, UK

**M. Faisal**
Center of Nanoscience and Technology (CNT), Nile University, Nile Avenue, Giza, Egypt

**Gaurav Gupta**
School of Pharmacy, Suresh Gyan Vihar University, Jagatpura, Jaipur – 302017, India

**Jaison Jeevanandam**
Department of Chemical Engineering, Faculty of Engineering and Science, Curtin University,
CDT 250, Miri – 98009, Sarawak, Malaysia, E-mail: jaison.jeevanandam@gmail.com

**Kuruvilla Joseph**
Department of Chemistry, Indian Institute of Space Science and Technology, Valiyamala,
Thiruvananthapuram, Kerala, India, E-mail: sarithatvla@gmail.com

**Deepak N. Kapoor**
School of Pharmaceutical Sciences, Shoolini University of Biotechnology and Management
Sciences, Solan – 173229, India

**Yokraj Katre**
Department of Chemistry, Kalyan PG College, Bhilai Nagar, Durg – 490006, Chhattisgarh, India

**Bala S. C. Koritala**
Department of Pharmaceutical Sciences, College of Pharmacy and Pharmaceutical Sciences,
Washington State University, Spokane, WA – 99202, USA; Sleep and Performance Research Center,
Washington State University, Spokane, WA – 99210, USA

**Mannam Krishnamurthy**
Department of Chemistry (PG Studies), Shree Velagapudi Rama Krishna Memorial College,
Nagaram – 522268, Guntur District, Andhra Pradesh, India; Varsity Education Management Limited,
Ayyappa Society Main Road, Hyderabad – 500081, Telangana, India

**Anil Kumar**
Department of Biotechnology, Government V.Y.T. PG. Autonomous College, Durg – 491001,
Chhattisgarh, India

**Enamala Manoj Kumar**
Bioserve Biotechnologies (India) Private Ltd., Hyderabad, A Reprocell Company, 3-1-135/1A,
CNR Complex, Genome Valley Main Road, R.R. District, Mallapur, Hyderabad – 500076,
Telangana, India

**Meegle S. Mathew**
Department of Chemistry, Indian Institute of Space Science and Technology, Valiyamala,
Thiruvananthapuram, Kerala, India, E-mail: meeglesmathew@gmail.com

**Vijay Mishra**
School of Pharmaceutical Sciences, Lovely Professional University, Phagwara, Punjab – 144411,
India

**Poonam Negi**
School of Pharmaceutical Sciences, Shoolini University of Biotechnology and Management
Sciences, Solan – 173229, India

**Mohammad A. Obeid**
Department of Pharmaceutical Science, Faculty of Pharmacy, Yarmouk University, Irbid, Jordan

**Kaushik Pal**
Laboratório de Biopolímeros e Sensores, Instituto de Macromoléculas,
Universidade do Rio de Janeiro, Rio de Janeiro – RJ, 21941-901, Brazil,
E-mails: kaushikpal@whu.edu.cn; kaushikphysics@gmail.com

**Parteek Prasher**
Department of Chemistry, University of Petroleum and Energy Studies, Dehradun – 248007, India

**I. Samy**
Assistant Professor, Engineering Department, Nile University, Cairo, Egypt; Center of Nanoscience
and Technology (CNT), Nile University, Nile Avenue, Giza, Egypt; Department of Industrial
Engineering and Service Management, School of Engineering, Nile University, Nile Avenue, Giza,
Egypt; Smart Engineering Systems Research Center, Nile University, Nile Avenue, Giza – 116453,
Egypt, E-mail: isamy@nu.edu.eg

**Appukuttan Saritha**
Department of Chemistry, School of Arts and Sciences, Amrita Vishwa Vidyapeetham, Amritapuri,
Clappana, Kollam, Kerala, India, E-mails: kjoseph.iist@gmail.com; sarithatvla@gmail.com

**Saurabh Satija**
School of Pharmaceutical Sciences, Lovely Professional University, Phagwara, Punjab – 144411,
India

**Ajaya Kumar Singh**
Department of Chemistry, Government V.Y.T. PG. Autonomous College, Durg – 491001,
Chhattisgarh, India, E-mail: ajayaksingh_au@yahoo.co.in

**S. Sreevidya**
Department of Chemistry, Kalyan PG College, Bhilai Nagar, Durg – 490006, Chhattisgarh, India

**Kirtana Sankara Subramanian**
Department of Food Science, Faculty of Veterinary and Agriculture Science,
University of Melbourne, Melbourne, Australia

**Malakondaiah Suresh**
Loyola Institute of Frontier Energy, Post Graduate and Research Department of Advanced Zoology
and Biotechnology, Loyola College, Chennai – 600034, Tamil Nadu, India

**Murtaza M. Tambuwala**
SAAD Center for Pharmacy and Diabetes, School of Pharmacy and Pharmaceutical Science,
Ulster University, Coleraine, UK

**Aparna Tirumalasetti**
Department of Chemistry, International Institute of Information Technology (IIIT), Nuzvid Campus,
Rajiv Gandhi University of Knowledge Technologies, Nuzvid (RGUKTN)-AP, Mylavaram Road,
Nuzvid – 521202, Krishna District, Andhra Pradesh, India

**Tean Zaheer**
Department of Parasitology, University of Agriculture, Faisalabad, Pakistan,
E-mail: teanzaheer942@gmail.com

**Mazhar S. Al Zoubi**
Department of Basic Medical Studies, Yarmouk University, Irbid, Jordan

# Abbreviations

| | |
|---|---|
| ACh | acetylcholine |
| AChE | acetylcholinesterase |
| AD | Alzheimer's disease |
| ADSCs | adipose-derived stem cells |
| AFM | atomic force microscopy |
| Ag | Argentum |
| AgNO$_3$ | silver nitrate |
| Al | aluminum |
| ALP | alkaline phosphatase |
| AMPs | antimicrobial peptides |
| APTE | 3-aminopropyltriethoxysilane |
| ASE | accelerated solvent |
| Au | aurum |
| BA | bio-active |
| BCP | biphasic calcium phosphate |
| Bi | bismuth |
| BSA | bovine serum albumin |
| BTE | bone tissue engineering |
| C | carbon |
| C | chromatographic |
| CaP | calcium phosphates |
| Cat-CS | catechol modified-chitosan |
| CBD-BDNF | collagen-binding neurotrophic factors |
| CeO$_2$ | cerium dioxide |
| CHyA | collagen–HyA |
| CO | carbon monoxide |
| Co | cobalt |
| CO$_2$ | carbon dioxide |
| COSs | chitooligosaccharides |
| CSD | chitosan derivatives |
| CTAB | cetyltrimethylammonium bromide |
| Cu | copper |
| DAD | diode array detector |

| | |
|---|---|
| DD | degree of deacetylation |
| DDAB | di-dodecyl dimethylammonium bromide |
| DHS | dry heat |
| DLS | dynamic light scattering |
| DNA | deoxyribonucleic acid |
| DOX | doxorubicin |
| DP | degree of polymerization |
| E | extraction |
| ECM | extracellular matrix |
| ESBL | extended-spectrum beta-lactamase |
| EtO | ethylene oxide |
| Fe | iron |
| FHB | fibroblasts |
| FL-Na | fluorescein Na |
| FN | facial nerve |
| FT-IR | Fourier transform infrared |
| GA | glutaraldehyde |
| GAGs | glycosaminoglycans |
| GFAAS | graphite furnace atomic absorption spectroscopy |
| GlcNAc | N-acetyl-d-glucosamine |
| GluN | d-glucosamine |
| GNPs | green nanoparticles |
| GO | graphene oxide |
| GSH | glutathione |
| HA | hydroxyapatite |
| HaCaT | human keratinocyte |
| HPV | human papillomavirus |
| I | ion |
| ICC | inverted colloidal crystals |
| ICPES | inductively coupled plasma-optical emission spectrometry |
| ICPMS | inductively coupled plasma-mass spectrometry |
| IFE | inner filter effect |
| In | indium |
| iPS | induced pluripotent stem |
| ISCOMS | immune-stimulating complexes |
| LIBS | laser-induced breakdown detection technique |
| MB | methylene blue |
| MDR-TB | multidrug-resistant tuberculosis |

| | |
|---|---|
| Mg | magnesium |
| MIC | minimum inhibitory concentration |
| MP | mobile phase |
| MRSA | methicillin-resistant Staphylococcus aureus |
| MRSE | methicillin-resistant Staphylococcus epidermidis |
| MSNs | mesoporous silica nanoparticles |
| MTA | mineral trioxide aggregate |
| MTX | methotrexate |
| MW | molecular weight |
| MWCNT | multiwalled carbon nanotubes |
| N | nitrogen |
| NADH | nicotinamide adenine dinucleotide |
| NADPH | nicotinamide adenine dinucleotide phosphate |
| NDDS | nano-sized drug delivery systems |
| NGF | nerve growth factor |
| Ni | nickel |
| NMQC | noble metal quantum clusters |
| NMR | nuclear magnetic resonance |
| NP | nanoparticle |
| NS/PCs | neural stem/progenitor cells |
| NSCs | neural stem cells |
| PA | polyamide |
| Pb | lead |
| PC | polycarbonates |
| PCL | polycaprolactone |
| PCs | phytoconstituents |
| Pd | palladium |
| PDA | polydopamine |
| PDS | polydioxanone |
| PDT | photodynamic therapy |
| PE | polyethylene |
| PEG | poly(ethylene glycol) |
| PEO | poly(ethylene oxide) |
| PET | polyethylene terephthalate |
| PGA | polyglycolide |
| PHA | polyhydroxyalkanoate |
| PHB | poly(4-hydroxybutyrate) |
| PHV | poly-hydroxyvalerate |

| PLA | poly(lactic acid) |
| PLGA | poly(lactic-co-glycolic acid) |
| PMA | polymethacrylates |
| PP | polypropylene |
| PPF | polypropylene fumigates |
| PS | polystyrene |
| PSC | pepsin-solubilized collagen |
| PSNP | polystyrene nanoparticle |
| Pt | platinum |
| PTFE | polytetrafluoroethylene |
| PTT | photothermal therapy |
| PU | polyurethane |
| PVC | polyvinyl chloride |
| PVP | polyvinylpyrrolidone |
| R&S | reducer and a stabilizer |
| RNA | ribonucleic acid |
| ROS | reactive oxygen species |
| RP | rapid prototyping |
| RP | reverse phase |
| RSCs | rat Schwann cells |
| S | spectrophotometry |
| S | sulfur |
| SAPN | self-assembling protein nanoparticle |
| Sb | antimony |
| SCF | super critical-fluid |
| Se | selenium |
| SE | soxhlet |
| SF | silk fibroin |
| Si | silicon |
| SiRNA | short interfering RNA |
| SP | stationary phase |
| SSZ | sulphasalazine |
| STE | skin tissue engineering |
| STM | scanning tunneling microscopy |
| STS | scanning tunneling spectroscopy |
| Te | tellurium |
| TEM | transmission electron microscope |
| TG | thermogravimetric |

| TGF-$\beta$ | transforming growth factor $\beta$ |
|---|---|
| Ti | titanium |
| Tm | temperatures |
| USWAE | ultrasonic-wave-assisted extraction |
| UV | ultraviolet |
| VH | venlafaxine HCl |
| XRD | x-ray diffraction analysis |
| Zn | zinc |

# Preface

The green nanomaterials synthetic approach of technology-based spectroscopic investigations in order to create the innovations that sustainably boost the competitiveness of the industry is a blessing to the modern industrialized world. By adopting a nanotechnological methodology and by using traditional methods, we can reduce the scarcity of natural resources and reduce environmental pollution. Therefore, in terms of environmental sustainability, the technology industries are embracing change. They are changing to avoid negative consequences or to meet green demand, or to achieve both. Whatever their motivation, they are incontrovertibly shifting toward evergreen.

It's my immense pleasure to introduce a platform for the development of eco-friendly technologies in a green material synthesis that is of considerable importance to expand easily and successfully through this book, titled *Green Nanomaterials*: *Sustainable Technologies and Applications*. My best knowledge of green fabrication is based on more than 20 years of experimentation in a wide array of disciplines, ranging from art to applied physics, chemistry, biology, nanotechnology, and materials science.

Nowadays, a variety of green nanomaterials with well-defined chemical composition, size, and morphology have been synthesized by various cost-effective techniques, and their significant applications in many cutting-edge technological areas have been explored. The recent technological advancement in green nanotechnology has opened a brand new avenue for research and development in the field of medicinal plants mediated nanoparticles, biopolymers, biotechnology, antimicrobials, and biomedicals. Green nanotechnology is basically about making green nanoproducts in the maintenance of sustainability.

The meaning of green technology is a technology that is environmental friendly and developed in such a way that it doesn't disturb our environment while also conserving natural resources. The objectives of nanotechnology are to create eco-friendly processes and products.

Conflicting with this positive message is the growing body of research that raises questions about the potentially negative effects of engineered nanoparticles on human health and the environment. The major goal of a continuously evolving group of methods and materials, from techniques for generating energy to non-toxic cleaning products is explored in the book chapters. However, spectroscopy is used as a tool for studying the structures of nanomaterials. The large number of wavelengths emitted by these systems makes it possible to investigate their structures in detail, including the electronic configurations of the ground and various excited states. Spectroscopy also provides a precise analytical method for finding the constituents in a material having an unknown chemical composition and elements.

The pace of green nanotechnology is a major challenge that this book deals with in seven significant chapters. Chapter 1 investigates a variety of green nanoparticles (GNPs) with certain chemical compositions, dimensions, and structures manufactured with numerous techniques and their applications in varied areas of technological areas. It also considers eco-friendly routes in the fabrication of material, which is of substantial importance to broaden their biotic purposes.

Chapter 2 is establishes a capable approach to fabricate green polymer nanocomposites from waste, such as natural fibers such as chitin fiber, chitin whisker fiber, cellulose fiber, nano cellulose fiber, eggshells, and cotton waste. Chapter 3 deals with the green chemistry synthesis of nanomaterials that has emerged as an eco-friendly and alternative approach for the synthesis of novel nanomaterials with great potential in medical and pharmaceutical applications.

Chapter 4 addresses the biomedical applications of chitosan and collagen towards the generation of fibrous scaffolds for tissue engineering (bone tissue, cartilage tissue, skin tissue, and neural tissue) with respect to chitosan and collagen scaffolds, their enzyme immobilization via chitosan and collagen matrices and matrix drug delivery mechanisms via chitosan and collagen matrices. Chapter 5 discusses the advent of green initiatives in nanotechnology, which has revolutionized the biosensor and drug delivery arena, as well as various green strategies used for the fabrication of potential nanoclusters that could be employed in the field of bio-detection. We also may predict that biosensor technology will revolutionize development in the food technology, agricultural, and packaging industries in the coming years.

Chapter 6 stresses that it is imperative to further investigate the mechanisms of target pathogen toxicity and development of therapeutic windows, as well as the development and standardization of model biological organisms for use in diagnostic toxicity assays.

An overview of various green synthetic approaches used for the production of silver nanoparticles and their efficacy in exhibiting antimicrobial activity is illustrated in Chapter 7. Finally, Chapter 8 reflects that the cost-effective biosensors that can simultaneously detect two toxins are more challenging and are yet to become a reality. Herein, single-step synthesis of reduction of inorganic metallic salt ions to nanoparticles by the organic PCs from the plant source is efficiently used in a user-friendly manner. With the uniqueness of bio-degradability, these protecting Sec-Met from the plant kingdom function as operative bio-reduction and bio-stabilization procedures, commanding non-toxicities and non-expensive etiquettes. Assorted segments involved in operations, stabilization, and application forms of nanoparticles by green nano-trends are also discussed.

**— Kaushik Pal, PhD., & DSc**

# Introduction

Green nanotechnology is the study of nanoscience and its various uses in the environment. With the help of this technology, a number of applications are invented for recycling of products, using eco-friendly raw materials for various productions, minimizing the polluting agents during manufacturing, reducing cost and energy, and various other such concerning matters. Green nanotechnology applications are expected to solve many environmental problems such as saving energy, water treatment, waste management, etc. Recent research and development have led to the innovation of green nanomaterials applications, which will save us from the energy crisis. The novel book Green nanotechnology and applied spectroscopy is an outstanding platform for researchers/scientists with the interests of inter- and cross-multidisciplinary across the whole of green chemistry of nanoengineering and green nanotechnology application in materials research. The book is a unique mixture of exclusive ideas from peer-reviewed regular articles, the latest research newsletters, mini-reviews, and invited papers on key developments. The book also provides comprehensive coverage of this exciting and dynamic new field as well as primary ideas of fundamental of soft-nanomaterials fabrication and brand new spectroscopic integration. Apple Academic Publishers undertook the mission of shaping the future of nanoscience by green synthetic approach, bringing together the latest technologies and most remarkable innovations.

# CHAPTER 1

# Bio-Inspired Self-Assembly Green Nanomaterials for Multifunctional Applications

S. I. ASIYA[1,3] and KAUSHIK PAL[2,3]

[1]*Bharath Institute of Higher Education and Research,*
*Bharath University, 173 Agharam Road, Selaiyur, Chennai – 600073,*
*Tamil Nadu, India*

[2]*Laboratório de Biopolímeros e Sensores, Instituto de Macromoléculas,*
*Universidade do Rio de Janeiro, Rio de Janeiro – RJ, 21941-901, Brazil*

[3]*International and Inter University Centre for Nanoscience and*
*Nanotechnology (IIUCN), School of Energy Materials,*
*Mahatma Gandhi University, Kottayam, Kerala- 686560, India.*

## ABSTRACT

As the understanding of the necessity of a healthy society and environment develops, so does the necessity of green materials and its development. Green nanotechnology has significant value since it minimizes nanoparticle toxicity and expands the biomedical applications of nanoparticles by using environmentally acceptable and natural sources. Green chemistry research focuses on the production of nanomaterials using biological systems such as plants, marine algae, fungus, and bacteria, where the extracts act as reducing and stabilizing agents, making biosynthesized nanoparticles more biocompatible. This novel class of green nanomaterials will have a wide range of environmental and biological uses due to its inherent biocompatibility, biodegradability, and carbon neutrality. The primary factors for selecting a green synthesis approach are usually an environmentally friendly, reducing agent, a non-hazardous capping agent, and an ecologically compatible solvent system. This chapter examines the plant extracts facilitated green synthesis of nanomaterials, where plant extracts from various parts such as leaf, root, latex, seed and stem act as a stabilizing or reducing agent in the biosynthesis of nanoparticles. Microorganisms such as bacteria, fungus, and yeast can also be used to make green nanoparticles by exploiting their defense mechanisms. The vast applications for green manufactured nanomaterials employing either plant extracts or microbes in the fields of medicine, biomedical metals materials, and biosensors are also thoroughly examined.

## 1.1 INTRODUCTION

Nanotechnology is of enormous interest in the area of both academia and industry as it involves the design and utilization of materials with at least one dimension limited to between 1 nm and 100 nm. The structural features of nanomaterials exhibiting distinct physical and chemical properties can be tailored to attain novel functions that find innumerable potential applications in various fields of science and engineering [1]. The properties of materials with nanometric dimensions differ considerably from their bulk counterparts. In contrast to bulk materials, relatively less raw materials, cost, and energy are involved in nanomaterials to achieve the same aim [2]. Research efforts geared towards the manipulation of these nanoparticles into well-designed functional materials has generated huge excitement in the area of nanotechnology. Novel and improved properties are exhibited by nanoparticles on the basis of their nanoscale dimension, molecular distribution, and morphology. Their reduced size and the unique characteristics they possess attract their presence in chip technology, and the ability to fine-tune the nanomaterial properties offers extensive applications in optoelectronics, photovoltaic, biomedical, and thermoelectric field [3].

Nanoparticles such as $ZnO$, $FeO$, $SiO_2$, $CeO_2$, and $TiO_2$, often find application due to their superior photocatalytic properties. Nanomaterials of Ag, Au, Fe, Cu, Pt, Pd, Ni, and Co- in are extensively used for antimicrobial, optical catalytic, electronic, sensing purposes, and as doping agents. Few metal-oxide nanoparticles are used as ingredients of rubber additives, catalytic converters, biomedical imaging, photovoltaic cells, and sensors and for environmental remediation (paints, cosmetics, and plastics products) [4–7].

The significance of nanotechnology in today's world has been emphasized in the development of nanoparticles with various sizes, shapes, and chemical compositions. Nanoparticles can be synthesized using various traditional chemical and physical methods like chemical vapor deposition, laser ablation, etching, supercritical fluid, sol-gel technique, pyrolysis, and electrodeposition. Chemical synthesis of nanoparticles is achieved by chemical reduction using several metals and chemicals like sodium citrate, ascorbate, sodium borohydride, etc. Though the nanoparticles so synthesized exhibit copious applications, these synthesis methods suffer certain drawbacks such as energy consumption is too high, use of environmentally hazardous chemicals, high cost, form toxic byproducts, need complex instruments, and low production rate [2, 8]. Researchers have also recommended that nanoparticles have hazardous effects at the cellular, subcellular, and molecular levels [9, 10], and the health risk and environmental impact of direct and indirect exposure to nanoparticles have to be addressed quickly. The probability of chemical precursors being absorbed onto the surface of nanoparticles hinders the chemically synthesized nanoparticles in biomedical applications. These factors urged the exploration of novel methods and materials for the development of nanoparticles with reduced environmental impact based on the principles of green chemistry, which is a set of principles that boosts the production of nanomaterials eliminating the usage of toxic chemical substances and involving the usage of natural sources, nontoxic solvents, and energy-efficient synthesis procedures [11, 12]. Green nanotechnology owns remarkable value as the usage of ecofriendly and natural sources reduces the toxicity of nanoparticles and provides a tremendous increase in the biomedical applications of nanoparticles. Green chemistry researches are focused towards nanomaterial synthesis expending biological systems such as plants, marine algae, fungi, and bacteria where the extract function as reducing and stabilizing agents rendering more biocompatibility to biosynthesized nanoparticles [13]. It has been observed that the green synthesis of nanoparticles using plant extract has gained huge interest as it is faster, simpler, and more cost-effective than using microbes, enabling the synthesis of green nanomaterials with better size and morphology [7, 14, 15]. The microorganisms are considered as potential bio-factories for the green synthesis of metal nanoparticles due to the extensive range of microorganisms that respond in a diverse way with the metal ions for the synthesis of metal nanoparticles. Microbial metal nanoparticles of enormous morphology have been described in various species of bacteria, fungi, and yeasts due to their improved growth rate, easy cultivation, and their ability to grow under various conditions of temperature, pH, and pressure [16, 17]. Thus, green nanotechnology is considered as the combination of nanotechnology and green chemistry principles, which plays a vital role in constructing an ecologically sustainable society.

## 1.2  GREEN SYNTHESIS OF NANOMATERIALS

Nanoparticles find promising applications in numerous products ranging from health care products to high-performance composites. Few important and widely recognized applications of nanomaterials include developing a catalyst for environmental remediation, efficient photovoltaic, thermoelectric materials, energy-conserving nanocomposite material for automobiles, and nanosensors [18]. To understand new nanotechnologies that cause little harm to human health or the environment and to cultivate technologies that can be used to safeguard the environment, it is appropriate to design and develop greener nanoproduction methods. Green chemistry is defined as the exploitation of a set of principles that diminishes or eradicates the usage or production of harmful substances in the design, fabrication, and application of chemical products [19]. Hence, various synthetic approaches for the fabrication of nanoparticles with different sizes and shapes as depicted schematics diagram in Figure 1.1.

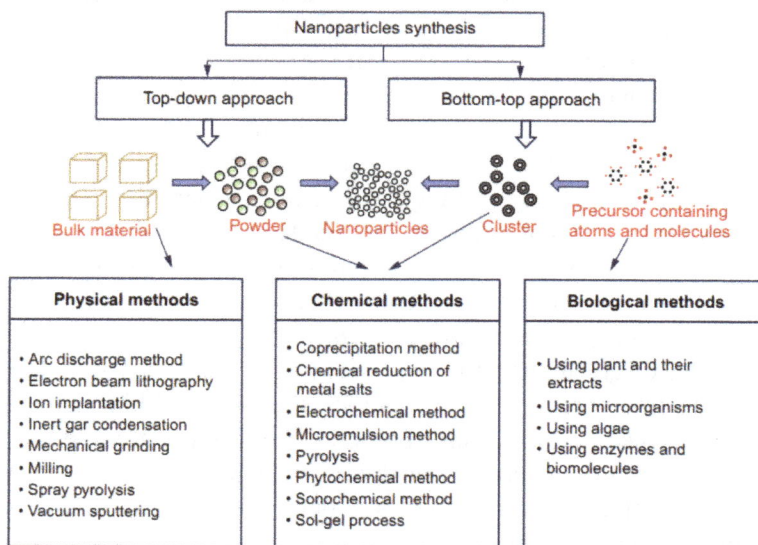

**FIGURE 1.1**   Different approaches for the synthesis of nanoparticles.
*Source:* Reprinted with permission from Ref. [20], Copyright ©2018, Synthesis of inorganic nanomaterials, Elsevier.

Green routes of synthesis have been widely used in the design of a wide range of nanoparticles to prevent pollution, reduce waste, and protect health and the environment from harmful chemicals. Green synthesis of nanomaterials is a bottom-up procedure where the core reaction-taking place is the oxidation or reduction [18]. The twelve principles of green chemistry are as follows:

1. Prevent/reduce waste;
2. Atom economy;
3. Nontoxic synthesis methodology;
4. Designing safer chemicals;
5. Safer solvents;
6. Energy efficiency;
7. Use of renewable feedstock;
8. Reduce/eliminate derivatives;
9. Catalysis;
10. Design for degradation;
11. Real-time analysis for pollution prevention;
12. Inherently safer method for preventions of accidents.

The oxidizing/reducing properties of plant extracts are highly applicable for the reduction of metal compounds into their corresponding nanoparticles. Synthesis of nanoparticles using various types of microorganisms is found to be safer and cost-effective besides the biocompatibility of green nanomaterial due to the coating of biological molecules on the surface of nanoparticles [21]. These bio-inspired nanoparticles find remarkable applications in biomedicines and associated fields.

Green synthesis is appreciable compared to the conventional chemical and physical method as this method is eco-friendly, economical, free from harmful chemicals, high pressure, high energy, and rise in temperature [22]. Green synthesis of nanomaterials offers better management, regulation over crystal growth, and their stabilization. Enormous chemical substances are available in nature that can act as an appropriate reducing agent for the synthesis of green nanomaterials such as plant extracts, biopolymers, microbes, vitamins, proteins, etc., [23, 24]. Abundantly available plant extracts are considered as one of the best favorable natural reducing agents [25]. Usually, an environmental friendly, reducing agent, a nonhazardous capping agent, and an ecologically compatible solvent system are the main principles for choosing the green synthesis strategy [26].

### 1.2.1   *PLANT EXTRACTS FACILITATED GREEN SYNTHESIS OF NANOMATERIALS*

Plant extracts from various parts such as leaf, root, latex, seed, and stem act as a stabilizing or reducing agent in the biosynthesis of nanoparticles. For example, leaf extracts of *Jasminum sambac* is used for the preparation of Au, Ag, Au-Ag alloy nanoparticles [27]. *Olive leaf* extract with hot water at high reaction temperature is used for the synthesis of various morphologies of gold nanoparticles [28]. Iron-polyphenol nanoparticles were synthesized using leaves of *Eucalyptus tereticornis, Melaleuca nesophila,* and *Rosemarinus officinalis* [29]. Nanoparticle synthesis using green tea leaf extract [30], extract of *Terminalia chebula* fruit [31], Oolong, and black tea leaf extract [32], banana peel along with *Colocasia esculenta* leaves extract [33], sorghum bran extract [34], eucalyptus leaf extract [35], and *Tridax procumbens* [36] have been carried out. In addition, Figure 1.2 illustrates the synthesis of nanoparticles of some of the plant parts from a natural source by green chemistry assisted process.

The morphology of nanoparticles can be organized by a slight modulation in pH and reaction temperature. An extensive range of metal nanoparticles such as gold, silver, platinum, palladium, titanium, copper, and iron have been synthesized using plant extracts. Researches confirm that the reducing property of the plant extracts and their biomolecules shows a remarkable role in the reduction of nanoparticles [37]. It has been observed that stable metal nanoparticles can be synthesized easily using plant extract owing to the high reduction capability of metal ions using plant extracts. Biologically active compounds found in plants such as phenolic acid, amino acid, polyphenol, saponin, protein, flavone, sugar, terpenoid, etc., self-assemble to act as capping and stabilizing agent for the synthesis of metal nanoparticles [7]. The processes involved in the plant extracts-mediated synthesis of nanoparticles start with the preparation of plant extracts using different plant parts/whole plant followed by the preparation of the metal salt solution and then mixing and incubation of plant extract and metal salt solution at ambient conditions.

Indeed, the numerous processes involved in the synthesis of green nanoparticles (GNPs) from natural plant extract by green chemistry route, as demonstrated in Figure 1.3. Properties of the plant extract, such as its concentration, metal salt concentration, reaction time, the reaction solution pH, and temperature, influence the quality, size, and morphology of the synthesized nanoparticles.

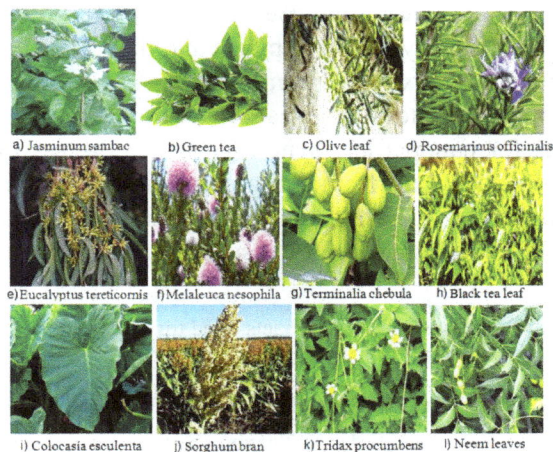

a) Jasminum sambac    b) Green tea    c) Olive leaf    d) Rosemarinus officinalis

e) Eucalyptus tereticornis    f) Melaleuca nesophila    g) Terminalia chebula    h) Black tea leaf

i) Colocasia esculenta    j) Sorghum bran    k) Tridax procumbens    l) Neem leaves

**FIGURE 1.2**  Displaying various plant parts as natural sources for the extraction of nanomaterials synthesis in green chemistry route.

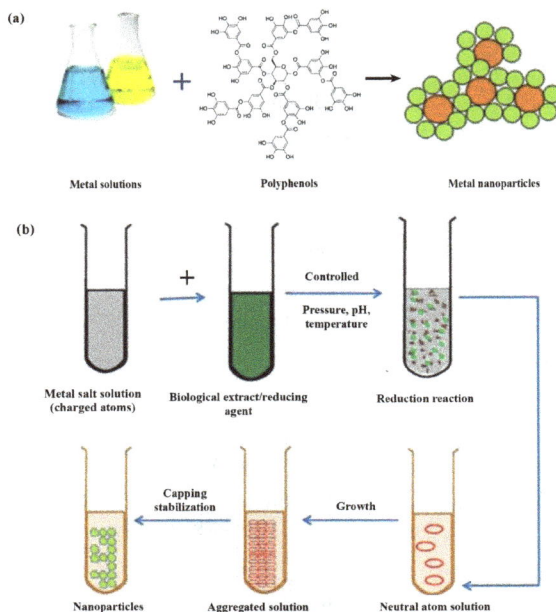

(a)

Metal solutions          Polyphenols          Metal nanoparticles

(b)

Controlled

Pressure, pH, temperature

Metal salt solution (charged atoms)    Biological extract/reducing agent    Reduction reaction

Capping stabilization    Growth

Nanoparticles    Aggregated solution    Neutral atom solution

**FIGURE 1.3**  (a) The chemical constituents of plant extract responsible for the bioreduction of metal ions, (b) various processes involved in the green synthesis of nanoparticles. *Source:* Reprinted with permission from Ref. [20], Copyright ©2018, Synthesis of inorganic nanomaterials, Elsevier.

In several last decades, scientists/researchers enormously trying to nanoparticles synthesis by applying plants and their parts are an effective method that is gaining extreme prominence in all the areas aiming at a greener environment. Extensive research work is carried out using plants and their parts for nanoparticle synthesis due to the ease in scaling up for larger production, apart from being cost-effective and environmental friendly. However, Table 1.1 attributes the detailed combination of metal solutions and leaf extracts used for the synthesis of nanoparticles.

**TABLE 1.1**    Metal Solutions and Leaf Extracts Used for the Synthesis of Nanoparticles

| Leaf | Particle Size | Precursor Used | References |
|------|--------------|----------------|------------|
| **Silver Nanoparticles from Leaf Extract** | | | |
| *Musa balbisiana* | Up to 200 nm | Silver nitrate | [38] |
| *Catharanthus roseus* | 35–55 nm | | [39] |
| *Phlomis leaf extract* | 27 nm | | [40] |
| *Saraca indica* | About 98 nm | | [41] |
| *Cymbopogan citratus* | 32 nm | | [42] |
| *Moringa oleifera* | 57 nm | | [43] |
| *Acalypha indica* | 20–30 nm | | [44] |
| **Zinc Nanoparticles from Leaf Extracts** | | | |
| *Moringa oleifera* | 13–61 nm | Zinc nitrate [Zn $(NO_3)_2$ $6H_2O$] | [45] |
| *Limonia acidissima* | 12–53 nm | | [46] |
| *Eichhornia crassipes* | 32 nm | | [47] |
| *Aloe barbadensis Miller* | 34 nm | | [48] |
| *Parthenium hysterophorous* | 16.1–58.6 nm | | [49] |
| *Lobelia leschenaultiana* | 20–65 nm | Zinc acetate | [50] |
| *Aspalathus linearis* | 1–8.5 nm | Zinc nitrate hexahydrate | [51] |
| **Gold Nanoparticles from Leaf Extract** | | | |
| *Magnolia kobus* and *Diopyros kaki* leaf extracts | 5–300 nm | Aqueous $HAuCl_4$ solution | [52] |
| *Coleus amboinicus* | 4.6 to 55.1 nm | | [53] |
| *Nepenthes khasiana* | 50 to 80 nm | Gold (III) chloride | [54] |
| *Allium cepa* (onion) | 100 nm | Aqueous chloro-auric acid ($HAuCl_4$) solution | [55] |
| *Terminalia arjuna* | 20–50 nm | | [56] |

**TABLE 1.1** *(Continued)*

| Leaf | Particle Size | Precursor Used | References |
|---|---|---|---|
| **Iron Nanoparticles from Leaf Extract** | | | |
| *Azadirachta indica, Magnifera indica, Murraya koenigii, Magnolia champaca* | 300–500 nm | Ferrous sulfate heptahydrate | [57] |
| *Sorghum* (plant) source bran | 50 nm Avg. | $FeCl_3$ | [34] |
| *Carica papaya* | 33 nm Avg. | $FeCl_3\ 6H_2O$ | [58] |
| *Terminalia chebula* | 80–100 nm | Ferrous sulfate $(FeSO_4\ 7H_2O)$ | [31] |
| Vine leaves, black tea leaves, and grape marc | 15–45 nm | Ferrous sulfate $(FeSO_4\ 7H_2O)$ | [59] |
| Oolong tea | 40–50 nm | | [60] |
| *Tridax procumbens* | 80–100 nm | $FeCl_3$ | [36] |
| **Copper Nanoparticles from Leaf Extract** | | | |
| *Tecoma castanifolia* leaf extract | 100 nm | Copper sulfate | [61] |
| *Murraya koenigii* leaf | 97 nm | | [62] |
| *Ginkgo biloba* L. leaf | | Copper chloride $[CuCl_2\ 2H_2O]$ | [63] |

## 1.2.2 MICROORGANISM MEDIATED GREEN SYNTHESIS OF NANOMATERIALS

Currently, biological resources have been often explored for the biosynthesis of metal or metal-based nanoparticles. These biological resources usually provide a versatile, economical, and eco-friendly method to synthesize metal nanoparticles [64] that exhibit interesting physical, chemical, and biological properties. An alternate way of producing GNPs is by using microorganisms such as bacteria, fungi, and yeast making use of their defense mechanism. The opposition caused by the bacterial cells for reactive ions in the environment is liable for the synthesis of nanoparticles. As the high ion concentration is hazardous for bacterial cells, the reactive ions are converted into stable atoms to prevent cell death. This property of bacteria is being utilized for the green synthesis of nanoparticles [65]. Various unicellular and multicellular microorganisms are able to synthesize metallic nanoparticles with attractive morphology [66]. Enormous enzymes are secreted, which hydrolyze metals and thus results in the enzymatic reduction of metal ions [67]. The intracellular route of synthesis comprises moving ions into the microbial cell to generate nanoparticles in the presence of enzymes, whereas in the extracellular route, ions are captured on the cell surfaces and are reduced to nanoparticles in the presence of enzymes. Though microbial synthesis of nanoparticles is ecological and compatible, the fabrications of nanoparticles are slow, and the productions of microbes are costly and prolonged.

These nanoparticles have been used in a wide array of applications, mostly for biomedical uses. Recently, silver nanoparticles that were synthesized using *Bacillus brevis* display excellent antimicrobial activities against the multidrug-resistant strains of *Staphylococcus aureus* and *Salmonella typhi* [68]. *Pseudomonas stutzeri* is another bacterial strain, which was found capable of accumulating silver nanoparticles using an intracellular mechanism [69]. The *Bacillus* sp. was also found to synthesize silver nanoparticles in the intracellular periplasmic space [70]. Two different isolated strains of *Pseudomonas aeruginosa* were used for the biosynthesis of gold nanoparticles, generating different sizes of it [71]. Among the actinomycetes, alkalo-tolerant (*Rhodococcus* sp.) and alkalo-thermophilic (*Thermomonospora* sp.) actinomycetes were used for the intracellular synthesis of gold nanoparticles [72].

Nanoparticle synthesis by using algae is gaining huge interest and *Sargassum wightiiis* being identified for the characteristics of a variety of applications. Among numerous nanoparticles that are available, only a few will be suitable to carry out the application part. Figure 1.4 displays some of the microbes involved in the green synthesis of nanomaterials.

Extracellular microbial enzymes are known to play a substantial role as reducing agents in the production of metal nanoparticles [72]. Studies suggest that cofactors such as nicotinamide adenine dinucleotide (NADH) and reduced form of nicotinamide adenine dinucleotide phosphate (NADPH) dependent enzymes both play vital roles as reducing agents via the transfer of the electron from NADH by NADH-reliant enzymes, which act as electron carriers [73]. Hence, Figure 1.5 indicates the role of NADH and NADH-dependent microbial enzymes in the synthesis of metal nanoparticles. *F. ocuminatum* isolated from infected ginger plants were also successfully used for the biosynthesis of silver nanoparticles [74].

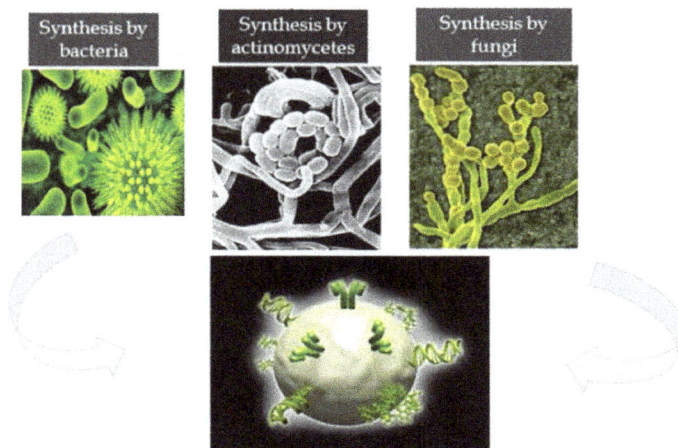

**FIGURE 1.4**    Microbes involved in the green synthesis of nanomaterials.
*Source:* Reprinted with permission from Ref. [75], Copyright ©2015, Green processes for nanotechnology, Springer Nature.

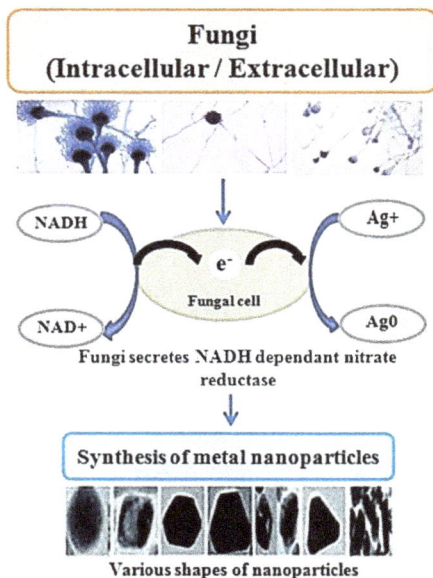

**FIGURE 1.5**    Synthesis of metal nanoparticles employing NADH and NADH-dependent microbial enzymes.
*Source:* Reprinted with permission from Ref. [76], Copyright ©2018, Journal of nanostructure in chemistry, Springer Nature, under the creative commons attribution license.

A list of microorganisms involved in the syntheses of some of the most widely used nanoparticles and their applications specifically summarize in Table 1.2.

**TABLE 1.2**  List of Microorganisms Involved in the Green Syntheses of Nanoparticles and Their Applications

| SL. No. | Microorganisms | Nanoparticle | Size/Shape | Application | References |
|---|---|---|---|---|---|
| | | **Bacteria** | | | |
| 1. | *Actinobacter* | Ag | 13.2 nm/ Spherical | Antibacterial | [77] |
| 2. | *Klebsiella pneumonia* | Au | 10–15 nm/ Spherical | Antibacterial | [78] |
| 3. | *Sinomonas mesophila* | Ag | 4–50 nm/ Spherical | Antibacterial | [79] |
| 4. | *Shewanella loihica* | Cu | 10–16 nm/ Spherical | Antibacterial | [80] |
| 5. | *Shewanella loihica* | Pt | 1–10 nm/ Spherical | Dye degradation | [81] |
| 6. | *Shewanella loihica* | Pd | 1–12 nm/ Spherical | Dye degradation | [81] |
| | | **Fungi** | | | |
| 7. | *Aspergillus niger* | ZnO | 53–69 nm/ Spherical | Antibacterial, dye degradation | [82] |
| 8. | *Trichoderma longibrachiatum* | Ag | 10 nm/ Spherical | Antifungal against phyto-pathogenic fungi | [83] |
| 9. | *Trichoderma harzianum* | Au | 32–44 nm/ Spherical | Antibacterial, dye degradation | [84] |
| 10. | *Fusarium oxysporum* | Ag | 21.3–37 nm/ Spherical | Antimicrobial | [85] |
| 11. | *Pleurotus ostreatus* | Au | 10–30 nm/ Spherical | Antimicrobial, anticancer | [86] |
| 12. | *Macrophomina phaseolina* | Ag/AgCl | 5–30 nm/ Spherical | Antibacterial | [87] |
| | | **Algae/Cyanobacteria** | | | |
| 13. | *Neochloris oleoabundans* | Ag | 40 nm/ Spherical | Antibacterial | [88] |
| 14. | *Cystoseira baccata* | Au | 8.4 nm/ Spherical | Anticancer | [89] |

**TABLE 1.2** *(Continued)*

| SL. No. | Microorganisms | Nanoparticle | Size/Shape | Application | References |
|---------|----------------|--------------|------------|-------------|------------|
| 15. | *Chlorella pyrenoidosa* | CdSe QD | 4–5 nm | Imatinib sensing | [90] |
| 16. | *Spirulina platensis* | Pd | 10–20 nm/ Spherical | Adsorbent | [91] |
| 17. | *Chlorella pyrenoidosa* | $TiO_2$ | 50 nm/ Spherical | Dye degradation | [92] |

## 1.3 APPLICATIONS OF GREEN NANOMATERIALS

Compared to the chemical-based fabrication of nanomaterials, green synthesized nanomaterials are found to have enormous applications in the area of medicine and biological system. Figure 1.6 illustrates the immense applications for green synthesized nanomaterials using either plant extract or microbes.

### 1.3.1 GREEN NANOMATERIAL IN THE FIELD OF MEDICINES

Problems allied with herbal medicines can be astounded with nano-sized drug delivery systems (NDDS) of herbal drugs, having a potential future for enhancing their activity. Hence, including nanocarriers as an NDDS in conventional medical systems would be necessary to combat more chronic diseases like diabetes, cancer, asthma, and others, with the aid of herbal drugs. Biomolecules available in plant extract synthesis stable nanoparticles, which in fact, increase their application in the field of medicines. Recent researches reveal that the plant-mediated nanoparticles are compatible for nanomedicine applications because of their high stability in different biological media [93]. Physiochemical applications also benefit the advantages of green nanomaterials. Biosynthesis of $In_2O_3$ exploiting 'Aloe vera' plant extract exhibits photoluminescence in the ultra-violet region.

The strong emissions of indium oxide are related to the radioactive recombination of an electron occupying oxygen vacancy with a photo-excited hole. Researches confirm the use of GNPs as fluorescence labels for the detection of various analytes. Leaf as well as fruit extracts of *Ricinus communis* were reported to display greater antiviral activity that acts upon virus and cell culture [95]. Studies have also revealed that the green synthesis of silver nanoparticles expending E. the prostrata leaf extract could show larvisidal activity against filariasis and malaria vectors. The optical properties of gold nanoparticles have been extensively used in cancer diagnostics and treatment.

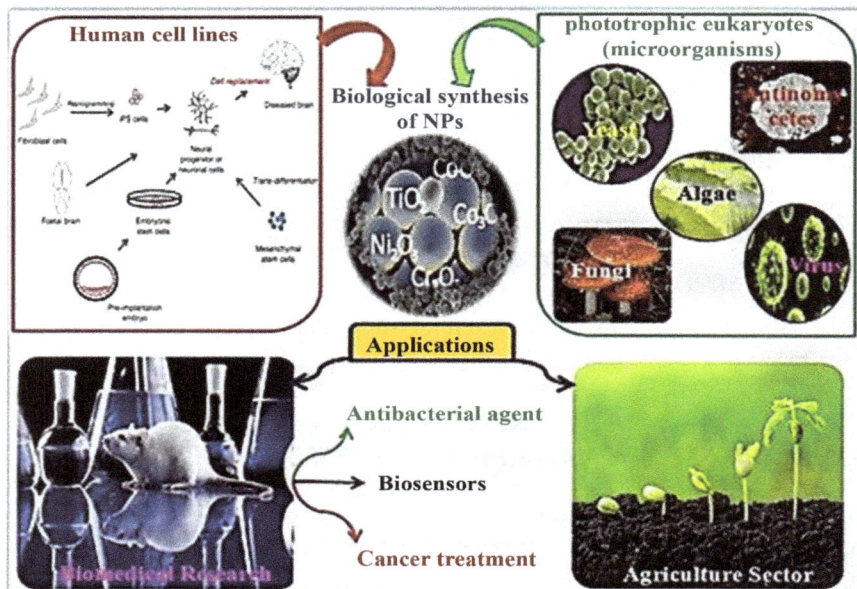

**FIGURE 1.6** Applications of biosynthesized nanoparticles.
*Source:* Reprinted with permission from Ref. [94], Copyright ©2018, Colloids, and surfaces B: Biointerfaces, Elsevier.

### 1.3.1.1 BIOMEDICAL METALLIC MATERIAL

As the life expectancy of human beings increased with the advancement in the field of medicines, there has been a huge demand for the reliable biomedical metallic material to offer a high-quality life for the aging population. Biomedical metallic materials are expected to meet high standards of performance at affordable cost and available manufacturing facilities. It is essential that the surgical implants maintain high strength, good biocompatibility, and chemical stability. The commonly used biomedical metallic materials include stainless steel, cobalt-based alloys, and commercially pure titanium or titanium-based alloys. For example, Titanium alloy has been chosen for fabricating implants owing to its good mechanical and corrosion characteristics [96]. However, wear fragments due to wear corrosion and release of metallic ions often leads to inflammations in the tissue or some allergy. Cytotoxicity concerns are mainly related to the presence of vanadium, but also high concentrations of titanium and aluminum ions can be dangerous [95, 97]. Biological coatings of tin and titanium oxides are employed to provide corrosion resistance, bioactivity, cytocompatibility, and bioconductivity. Like all the mechanical components, these biomedical metallic materials are also subjected to degradation that affects the life span of the implants. As the degraded implants need to be replaced through successive surgeries; thorough efforts were made to improve the durability of the implants, which led to the developments of enhanced metallic biomaterials. It has been observed that the wear and corrosion are interdependent in an intricate way. The wear on electrochemical behavior is influenced by frictional load, applied voltage, and pH of the solution [98]. Researches on the tribocorrosion of stainless steel pairs in a Ringer's solution under gross slip condition conclude that the presence of a corrosive lubricant causes mechanical energy dissipation and the wear and corrosion damage on the contact surfaces and is due to the electrochemical phenomenon caused by the electrolyte [99]. Investigations on titanium and its alloys at anodic potential under fretting corrosion demonstrate that the electrochemical response of the alloy to the wear and corrosion is significant in the presence of slip [100]. The wearing is also stimulated by the applied potential because of continuous oxidation of the surface layer formed by mechanical mixing of plastically deformed metal and oxide debris [101].

Life spans of biological adhesive joints are dependent on thin surface films that show indifferent properties compared to their bulk materials. The biological responses are influenced by the surface properties of the surface such as its chemistry, energy, and morphology due to the facts that (i) biomaterial surface is the only part that will be in touch with the bio environment; (ii) Morphology and composition of the surface varies with that of the bulk; (iii) surface characteristics of the biomaterials controls the biological responses; and (iv) topography of the biomaterial influence the mechanical stability of the implant-tissue interface [102]. Generally, the surgical implants fabricated using stainless steel, titanium alloys, and Cobalt-Chrome alloys have Young's module (100 to 200 GPa) much higher than the human bones (1–30 GPa) [103], resulting in aseptic loosening [104]. Cyclic motions between the implants and human tissues interrupt the protective surface coatings and cause wear debris, increasing the risks of immunological response. Green nanomaterials, particularly engineered nanostructures on the surface, plays a vital role in reducing/ preventing these bio complications by enhancing mechanical, chemical, and physical properties.

### 1.3.1.2 BIOSENSORS DEVICES

*Biosensors* are devices used to detect the presence or concentration of a biological analyte. These analytes are often of biological origin like DNAs (deoxyribonucleic acid) of bacteria or viruses, or proteins which are generated from the immune system (antibodies, antigens) of infected or contaminated living organisms. *Biosensors* consist of three parts: a component that recognizes the analyte and produces a signal, a signal transducer, and a reader device.

The electronic and optical sensing properties of the biomaterial surface are utilized in the fabrication of biosensors. The immobilization of biomolecule-nanoparticle conjugates on the surface provides a broad approach for the development of optical or electronic biosensors [75]. Gold or silver metal nanoparticles show plasmon absorbance bands in the visible spectral region, which can be governed by the particle size. Reduced particle size compared to the incident wavelength hinders the propagation of the oscillating electrons along the surface as the case for classic surface resonance setup. Ion detection and quantification of analytes are achieved by altering the optical behavior of the nanoparticles by binding them to distinct molecules. Agglomeration alters the absorption properties of gold nanoparticles significantly. Spectral shifts observed in agglomerated metal nanoparticles is the basic principle used in the fabrication of biosensors [105]. Polarization of the electron density takes place on one side of the particle where the plasmons oscillate in resonance with the incident light frequency and are strongly dependent on morphology and the dielectric constant of its environment. Each recognition event in the environment causes a change of the oscillating frequency leading to a change in the gold nanoparticles, which paves the foundation for the development of colorimetric biosensors for DNA or oligonucleotide detection, or immu-nosensors [106–108].

Other than optical properties, gold nanoparticles have an excellent ability to transfer electrons between a wide range of electroactive biological species and the electrode. This principle is principally used for redox enzyme biosensing, where the bioreceptor unit catalyzes the oxidation or reduction of the analyte. Gold nanoparticles act as electron shuttles, where the gold nanoparticles can approach to the redox center of the enzyme regenerating this biocatalyst by transferring the electrons involved in the redox reaction to the electrode.

### 1.3.1.3 DRUG DELIVERY

Incorporation of green nanotechnology with the drug delivery area has launched a novel realm of green nanomedicine. To attain targeted delivery and to avoid rapid degradation of drugs or protection from clearance, a glut of the precise drug delivery system has been developed. The significance of manipulating nanoparticles as powerful drug delivery system (for the prevention and therapy of different diseases) exist in their enhanced bioavailability; controlled and sustained drug release; high drug loading capacity; prolonged circulation time; enhanced intracellular penetration and targeted delivery to specific sites or organs; protection of the active ingredient against physiological pH, enzymes, and moisture; usage of various ways of administration, including parenteral, oral, nasal, intra-ocular; and many more [107].

Up till now, numerous nanocarriers, such as metal/metal oxide NPs, nonmetal NPs, quantum dots, polymeric NPs, silica NPs, carbon nano-materials, liposomes, dendrimers, nanostructured lipid carriers, solid lipid nanoparticles, etc., have been designed to carry diverse molecules, such as drugs, peptides, and proteins, DNA/RNA, antibodies, etc. Figure 1.7 illustrates the mechanism drug delivery by using liposomes as nanocar-riers consisting of nanocarriers to transport anticancer drugs to the cancer site, *targeting mechanisms* to pinpoint the cancerous site and *stimulus techniques* to discharge the drug at the pre-located cancer cell site.

To improve the quality of nanoparticles, a green synthesis route has been employed, which involves no harmful chemicals or toxic byproducts, highly efficient and cost-effective. Currently, biosynthesized green metal nanoparticles are used as a prospective drug delivery system due to their chemical surface properties and morphologies. Polymeric nanoparticles have gained remarkable attention due to their unique optical, electrical, and optoelectrical qualities, as well as interesting applications in biomedical sciences, sensing, drug delivery, and many more. Studies reveal that surface alteration of polymeric nanoparticles with hydrophilic polymers, like poly(ethylene glycol) (PEG), and poly(ethylene oxide) (PEO) has developed as a way to improve the solubility of hydrophobic medicines. Electroresponsive polymers are identified as a smart nanomaterial for drug delivery as they can shrink, swell, or bend in response to the electric field.

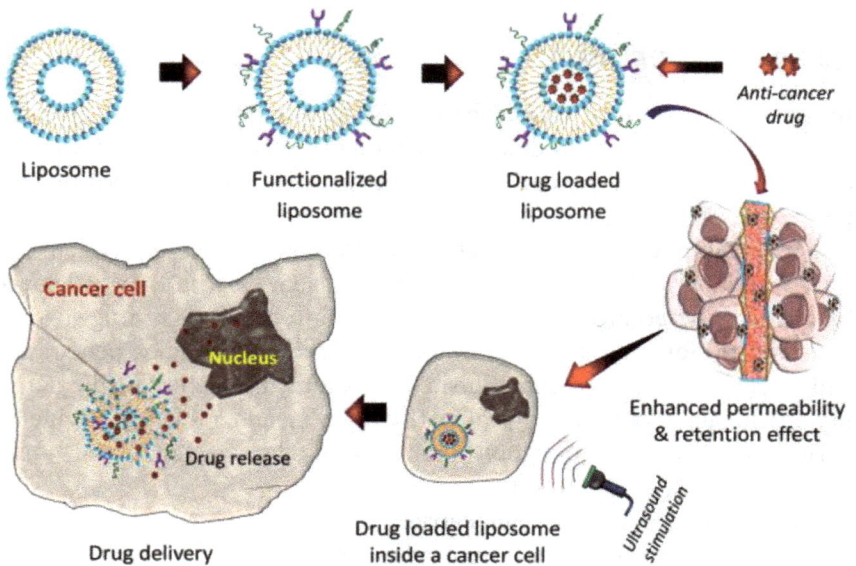

**FIGURE 1.7**    Mechanism of drug delivery system for cancer treatment.
*Source:* Reprinted with permission from Ref. [109], Copyright©2019, Journal of advanced research, Elsevier, under the creative commons attribution license.

Mesoporous silica nanoparticles (MSNs) are recommended to act as a drug delivery carrier as they possess large surface area, pore volume, and easily changeable surface properties. The most common mesoporous silica material includes MCM-48, MCM-41, and SBA-15 with a pore size of 2–10 nm, which have two/three-dimensional cubic characteristic features [110]. The channel in MSNs keeps the drug within the pores in an amorphous/noncrystalline state that facilitates the drug dissolution. Site-specific administration and long-term release are prerequisite to achieve sustainable drug delivery in the body. MSN fabricated using nonhazardous surfactants (didodecyldimethylammonium bromide (DDAB) and cetyltrimethylammonium bromide (CTAB)) prove that the drug delivery behavior is proportional to the size of particles, more precisely related to the pore channel length [111]. MSNs based on stimuli-responsive controlled drug delivery systems were developed by applying controls such as gatekeepers over the pore entrance due to which the drug cannot escape out from silica carriers unless the carriers are exposed to external stimuli (redox potential, temperature, and pH). The amino-modified MSNs are a potential bifunctional drug delivery system for cefazolin (an antibiotic drug). The MSNs (SBA-15) were formed via the greener sol-gel method, and further, the surface functionalization was carried out by post grafting synthesis and higher encapsulation with a slow and sustained release over 7 days was demonstrated. Furthermore, Figure 1.8 demonstrates the targeted delivery and controlled release of cisplatin drug molecules from doubly decorated MSNs, which were internally grafted with fluorescent conjugates and externally coated with polydopamine (PDA) and graphene oxide (GO) layers. The brush-like internal conjugates conferred fluorescent functionality and high capacity of cisplatin loading into MSNs, as well as contributing to a sustained release of the cisplatin through a porous channel with the assistance of external PDA layer [112].

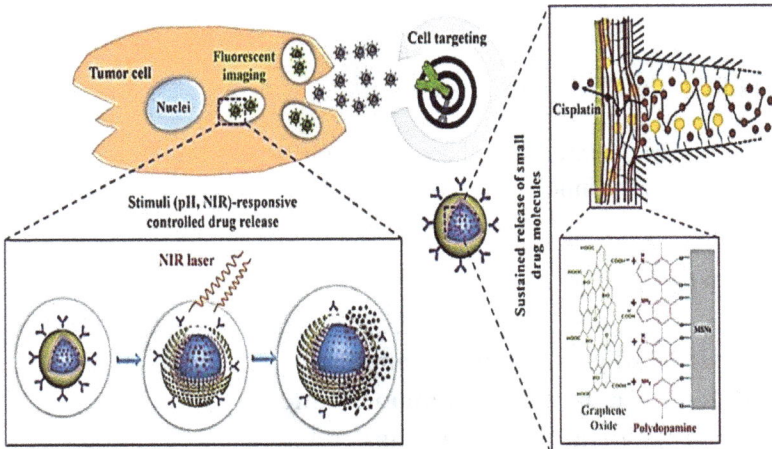

**FIGURE 1.8** Targeted delivery and controlled release of cisplatin drug molecules from doubly decorated MSNs.
*Source:* Reprinted with permission from Ref. [113], Copyright ©2018, Acta biometerialia, Elsevier.

## 1.4 CONCLUSIONS

Nanomaterials have engrossed distinct attention in the varied field of applied science and particularly rising attention has been witnessed in the biosynthesis of nanomaterials. The green route of nanomaterial synthesis leads to the utilization of ecological methods for the development of harmless and biocompatible nanomaterials. The growth of echo-friendly routes in the fabrication of material is of substantial importance to broaden their biotic purposes. Now, a variety of GNPs with certain chemical compositions, dimensions, and structures manufactured with the help of numerous techniques and their applications in varied areas of technologies technological areas have been observed. Eco-friendly methods for the development of metal nanomaterials have emerged as a boom to mankind due to its contribution in various fields closely related to manhood. Accordingly, the unsophisticated biosynthesis of nanoparticles with controlled dimensions and shapes by using molecular cloning and genetic engineering approaches and other photo-biological techniques will be a marvelous expansion in the nanobiotechnology area. Nanomaterials by renewable bioresources and biocompatible agents with exceptional physicochemical, optoelectronics, and electronic properties are of immense significance for wider purposes in the areas of chemistry, medicine, electronics, and agriculture.

## CONFLICT OF INTEREST

All the authors declared that there is no conflict of interest to publish the chapter as a recent innovation.

## KEYWORDS

- cetyltrimethylammonium bromide
- di-dodecyl dimethylammonium bromide
- mesoporous silica nanoparticles
- nano-sized drug delivery systems
- nicotinamide adenine dinucleotide phosphate
- poly(ethylene glycol)

## REFERENCES

1. Genther-Yoshida, P., Casassa, M., Shull, R., Pomrenke, G., Thomas, I., Price, R., Doe, B. V., et al., (1999). *National Science and Technology Council Committee on Technology the Interagency Working Group on Nanoscience, Engineering and Technology.* Washington, DC about the National Science and Technology Council.
2. Su, C., & Puls, R. W., (1999). Kinetics of trichloroethene reduction by zerovalent iron and tin: Pretreatment effect, apparent activation energy, and intermediate products. *Environmental Science and Technology, 33*(1), 163–168.
3. Koch, C. C., (2006). *Nanostructured Materials: Processing, Properties and Applications,* William Andrew.
4. Goswami, L., Kim, K. H., Deep, A., Das, P., Bhattacharya, S. S., Kumar, S., & Adelodun, A. A., (2017). Engineered nano particles: Nature, behavior, and effect on the environment, *Journal of Environmental Management, 196,* 297–315.
5. Hara, S. O., Krug, T., Quinn, J., Clausen, C., & Geiger, C., (2006). Field and laboratory evaluation of the treatment of DNAPL source zones using emulsified zero-valent iron. *Remediation Journal: The Journal of Environmental Cleanup Costs, Technologies and Techniques, 16*(2), 35–56.
6. Ghosh, S., Patil, S., Ahire, M., Kitture, R., Jabgunde, A., Kale, S., Pardesi, K., et al., (2011). Synthesis of gold nanoanisotrops using *Dioscorea bulbifera* tuber extract. *Journal of Nanomaterials.*
7. Mittal, A. K., Chisti, Y., & Banerjee, U. C., (2013). Synthesis of metallic nanoparticles using plant extracts. *Biotechnology Advances, 31*(2), 346–356.
8. Ponder, S. M., Darab, J. G., & Mallouk, T. E., (2000). Remediation of Cr (VI) and Pb (II) aqueous solutions using supported, nanoscale zero-valent iron. *Environmental Science and Technology, 34*(12), 2564–2569.
9. Lee, C., Kim, J. Y., Lee, W. I., Nelson, K. L., Yoon, J., & Sedlak, D. L., (2008). Bactericidal effect of zero-valent iron nanoparticles on *Escherichia coli. Environmental Science and Technology, 42*(13), 4927–4933.
10. García, A., Espinosa, R., Delgado, L., Casals, E., González, E., Puntes, V., Barata, C., et al., (2011). Acute toxicity of cerium oxide, titanium oxide and iron oxide nanoparticles using standardized tests. *Desalination, 269*(1–3), 136–141.
11. Anastas, P. T., Bartlett, L. B., Kirchhoff, M. M., & Williamson, T. C., (2000). The role of catalysis in the design, development, and implementation of green chemistry. *Catalysis Today 55*(1/2), 11–22.
12. Lu, Y., & Ozcan, S., (2015). Green nanomaterials: On track for a sustainable future. *Nano Today, 10*(4), 417–420.
13. Mohanpuria, P., Rana, N. K., & Yadav, S. K., (2008). Biosynthesis of nanoparticles: Technological concepts and future applications. *Journal of Nanoparticle Research, 10*(3), 507–517.
14. Makarov, V., Love, A., Sinitsyna, O., Makarova, S., Yaminsky, I., Taliansky, M., & Kalinina, N., (2014). "Green" nanotechnologies: Synthesis of metal nanoparticles using plants. *Acta Naturae (English version), 6*(1), 20.

15. Raveendran, P., Fu, J., & Wallen, S. L., (2003). Completely "green" synthesis and stabilization of metal nanoparticles. *Journal of the American Chemical Society, 125*(46), 13940–13941.

16. Barabadi, H., Ovais, M., Shinwari, Z. K., & Saravanan, M., (2017). Anticancer green bionanomaterials: Present status and future prospects. *Green Chemistry Letters and Reviews, 10*(4), 285–314.

17. Emmanuel, R., Saravanan, M., Ovais, M., Padmavathy, S., Shinwari, Z. K., & Prakash, P., (2017). Antimicrobial efficacy of drug blended biosynthesized colloidal gold nanoparticles from *Justicia* glauca against oral pathogens: A nanoantibiotic approach. *Microbial Pathogenesis, 113*, 295–302.

18. Naik, R. R., Stringer, S. J., Agarwal, G., Jones, S. E., & Stone, M. O., (2002). Biomimetic synthesis and patterning of silver nanoparticles. *Nature Materials, 1*(3), 169–172.

19. Anastas, P. T., & Warner, J. C., (1998). Principles of green chemistry. *Green Chemistry: Theory and Practice*, 29–56.

20. Devatha, C. P., & Thalla, A. K., (2018). Green synthesis of nanomaterials. *Synthesis of Inorganic Nanomaterials* (pp. 169–184). Elsevier.

21. Hakim, L. F., Portman, J. L., Casper, M. D., & Weimer, A. W., (2005). Aggregation behavior of nanoparticles in fluidized beds. *Powder Technology, 160*(3), 149–160.

22. Shankar, S. S., Rai, A., Ankamwar, B., Singh, A., Ahmad, A., & Sastry, M., (2004). Biological synthesis of triangular gold nanoprisms. *Nature Materials, 3*(7), 482–488.

23. Virkutyte, J., & Varma, R. S., (2011). Green synthesis of metal nanoparticles: Biodegradable polymers and enzymes in stabilization and surface functionalization. *Chemical Science, 2*(5), 837–846.

24. Iravani, S., (2011). Green synthesis of metal nanoparticles using plants. *Green Chemistry, 13*(10), 2638–2650.

25. Kumar, V., & Yadav, S. K., (2009). Plant-mediated synthesis of silver and gold nanoparticles and their applications. *Journal of Chemical Technology and Biotechnology: International Research in Process, Environmental and Clean Technology, 84*(2), 151–157.

26. Nadagouda, M. N., & Varma, R. S., (2006). Green and controlled synthesis of gold and platinum nanomaterials using vitamin B2: Density-assisted self-assembly of nanospheres, wires and rods. *Green Chemistry, 8*(6), 516–518.

27. Yallappa, S., Manjanna, J., & Dhananjaya, B., (2015). Phytosynthesis of stable Au, Ag and Au-Ag alloy nanoparticles using *J. sambac* leaves extract and their enhanced antimicrobial activity in presence of organic antimicrobials. *Spectrochimica Acta Part A: Molecular and Biomolecular Spectroscopy, 137*, 236–243.

28. Khalil, M. M., Ismail, E. H., & El-Magdoub, F., (2012). Biosynthesis of Au nanoparticles using olive leaf extract: 1st nano updates. *Arabian Journal of Chemistry, 5*(4), 431–437.

29. Wang, H., Li, Z., Yang, J., Li, Q., & Zhong, X., (2009). A novel activated mesocarbon microbead (aMCMB)/$Mn_3O_4$ composite for electrochemical capacitors in organic electrolyte. *Journal of Power Sources, 194*(2), 1218–1221.

30. Shahwan, T., Sirriah, S. A., Nairat, M., Boyacı, E., Eroğlu, A. E., Scott, T. B., & Hallam, K. R., (2011). Green synthesis of iron nanoparticles and their application

as a Fenton-like catalyst for the degradation of aqueous cationic and anionic dyes. *Chemical Engineering Journal, 172*(1), 258–266.

31. Kumar, K. M., Mandal, B. K., Kumar, K. S., Reddy, P. S., & Sreedhar, B., (2013). Biobased green method to synthesize palladium and iron nanoparticles using *Terminalia chebula* aqueous extract. *Spectrochimica Acta Part A: Molecular and Biomolecular Spectroscopy, 102*, 128–133.

32. Kuang, Y., Wang, Q., Chen, Z., Megharaj, M., & Naidu, R., (2013). Heterogeneous Fenton-like oxidation of monochlorobenzene using green synthesis of iron nanoparticles. *Journal of Colloid and Interface Science, 410*, 67–73.

33. Thakur, S., & Karak, N., (2014). One-step approach to prepare magnetic iron oxide/reduced graphene oxide nanohybrid for efficient organic and inorganic pollutants removal. *Materials Chemistry and Physics, 144*(3), 425–432.

34. Njagi, E. C., Huang, H., Stafford, L., Genuino, H., Galindo, H. M., Collins, J. B., Hoag, G. E., & Suib, S. L., (2011). Biosynthesis of iron and silver nanoparticles at room temperature using aqueous sorghum bran extracts. *Langmuir, 27*(1), 264–271.

35. Wang, T., Lin, J., Chen, Z., Megharaj, M., & Naidu, R., (2014). Green synthesized iron nanoparticles by green tea and eucalyptus leaves extracts used for removal of nitrate in aqueous solution. *Journal of Cleaner Production, 83*, 413–419.

36. Senthil, M., & Ramesh, C., (2012). Biogenic Synthesis of $Fe_3O_4$ nanoparticles using *Tridax* procumbens leaf extract and its antibacterial activity on pseudomonas aeruginosa. *Digest Journal of Nanomaterials and Biostructures (DJNB), 7*(4).

37. Jia, L., Zhang, Q., Li, Q., & Song, H., (2009). The biosynthesis of palladium nanoparticles by antioxidants in *Gardenia jasminoides* Ellis: Long lifetime nanocatalysts for p-nitrotoluene hydrogenation. *Nanotechnology, 20*(38), 385601.

38. Banerjee, P., Satapathy, M., Mukhopahayay, A., & Das, P., (2014). Leaf extract mediated green synthesis of silver nanoparticles from widely available Indian plants: Synthesis, characterization, antimicrobial property and toxicity analysis. *Bioresources and Bioprocessing, 1*(1), 3.

39. Ponarulselvam, S., Panneerselvam, C., Murugan, K., Aarthi, N., Kalimuthu, K., & Thangamani, S., (2012). Synthesis of silver nanoparticles using leaves of *Catharanthus roseus* Linn. G. Don and their antiplasmodial activities. *Asian Pacific Journal of Tropical Biomedicine, 2*(7), 574.

40. Allafchian, A., Mirahmadi-Zare, S., Jalali, S., Hashemi, S., & Vahabi, M., (2016). Green synthesis of silver nanoparticles using *Phlomis* leaf extract and investigation of their antibacterial activity. *Journal of Nanostructure in Chemistry, 6*(2), 129–135.

41. Perugu, S., Nagati, V., & Bhanoori, M., (2016). Green synthesis of silver nanoparticles using leaf extract of medicinally potent plant *Saraca indica*: A novel study. *Applied Nanoscience, 6*(5), 747–753.

42. Masurkar, S. A., Chaudhari, P. R., Shidore, V. B., & Kamble, S. P., (2011). Rapid biosynthesis of silver nanoparticles using *Cymbopogan citratus* (lemongrass) and its antimicrobial activity. *Nano-Micro Letters, 3*(3), 189–194.

43. Prasad, T., & Elumalai, E., (2011). Biofabrication of Ag nanoparticles using *Moringa oleifera* leaf extract and their antimicrobial activity. *Asian Pacific Journal of Tropical Biomedicine, 1*(6), 439.

44. Krishnaraj, C., Jagan, E., Rajasekar, S., Selvakumar, P., Kalaichelvan, P., & Mohan, N., (2010). Synthesis of silver nanoparticles using *Acalypha indica* leaf extracts and

its antibacterial activity against water borne pathogens. *Colloids and Surfaces B: Biointerfaces, 76*(1), 50–56.

45. Matinise, N., Fuku, X., Kaviyarasu, K., Mayedwa, N., & Maaza, M., (2017). ZnO nanoparticles via *Moringa oleifera* green synthesis: Physical properties and mechanism of formation. *Applied Surface Science, 406*, 339–347.

46. Patil, B. N., & Taranath, T. C., (2016). *Limonia acidissima* L. leaf mediated synthesis of zinc oxide nanoparticles: A potent tool against mycobacterium tuberculosis. *International Journal of Mycobacteriology, 5*(2), 197–204.

47. Vanathi, P., Rajiv, P., Narendhran, S., Rajeshwari, S., Rahman, P. K., & Venckatesh, R., (2014). Biosynthesis and characterization of phyto mediated zinc oxide nanoparticles: A green chemistry approach. *Materials Letters, 134*, 13–15.

48. Sangeetha, G., Rajeshwari, S., & Venckatesh, R., (2011). Green synthesis of zinc oxide nanoparticles by aloe barbadensis miller leaf extract: Structure and optical properties. *Materials Research Bulletin, 46*(12), 2560–2566.

49. Sindhura, K. S., Prasad, T., Selvam, P. P., & Hussain, O., (2014). Synthesis, characterization and evaluation of effect of phytogenic zinc nanoparticles on soil exo-enzymes. *Applied Nanoscience, 4*(7), 819–827.

50. Banumathi, B., Malaikozhundan, B., & Vaseeharan, B., (2016). *In vitro* acaricidal activity of ethnoveterinary plants and green synthesis of zinc oxide nanoparticles against *Rhipicephalus* (Boophilus) micro plus. *Veterinary Parasitology, 216*, 93–100.

51. Diallo, A., Beye, A., Doyle, T. B., Park, E., & Maaza, M., (2015). Green synthesis of $Co_3O_4$ nanoparticles via *Aspalathus linearis*: Physical properties. *Green Chemistry Letters and Reviews, 8*(3/4), 30–36.

52. Song, J. Y., Jang, H. K., & Kim, B. S., (2009). Biological synthesis of gold nanoparticles using *Magnolia kobus* and *Diopyros kaki* leaf extracts. *Process Biochemistry, 44*(10), 1133–1138.

53. Narayanan, K. B., & Sakthivel, N., (2010). Phytosynthesis of gold nanoparticles using leaf extract of *Coleus amboinicus* Lour. *Materials Characterization, 61*(11), 1232–1238.

54. Bhau, B., Ghosh, S., Puri, S., Borah, B., Sarmah, D., & Khan, R., (2015). Green synthesis of gold nanoparticles from the leaf extract of *Nepenthes khasiana* and antimicrobial assay. *Adv. Mater. Lett., 6*(1), 55–58.

55. Parida, U. K., Bindhani, B. K., & Nayak, P., (2011). Green synthesis and characterization of gold nanoparticles using onion (*Allium cepa*) extract. *World Journal of Nano Science and Engineering, 1*(04), 93.

56. Gopinath, K., Gowri, S., Karthika, V., & Arumugam, A., (2014). Green synthesis of gold nanoparticles from fruit extract of *Terminalia arjuna*, for the enhanced seed germination activity of gloriosa superba. *Journal of Nanostructure in Chemistry, 4*(3), 115.

57. Devatha, C., Thalla, A. K., & Katte, S. Y., (2016). Green synthesis of iron nanoparticles using different leaf extracts for treatment of domestic waste water. *Journal of Cleaner Production, 139*, 1425–1435.

58. Latha, N., & Gowri, M., (2014). Bio synthesis and characterization of $Fe_3O_4$ nanoparticles using caricaya papaya leaves extract. *Synthesis, 3*, 1551–1556.

59. Machado, S., Pinto, S., Grosso, J., Nouws, H., Albergaria, J. T., & Delerue-Matos, C., (2013). Green production of zero-valent iron nanoparticles using tree leaf extracts. *Science of the Total Environment, 445*, 1–8.

60. Huang, L., Weng, X., Chen, Z., Megharaj, M., & Naidu, R., (2014). Green synthesis of iron nanoparticles by various tea extracts: Comparative study of the reactivity. *Spectrochimica Acta Part A: Molecular and Biomolecular Spectroscopy, 130*, 295–301.

61. Sharmila, G., Thirumarimurugan, M., & Sivakumar, V. M., (2016). Optical, catalytic and antibacterial properties of phytofabricated CuO nanoparticles using *Tecoma castanifolia* leaf extract. *Optik, 127*(19), 7822–7828.

62. Mohanraj, S., Anbalagan, K., Rajaguru, P., & Pugalenthi, V., (2016). Effects of phytogenic copper nanoparticles on fermentative hydrogen production by *Enterobacter cloacae* and clostridium acetobutylicum. *International Journal of Hydrogen Energy, 41*(25), 10639–10645.

63. Nasrollahzadeh, M., & Sajadi, S. M., (2015). Green synthesis of copper nanoparticles using *Ginkgo biloba* L. leaf extract and their catalytic activity for the Huisgen [3+2] cycloaddition of azides and alkynes at room temperature. *Journal of Colloid and Interface Science, 457*, 141–147.

64. Ovais, M., Raza, A., Naz, S., Islam, N. U., Khalil, A. T., Ali, S., Khan, M. A., & Shinwari, Z. K., (2017). Current state and prospects of the phytosynthesized colloidal gold nanoparticles and their applications in cancer theranostics. *Applied Microbiology and Biotechnology, 101*(9), 3551–3565.

65. Ajitha, B., Reddy, Y. A. K., & Reddy, P. S., (2015). Green synthesis and characterization of silver nanoparticles using *Lantana camara* leaf extract. *Materials Science and Engineering: C, 49*, 373–381.

66. Dhillon, G. S., Brar, S. K., Kaur, S., & Verma, M., (2012). Green approach for nanoparticle biosynthesis by fungi: Current trends and applications. *Critical Reviews in Biotechnology, 32*(1), 49–73.

67. Mahendra, R., Alka, Y., Bridge, P., & Aniket, G., (2009). Myconanotechnology: A new and emerging science. *Applied Mycology*, 258–267.

68. Saravanan, M., Barik, S. K., MubarakAli, D., Prakash, P., & Pugazhendhi, A., (2018). Synthesis of silver nanoparticles from *Bacillus brevis* (NCIM 2533) and their antibacterial activity against pathogenic bacteria. *Microbial Pathogenesis, 116*, 221–226.

69. Klaus, T., Joerger, R., Olsson, E., & Granqvist, C. G., (1999). Silver-based crystalline nanoparticles, microbially fabricated. *Proceedings of the National Academy of Sciences, 96*(24), 13611–13614.

70. Salam, H. A., Rajiv, P., Kamaraj, M., Jagadeeswaran, P., Gunalan, S., & Sivaraj, R., (2012). Plants: Green route for nanoparticle synthesis. *Int. Res. J. Biol. Sci., 1*(5), 85–90.

71. Husseiny, M., El-Aziz, M. A., Badr, Y., & Mahmoud, M., (2007). Biosynthesis of gold nanoparticles using Pseudomonas aeruginosa. *Spectrochimica Acta Part A: Molecular and Biomolecular Spectroscopy, 67*(3/4), 1003–1006.

72. Ahmad, A., Senapati, S., Khan, M. I., Kumar, R., Ramani, R., Srinivas, V., & Sastry, M., (2003). Intracellular synthesis of gold nanoparticles by a novel alkalotolerant actinomycete, *Rhodococcus* species. *Nanotechnology, 14*(7), 824.

73. Ovais, M., Khalil, A. T., Ayaz, M., Ahmad, I., Nethi, S. K., & Mukherjee, S., (2018). Biosynthesis of metal nanoparticles via microbial enzymes: A mechanistic approach. *International Journal of Molecular Sciences, 19*(12), 4100.

74. Ingle, A., Gade, A., Pierrat, S., Sonnichsen, C., & Rai, M., (2008). Mycosynthesis of silver nanoparticles using the fungus *Fusarium acuminatum* and its activity against some human pathogenic bacteria. *Current Nanoscience, 4*(2), 141–144.

75. Razavi, M., Salahinejad, E., Fahmy, M., Yazdimamaghani, M., Vashaee, D., & Tayebi, L., (2015). Green chemical and biological synthesis of nanoparticles and their biomedical applications. *Green Processes for Nanotechnology* (pp. 207–235). Springer.

76. Khandel, P., & Shahi, S. K., (2018). Mycogenic nanoparticles and their bio-prospective applications: Current status and future challenges. *Journal of Nanostructure in Chemistry, 8*(4), 369–391.

77. Wypij, M., Golinska, P., Dahm, H., & Rai, M., (2016). Actinobacterial-mediated synthesis of silver nanoparticles and their activity against pathogenic bacteria. *IET Nanobiotechnology, 11*(3), 336–342.

78. Prema, P., Iniya, P., & Immanuel, G., (2016). Microbial mediated synthesis, characterization, antibacterial and synergistic effect of gold nanoparticles using *Klebsiella pneumoniae* (MTCC-4030). *RSC Advances, 6*(6), 4601–4607.

79. Manikprabhu, D., Cheng, J., Chen, W., Sunkara, A. K., Mane, S. B., Kumar, R., Hozzein, W. N., Duan, Y. Q., & Li, W. J., (2016). Sunlight mediated synthesis of silver nanoparticles by a novel actinobacterium (*Sinomonas mesophila* MPKL 26) and its antimicrobial activity against multi drug resistant *Staphylococcus aureus*. *Journal of Photochemistry and Photobiology B: Biology, 158*, 202–205.

80. Lv, Q., Zhang, B., Xing, X., Zhao, Y., Cai, R., Wang, W., & Gu, Q., (2018). Biosynthesis of copper nanoparticles using *Shewanella loihica* PV-4 with antibacterial activity: Novel approach and mechanisms investigation. *Journal of Hazardous Materials, 347*, 141–149.

81. Ahmed, E., Kalathil, S., Shi, L., Alharbi, O., & Wang, P., (2018). Synthesis of ultra-small platinum, palladium and gold nanoparticles by *Shewanella loihica* PV-4 electrochemically active biofilms and their enhanced catalytic activities. *Journal of Saudi Chemical Society, 22*(8), 919–929.

82. Kalpana, V., Kataru, B. A. S., Sravani, N., Vigneshwari, T., Panneerselvam, A., & Rajeswari, V. D., (2018). Biosynthesis of zinc oxide nanoparticles using culture filtrates of *Aspergillus niger*: Antimicrobial textiles and dye degradation studies. *Open Nano, 3*, 48–55.

83. Elamawi, R. M., Al-Harbi, R. E., & Hendi, A. A., (2018). Biosynthesis and characterization of silver nanoparticles using *Trichoderma longibrachiatum* and their effect on phytopathogenic fungi. *Egyptian Journal of Biological Pest Control, 28*(1), 28.

84. Tripathi, R. M., Shrivastav, B. R., & Shrivastav, A., (2018). Antibacterial and catalytic activity of biogenic gold nanoparticles synthesized by *Trichoderma harzianum*. *IET Nanobiotechnology, 12*(4), 509–513.

85. Ahmed, A. A., Hamzah, H., & Maaroof, M., (2018). Analyzing formation of silver nanoparticles from the filamentous fungus *Fusarium oxysporum* and their antimicrobial activity. *Turkish Journal of Biology, 42*(1), 54–62.

86. Domany, E. B. E., Essam, T. M., Ahmed, A. E., & Farghali, A. A., (2018). Biosynthesis physico-chemical optimization of gold nanoparticles as anticancer and synergetic antimicrobial activity using *Pleurotus ostreatus* fungus. *J. Appl. Pharm. Sci.,* 8.
87. Spagnoletti, F. N., Spedalieri, C., Kronberg, F., & Giacometti, R., (2019). Extracellular biosynthesis of bactericidal Ag/AgCl nanoparticles for crop protection using the fungus *Macrophomina phaseolina. Journal of Environmental Management, 231,* 457–466.
88. Bao, Z., & Lan, C. Q., (2018). Mechanism of light-dependent biosynthesis of silver nanoparticles mediated by cell extract of *Neochloris oleoabundans. Colloids and Surfaces B: Biointerfaces, 170,* 251–257.
89. González-Ballesteros, N., Prado-López, S., Rodríguez-González, J., Lastra, M., & Rodríguez-Argüelles, M., (2017). Green synthesis of gold nanoparticles using brown algae *Cystoseira baccata*: Its activity in colon cancer cells. *Colloids and Surfaces B: Biointerfaces, 153,* 190–198.
90. Zhang, Z., Chen, J., Yang, Q., Lan, K., Yan, Z., & Chen, J., (2018). Eco-friendly intracellular microalgae synthesis of fluorescent CdSe QDs as a sensitive nanoprobe for determination of imatinib. *Sensors and Actuators B: Chemical, 263,* 625–633.
91. Sayadi, M. H., Salmani, N., Heidari, A., & Rezaei, M. R., (2018). Bio-synthesis of palladium nanoparticle using spirulina platensis alga extract and its application as adsorbent. *Surfaces and Interfaces, 10,* 136–143.
92. Sharma, M., Behl, K., Nigam, S., & Joshi, M., (2018). $TiO_2$-GO nanocomposite for photocatalysis and environmental applications: A green synthesis approach. *Vacuum, 156,* 434–439.
93. Maensiri, S., Laokul, P., Klinkaewnarong, J., Phokha, S., Promarak, V., & Seraphin, S., (2008). Indium oxide ($In_2O_3$) nanoparticles using Aloe vera plant extract: Synthesis and optical properties. *J. Optoelectron Adv. Mater., 10*(3), 161–165.
94. Saratale, R. G., Karuppusamy, I., Saratale, G. D., Pugazhendhi, A., Kumar, G., Park, Y., Ghodake, G. S., et al., (2018). A comprehensive review on green nanomaterials using biological systems: Recent perception and their future applications. *Colloids and Surfaces B: Biointerfaces, 170,* 20–35.
95. Ben, S. A. N., Zyed, R., Lassoued, M. A., Nidhal, S., Sfar, S., & Mahjoub, A., (2012). Plant-derived nanoparticles enhance antiviral activity against Coxsackievirus B3 by acting on virus particles and Vero cells. *Digest Journal of Nanomaterials and Biostructures, 7*(2), 737–744.
96. Khan, M., Williams, R., & Williams, D., (1996). *In-vitro* corrosion and wear of titanium alloys in the biological environment. *Biomaterials, 17*(22), 2117–2126.
97. McKay, G., Macnair, R., MacDonald, C., & Grant, M., (1996). Interactions of orthopedic metals with an immortalized rat osteoblast cell line. *Biomaterials, 17*(13), 1339–1344.
98. Okazaki, Y., (2002). Effect of friction on anodic polarization properties of metallic biomaterials. *Biomaterials, 23*(9), 2071–2077.
99. Duisabeau, L., Combrade, P., & Forest, B., (2004). Environmental effect on fretting of metallic materials for orthopedic implants. *Wear, 256*(7/8), 805–816.
100. Barril, S., Mischler, S., & Landolt, D., (2004). Influence of fretting regimes on the tribocorrosion behavior of Ti6Al4V in 0.9 wt.% sodium chloride solution. *Wear, 256*(9/10), 963–972.

101. Barril, S., Mischler, S., & Landolt, D., (2005). Electrochemical effects on the fretting corrosion behavior of Ti-6Al-4V in 0.9% sodium chloride solution. *Wear, 259*(1–6), 282–291.

102. Guo, K. W., & Tam, H. Y., (2015). Green techniques for biomedical metallic materials with nanotechnology. *Green Processes for Nanotechnology* (pp. 35–73). Springer.

103. Duerig, T., Pelton, A., & Stöckel, D., (1999). An overview of nitinol medical applications. *Materials Science and Engineering: A, 273*, 149–160.

104. Narayan, R., (2009). *Biomedical Materials*. Springer Science & Business Media..

105. Huo, Q., (2007). A perspective on bioconjugated nanoparticles and quantum dots. *Colloids and Surfaces B: Biointerfaces, 59*(1), 1–10.

106. Reynolds, R. A., Mirkin, C. A., & Letsinger, R. L., (2000). Homogeneous, nanoparticle-based quantitative colorimetric detection of oligonucleotides. *Journal of the American Chemical Society, 122*(15), 3795–3796.

107. Khosa, A., Reddi, S., & Saha, R. N., (2018). Nanostructured lipid carriers for site-specific drug delivery. *Biomedicine and Pharmacotherapy, 103*, 598–613.

108. Oldenburg, S. J., Genick, C. C., Clark, K. A., & Schultz, D. A., (2002). Base pair mismatch recognition using plasmon resonant particle labels. *Analytical Biochemistry, 309*(1), 109–116.

109. Hossen, S., Hossain, M. K., Basher, M., Mia, M., Rahman, M., & Uddin, M. J., (2019). Smart nanocarrier-based drug delivery systems for cancer therapy and toxicity studies: A review. *Journal of Advanced Research, 15*, 1–18.

110. Kao, K. C., & Mou, C. Y., (2013). Pore-expanded mesoporous silica nanoparticles with alkanes/ethanol as pore expanding agent. *Microporous and Mesoporous Materials, 169*, 7–15.

111. Qu, F., Zhu, G., Lin, H., Zhang, W., Sun, J., Li, S., & Qiu, S., (2006). A controlled release of ibuprofen by systematically tailoring the morphology of mesoporous silica materials. *Journal of Solid State Chemistry, 179*(7), 2027–2035.

112. Kanwar, R., Rathee, J., Salunke, D. B., & Mehta, S. K., (2019). Green nanotechnology-driven drug delivery assemblies. *ACS Omega, 4*(5), 8804–8815.

113. Tran, A. V., Shim, K., Thi, T. T. V., Kook, J. K., An, S. S. A., & Lee, S. W., (2018). Targeted and controlled drug delivery by multifunctional mesoporous silica nanoparticles with internal fluorescent conjugates and external polydopamine and graphene oxide layers. *Acta Biomaterialia, 74*, 397–413.

# CHAPTER 2

# Fabrication of Green Biopolymeric Nanocomposites

I. SAMY,[1,2,3] KAREEM M. ABD EL-RAHMAN,[4] AMAL ELHUSSIENY,[1] M. FAISAL,[1] and NICOLA. M. EVERITT[5]

[1]Center of Nanoscience and Technology (CNT), Nile University, Nile Avenue, Giza, Egypt

[2]Department of Industrial Engineering and Service Management, School of Engineering, Nile University, Nile Avenue, Giza, Egypt

[3]Smart Engineering Systems Research Center, Nile University, Nile Avenue, Giza – 116453, Egypt

[4]Department of Materials Science, Institute of Graduate Studies and Research, Alexandria University, Alexandria, Egypt

[5]Bioengineering Research Group, Faculty of Engineering, University of Nottingham, University Park, Nottingham NG7 2RD, UK

## ABSTRACT

In this study, chitosan and nano-chitosan were reinforced by using several types and concentrations of wastes; natural fibers such as chitin fiber, chitin whisker fiber, cellulose fiber, nano cellulose fiber, eggshells, and cotton waste. The chitin fibers were extracted from shrimp shell waste, and cellulose fibers were extracted from rice straw waste, while cotton waste was extracted from cotton stalks. The chitosan and nano-chitosan polymer were the matrices, and the different fillers acted as the reinforcement to form the green polymeric nanocomposites. Nano-chitosan was prepared by the cross-linker method to optimize the particle size of nano-chitosan and study the effect of different particle size on the physical properties of prepared films. Nanocomposite films were prepared from chitosan and nano-chitosan by solution casting after incorporating with fillers. Mechanical characterization was performed on all synthesized films. Furthermore, nanoindentation tests were performed to investigate the mechanical properties of the fabricated nanocomposite. The addition of fillers enhanced the elongation at break and the tensile strength, while the hardness and the reduced modulus decreased upon the addition of fillers.

## 2.1 INTRODUCTION

Since the 1950s, the production and expenditure of synthetic plastic materials have been thriving rapidly and outpacing any other material [1]. In 2018, the worldwide production of plastics attained 360 million tonnes, which is distributed, as shown in Figure 2.1 [2]. Conventional plastic products that are frequently used include polyethylene (PE), polypropylene (PP), polyethylene terephthalate (PET), polyvinyl chloride (PVC), and polystyrene (PS); they are all derived from petroleum resources [2].

Conventional polymers have superior mechanical properties, excellent thermal stability, and low cost, so they are consumed in a broad range of applications like pipes, containers, electrical conduits, and the packaging industry (films, bottles, plastic bags, etc.). Packaging activities consume 40% of the consumed, and they end up in landfills or litter in the oceans [3].

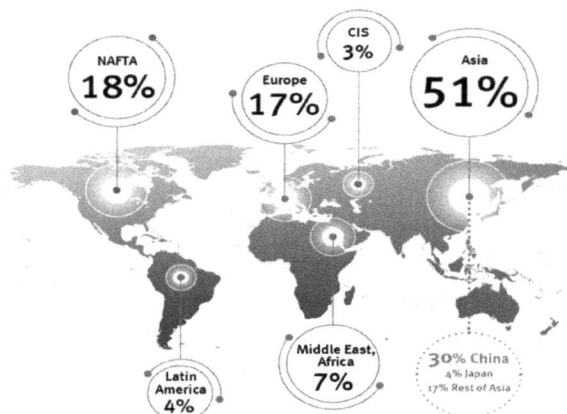

**FIGURE 2.1**   Distribution of global plastics production.
*Source:* Copyright permissions ©Plastics Europe Market Research Group (PEMRG) and Conversio Market and Strategy GmbH [2].

This huge consumption of petroleum-based conventional plastics resulted in ongoing waste accumulation all over the world. Over the last seven decades, plastic wastes reached 300 million tons; reflecting the current waste management pattern [1], due to the difficulty of collecting, low recycling percentage, reusing, and the resistance of the conventional plastics to bio-degradation as the majority of the plastic wastes consists of non-biodegradable synthetic plastics originated from a petroleum source. Thus, they accumulate in the environment for hundreds of years, becoming a significant part of solid waste and a serious disaster called "plastic pollution" [3, 4].

Plastic pollution is now clearly observed on land; thousands of animals and birds were killed due to eating plastic. Around 4.7 to 12.7 tons of waste was abandoned in oceans from 192 countries with coastal borders each year (according to the last report in 2016 by Imperial College, London) [5, 6]. The fisheries are not far from the consequences of this massive amount of plastics, unfortunately, caused entanglement accidents for 344 species, including marine turtles, seabirds, whales, and fish, resulting in at least $13 billion in total economic damage in the world's marine every year [1].

The ecosystem was massively damaged during the burning of plastics, destructive gases such as regular carbon dioxide ($CO_2$) with carbon $^{12}C$, carbon monoxide (CO), and dioxins are released. These harmful gases cause pollution and lead to the weakening of the ozone layer, causing climate change [3]. Thus some countries issued bans and levies to the imported conventional plastics [1, 7].

Researchers are currently developing sustainable methods to mitigate these problems and to overcome the drawbacks of the conventional non-biodegradable polymers by using biopolymers and bio-composites of biodegradable-bio-based polymers and natural fillers as an effective way to reduce the volume of plastic waste. Biopolymers refer to either biodegradable polymers or bio-based polymers; the biodegradable polymers undergo a biodegradation mechanism that takes place through microorganisms such as bacteria, fungi, and algae, with enzymatic activities that lead to a chain cleavage of the polymer to monomers and then decomposes into $CO_2$, water, methane, and biomass, according to the type of the biodegradation process. While, the bio-based polymers are made from organic renewable resources, as shown in Figure 2.2 [8–10].

By tailoring biodegradable bio-based composites (biocomposites), optimized characteristics can be gained, not only the biodegradation advantages such as reducing plastic accumulation and saving animals and fisheries, but also the bio-based advantages. Bio-based polymers mainly consist of $^{14}C$, which drives them to become a part of the natural carbon cycle. Carbon 14 or $^{14}C$ is the modern isotope of carbon; it is emitted in the form of $CO_2$ when the products are incinerated or biodegraded and capable of participating in the photosynthesis process during the biomass growth. Conversely, the other carbon isotope $^{12}C$ or old carbon, which originates from fossil fuels, is not capable of joining the natural carbon cycle or participating in the photosynthesis process. Thus, the polymers consisting of $^{14}C$ are exemplifying the concept of "zero-emission," which would have a vital role in preserving the climate and striving the global warming [11].

Unfortunately, substituting the traditional polymers totally by biodegradable polymers would be limited by the biodegradable polymers' high cost and poor mechanical properties. Preparation of bio-composites that contain biodegradable polymers and natural fillers as a renewable bio-based reinforcement can reduce the cost and enhance the mechanical properties through an ecofriendly plastic product [12].

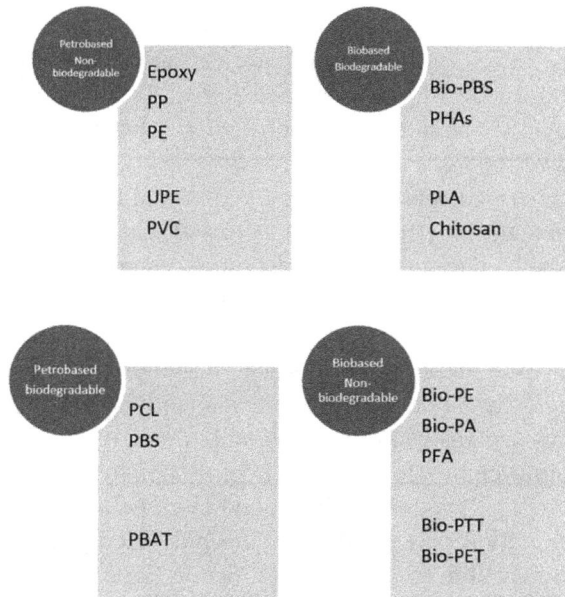

**FIGURE 2.2**   Types of polymers for bio-composites [12].
*Source:* Adapted from Ref. [12].

Advanced resources such as bio reinforcement materials, wastes, industrial coproducts, and reprocessed materials, agricultural waste can be used as both the matrix and reinforcement in biocomposites to minimize the use of nonrenewable resources, especially for wastes that suffer from the difficulty of removing from the environment [12]. The purpose of this research is not only using environmentally friendly materials to aid environment preservation; it is an attempt to represent a full model of waste management.

Waste management is the system of treating stable wastes and finding a variety of solutions for recycling objects. An effective waste management process accomplishes valorization of waste and attains a circular economy model where materials reuse in other applications and provide environmental and societal benefits. In this paper, resource recovery is attained as one of the waste management techniques, where useful discarded waste is processed to extract the reinforcements used in fabricating green polymeric composites. This circular economic model decreases pollution since large amounts of dry waste stored in hot climates like Egypt can cause fire hazards and contaminate the surface or ground waters. The move to a more sustainable society requires greater refinement to control waste [13].

Natural polymers are used in this research since they are biodegradable [14]. Chitosan is a natural polymer extracted from chitin, a polysaccharide that exists in exoskeletons of crustaceans such as shrimp, lobster, and crabs [15]. Chitosan is used for wound healing, filtration, and food packaging [16]. Nevertheless, it has weak mechanical properties that restrict its applications. Natural fillers are added to chitosan to improve its properties [17]. The mechanical properties of chitosan films vary according to the deacetylation rate, chemical structure, and molecular size. [18].

The selection of fillers depends on the application for green polymeric nanocomposites. In this topical research, cellulose, nano-cellulose, chitin, and chitin whiskers were selected as fillers. They improved the mechanical properties of chitosan when used as a sustainable material for shopping bags [18]. According to Giacomo D'Angelo et al., the percentage of filler that improved the mechanical properties of chitosan was 25, and 35% of fillers exhibited the highest fracture strength [18]. In this research, the same percentage fillers will be analyzed, but with nano-chitosan as a matrix. Nano-chitosan films are fabricated by crosslinking of chitosan.

Crosslinking significantly increases the elongation percentage due to the formation of strong covalent bonds. Further, crosslinking maintains the strength of the polymer [19].

Another successful application is using chitosan in food packaging applications due to its film formation property, biodegradability, and selective permeability to gases, and anti-bacterial effect. It functions as a matrix for combining fillers to enhance the mechanical properties [21]. Fillers such as cotton waste and eggshells waste were added in this study to improve the mechanical strength for the food packaging application. The reason for choosing cotton waste as filler is due to the excessive yearly harvest of 432,480 tons/ month of cotton in Egypt. Thus, the amount of waste collected could be around 360 tons of cotton waste per month, if only 1% of cotton is regarded as waste [22]. Regarding eggshells, they act as a sustainable material in food packaging, and their usage results in savings for food manufacturers that use large amounts of eggs and need to dispose of their waste. A mayonnaise manufacturer utilizes 1.3 million eggs every week, and pays £ 30,000 a year for eggshell disposal [23].

## 2.2   MATERIALS AND METHODS

### 2.2.1   MATERIALS

The shrimp shell waste, rice straw waste, and cotton waste were bought from local markets and farms in Egypt. Eggshell waste was collected from home waste. Chemicals used in the treatment of waste were bought from Sigma Aldrich, such as hydrochloric acid, sodium hydroxide, and acetic acid.

### 2.2.2   PREPARATION OF CHITOSAN AND NANO-CHITOSAN

Chitosan was obtained from shrimp shell waste by a deproteinization step, and a demineralization step to generate chitin. To produce nano-chitosan, chitosan was first dispersed into 2% acetic acid. Sodium tripolyphosphate was added to the chitosan solution dropwise [18, 24].

## 2.2.3   PREPARATION OF FILLERS

The cellulose was removed from the rice straw waste after removing lignin using alkali treatment. It was sonicated using ultrasonication to produce nano cellulose. 3 N of HCL was used to produce both chitin and chitin whiskers from shrimp shell waste [6]. The eggshell powder was prepared after collecting eggshells and washing by both DI water and ethanol, then oven drying. After drying, they were ground and sieved with a 40-micron mesh sieve. For cotton and nanocotton, cotton stalks were collected and shredded into small pieces about 0.1–1 cm in size. 200 g of shredded cotton stalks were added to a solution of 15% by weight NaOH and stirred at 1500 RPM at room temperature for 2 hrs. Cotton stalks were separated using a NaOH solution and washed thoroughly with purified water till neutralization. 380 mL of 1 M HCl was added to the cotton stalk fibers at 80°C, and magnetically stirred at 1500 RPM for 2 hrs. Cotton stalk fibers were removed using HCl solution and washed thoroughly with distilled water till neutralization. Cotton was extracted at this step; then, a chemical treatment was performed to produce nanocotton [25].

## 2.2.4   PREPARATION OF COMPOSITES

Each sample contained a matrix of chitosan or nano-chitosan and filler in different quantities, according to Table 2.1. The solutions were emptied into smooth plastic containers till it was completely dry.

**TABLE 2.1**   Combinations of the Synthesized Composites

| Sample | Matrix | Reinforcement | Percentage Reinforcement | Code |
|--------|--------|---------------|--------------------------|------|
| 1. | Chitosan | | | CS |
| 2. | Chitosan | Cotton waste | 5 | CS-5COT |
| 3. | Chitosan | Cotton waste | 15 | CS-5COT |
| 4. | Chitosan | Cotton waste | 25 | CS-5COT |
| 5. | Chitosan | Nanocotton waste | 5 | CS-5NCOT |
| 6. | Chitosan | Nanocotton waste | 15 | CS-15NCOT |
| 7. | Chitosan | Nanocotton waste | 25 | CS-25NCOT |

**TABLE 2.1**    *(Continued)*

| Sample | Matrix | Reinforcement | Percentage Reinforcement | Code |
|--------|--------|---------------|--------------------------|------|
| 8. | Chitosan | Eggshells | 5 | CS-5ES |
| 9. | Chitosan | Eggshells | 15 | CS-15ES |
| 10. | Chitosan | Eggshells | 25 | CS-25ES |
| 11. | Nano-chitosan | | | NC |
| 12. | Nano-chitosan | Nano rice straw | 5 | NC-5NRS |
| 13. | Nano-chitosan | Nano rice straw | 15 | NC-15NRS |
| 14. | Nano-chitosan | Nano rice straw | 25 | NC-25NRS |
| 15. | Nano-chitosan | Nano rice straw | 35 | NC-35NRS |
| 16. | Nano-chitosan | Chitin | 5 | NC-5 chitin |
| 17. | Nano-chitosan | Chitin | 15 | NC-15 chitin |
| 18. | Nano-chitosan | Chitin | 25 | NC-25 chitin |
| 19. | Nano-chitosan | Chitin | 35 | NC-35 chitin |
| 20. | Nano-chitosan | Chitin Whisker | 15 | NC-15 chitin whiskers |
| 21. | Nano-chitosan | Chitin Whisker | 35 | NC-35 chitin whiskers |

## 2.3   CHARACTERIZATION TECHNIQUES

Mechanical properties show the material's capability to withstand deformation, thus the limits of the material's functionality. Tensile tests were performed using the Instron machine, 50 kN maximum load for the chitosan reinforced composites. The specimens were cut and placed between the grips. Load and displacement were recorded [6]. For the nano-chitosan composites, nanoindentation was executed on a nanotest equipment. Nano-chitosan composites films were cut ($15 \times 15$ mm$^2$). A spherical 10 μm diameter indenter was used (20 indentations per sample) because it offers a smooth transition from elastic to elastic-plastic interaction. The intensity of penetration was documented when load is employed to the indenter. The Reduced modulus (E) and hardness values (H) were calculated [26].

## 2.4 RESULTS AND DISCUSSIONS

In a typical analysis, Figure 2.3 shows Young's modulus of the films with different compositions compared to pure CS films, CS-NCOT, and CS-ES composite films displayed higher modulus while CS-COT exhibited a lower value. Adding 15%, NCOT increased the value reaching 2466 MPa, while 15% ES exhibited 2752.89 MPa. Adding COT decreased Young's modulus of 921.0 MPa than Pure CS film (1374.73 MPa). Moreover, the increase in the filler wt.% at 25% demonstrated a decline in Young's modulus owing to the agglomeration of the excess percentage of fillers. Although NCOT and ES had enhanced Young's Modulus, but the elongation at break for NCOT and ES showed a poor performance. Young's modulus is an indication of the stiffness of composites. The addition of natural fillers improves the stiffness of the composites and reduces the elongation at break.

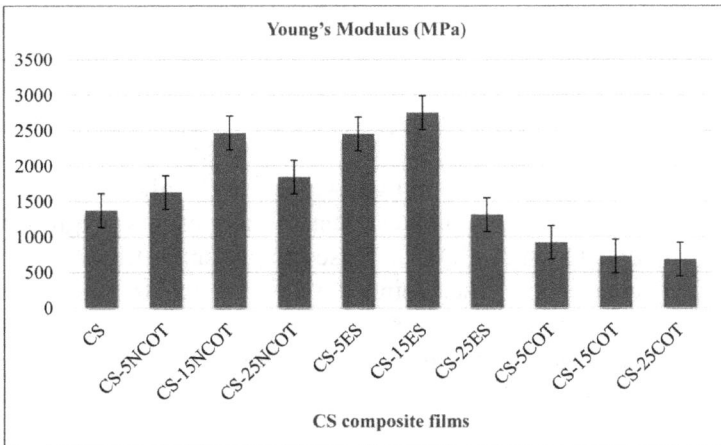

**FIGURE 2.3** Effect of type and composition of fillers on the Young's Modulus of CS films.

Hence, 25 wt.% of ES indicated the lowest elongation at break, which was 0.8%, as displayed in Figure 2.4. For the NCOT, it didn't not enhance the elongation compared to CS films, which was 4.2%. The addition of 5 wt.% and 15 wt.% of COT improved the elongation at break, extending the elongation at break to 35%. Thus, the CS-COT composite could be suitable for applications of stretch films for food packaging. NCOT and ES had low elongation at break percentage and a brittle behavior at room temperature due to the poor interfacial adhesion with the polymer. COT had an improved elongation at break due to the decrease in tensile strength. Therefore, the elongation at break increased. The composites were flexible due to the addition of cotton and broke at higher deformation.

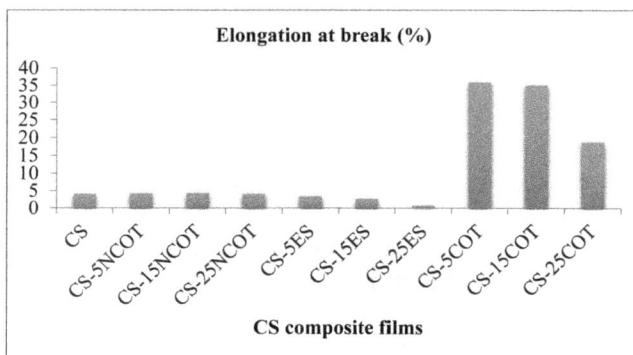

**FIGURE 2.4**   Effect of type and composition of fillers on the elongation at break of CS films.

The addition of different composition of fillers enhanced the tensile strength of chitosan reaching its highest value by adding 15 wt.% ES [27]. It showed the highest tensile strength 47.91 MPa, while 15 wt.% NCOT filler revealed a significant enhancement in the tensile strength reaching 41.95 MPa [28]. 15 wt.% COT increased the strength till 31 MPa but it started to decrease upon increasing the filler concentration. Increasing the addition fillers content in the matrix indicated higher tensile strength. The dispersion of the filler was better and the mixing of the matrix and filler was successfully done. The tensile strength decreased at a higher percentage. At 25 wt.%, the films were brittle, which was attributed to the agglomeration of fillers inside the matrix as shown in Figure 2.5 [29]. The agglomerations led to less interfaces between fillers and matrix.

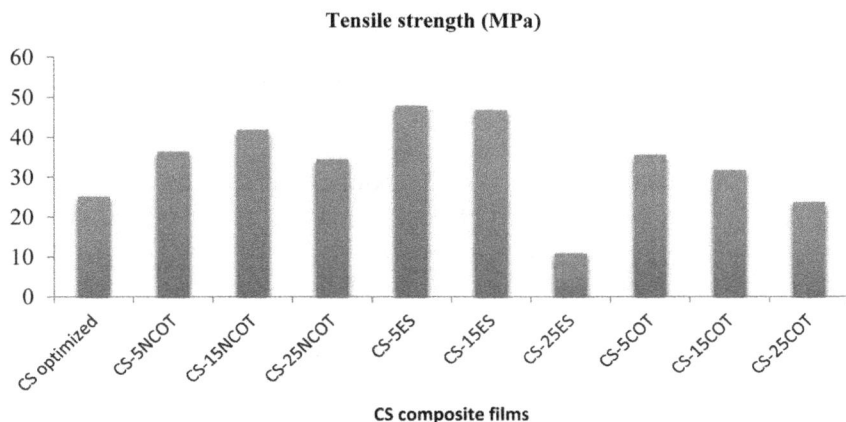

**FIGURE 2.5** Effect of type and composition of fillers on the tensile strength of CS [29]. *Source:* Copyright ©2017, Journal of thermal analysis and calorimetry, Springer.

The results showed in Table 2.2 that composite films have superior tensile and young's modulus compared to the neat chitosan due to reinforcement from the particles of the fillers to the chitosan interface. Moreover, mechanical properties of natural filler composites largely depend on the type of matrix, type, and composition of filler. Hence, the usage of plant-based fibers reinforced produced a composite with better strength and rigidity.

**TABLE 2.2** Summary of Results of the Mechanical Testing of CS and CS Composite Film

| Film | Young's Modulus (MPa) | Tensile Strength (MPa) | Elongation at Break (%) |
|------|------------------------|-------------------------|--------------------------|
| CS | 1374.73 MPa | 25.15 MPa | 4.2% |
| CS-5NCOT | 1627.91 MPa | 36.41 MPa | 4.3% |
| CS-15NCOT | 2466.48 MPa | 41.95 MPa | 4.4% |
| CS-25NCOT | 1844.26 MPa | 34.59 MPa | 4.2% |
| CS-5ES | 2451.75 MPa | 47.91 MPa | 3.5% |
| CS-15ES | 2752.89 MPa | 46.89 MPa | 2.8% |
| CS-25ES | 1313.58 MPa | 10.90 MPa | 0.8% |
| CS-5COT | 921.0 MPa | 35.73 MPa | 36.01% |

Nanoindentation experiments were conducted since they are less destructive than tensile testing. The direct results from a nanoindentation experiment are load versus displacement. The hardness is the calculated mean stress using the highest load value and the residual indentation area of the tip. For as spherical indenture, it changes as a function of penetration depth. Furthermore, the reduced modulus is calculated at the beginning of the unloading process. Hardness (H) and reduced modulus (E) were calculated for pure nano-chitosan and nano-chitosan composites. It demonstrated that pure NC films displayed the maximum value in hardness and reduced modulus 0.38 GPa and 12.500 GPa, respectively among all other combinations. This indicated there is an improvement in hardness or reduced modulus by adding fillers. The NC-25NRS and NC-35NRS presented inferior results than the NCS film, as revealed in Figures 2.6 and 2.7.

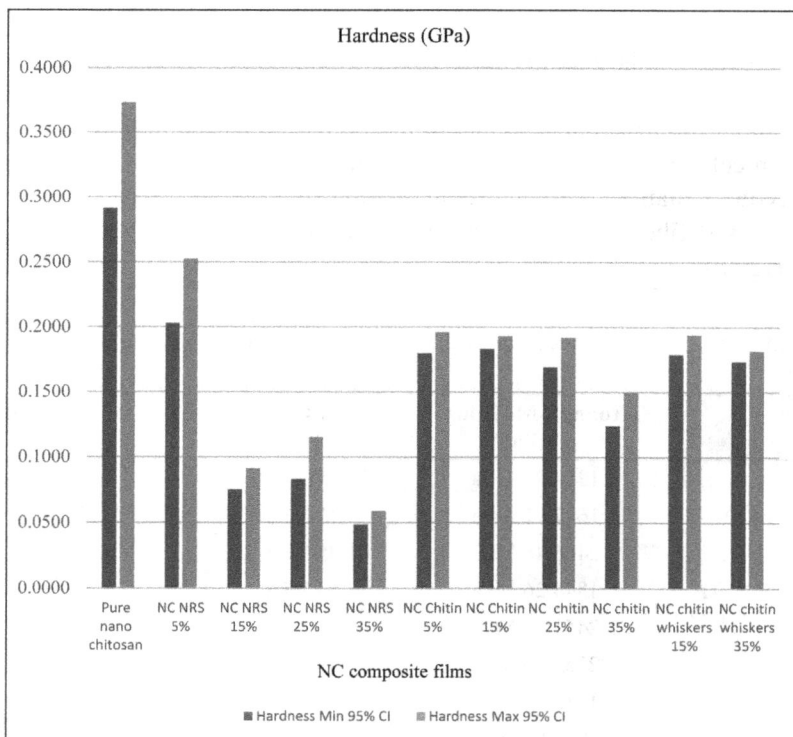

**FIGURE 2.6** Hardness of nano-chitosan and nano-chitosan composites.

The mean values of reduced modulus using the spherical tip suggested that the nanofilms are stiff and brittle. At the same time, NC-25 chitin whiskers and NC-25 chitin showed improvement in hardness and reduced modulus compared to other fillers due to the homogeneous dispersion of chitin and chitin whickers within the polymer as shown in Figures 2.6 and 2.7.

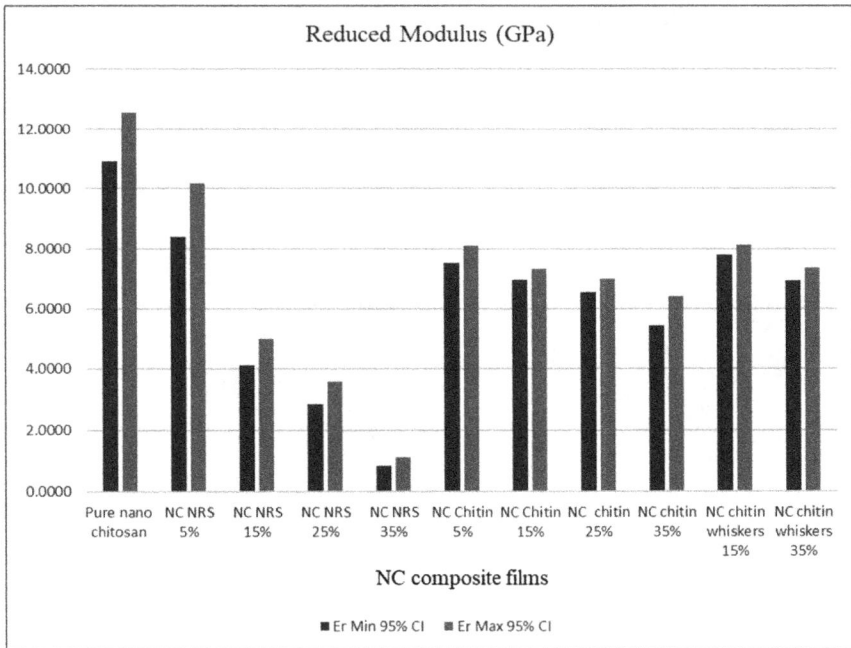

**FIGURE 2.7**    Reduced modulus of nano-chitosan and nano-chitosan composites.

The pure NC film showed homogeneity in the form of smooth surfaces without cracks or pores, indicating good miscibility in the synthesized films (Figure 2.8(a)). At the same time, a low interaction was observed (Figures 2.8(b) and 2.8(c)). Also, due to the resemblance between cellulose and chitosan structures,' a few chains overlapped between the matrix and the filler and deformation since the fibers were not well dispersed causing clusters as shown in Figure 2.8(d). Moreover, the nanofibers formed chains, which were surrounded by the NC layer. These chains were formed due to the high concentration of $NH_2$ in NC [30]. NC-25 chitin had a hard surface with whirls, with non-homogeneous particles of chitin and chitosan, which were not mixed, causing the formation of weak, cracked films. While, NC-25 chitin whiskers composite showed even dispersion of whisker within chitosan, forming a fibrous network structure in random orientation, but tight network showed in Figure 2.8(e).

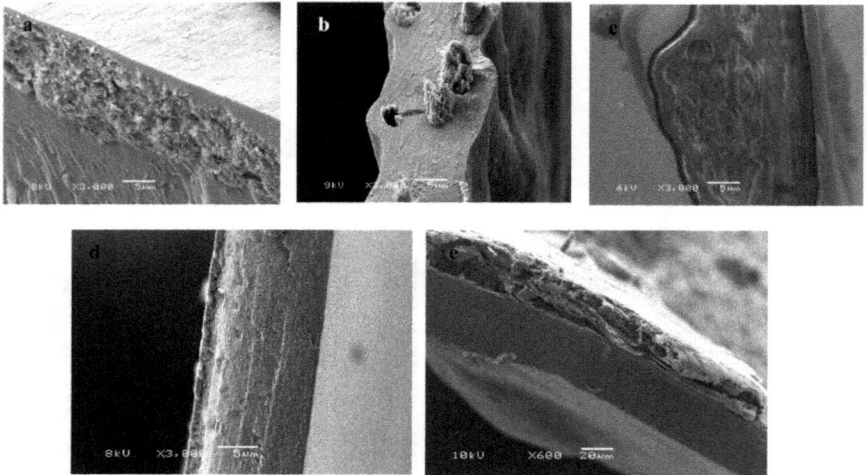

**FIGURE 2.8** Typical SEM image of (a) NC, (b) NC-25RS, (c) NC-25NRS, (d) NC-25 chitin, and (e) NC-chitin Whsiker.

## 2.5 CONCLUSIONS

The current study established a capable approach to fabricate green polymer nanocomposites from waste. The results attained for nano-chitosan showed that the hardness and reduced modulus are higher than the ones for composites. At the same time, the mechanical properties of the chitosan composites films were improved by the addition of 15 wt.% filler. Increasing the wt.% of fillers caused a decline in mechanical properties. This study is not only using eco-friendly materials to save the environment, but it is an attempt to represent a full model of waste management where the fillers are fabricated out of waste. Additionally, the selected natural fillers degrade naturally in the soil. Chitin is the waste byproduct after extracting chitosan, while rice straw was burnt after rice cultivation, and eggshells and cotton waste are also considered a type of waste, which is reused in a beneficial way. This investigation focuses on the biological production and biocompatibility of the chitosan reinforced with rice straw fibers, and chitin are favorable features for food packaging bag applications, which provide the suitable mechanical performance and biodegradability needed for biodegradable, eco-friendly food packaging bags.

## KEYWORDS

- **biopolymers**
- **mechanical properties**
- **nanocomposites**
- **natural fibers**
- **natural fillers bio-composites**
- **polyethylene**

## REFERENCES

1. Giacovelli, C., (2018). *Single-Use Plastics: A Roadmap for Sustainability.*
2. Plastics Europe, (2019). *Plastics-the Facts 2019: An Analysis of European Plastics Production, Demand and Waste Data.* www.plasticseurope.org (accessed on 9 November 2020).
3. Gumede, T., Luyt, A., & Müller, A., (2018). Review on PCL, PBS and PCL/PBS blends containing carbon nanotubes. *Express Polymer Letters, 12*(6).
4. Kale, S. K., Deshmukh, A. G., Dudhare, M. S., & Patil, V. B., (2015). Microbial degradation of plastic: A review. *Journal of Biochemical Technology, 6*(2), 952–961.
5. Nunes, P. A., Svensson, L. E., & Markandya, A., (2017). *Handbook on the Economics and Management of Sustainable Oceans.* Edward Elgar Publishing.
6. Van, S. E., Spathi, C., & Gilbert, A., (2016). The ocean plastic pollution challenge: Towards solutions in the UK. *Grant Brief Pap., 19*, 1–16.
7. Ahmadi, M., Behzad, T., Bagheri, R., & Heidarian, P., (2018). Effect of cellulose nanofibers and acetylated cellulose nanofibers on the properties of low-density polyethylene/thermoplastic starch blends. *Polymer International, 67*(8), 993–1002.
8. Madhu, G., Bhunia, H., Bajpai, P. K., & Nando, G. B., (2016). Physico-mechanical properties and biodegradation of oxo-degradable HDPE/PLA blends. *Polymer Science Series A, 58*(1), 57–75.

9. Leja, K., & Lewandowicz, G., (2010). Polymer biodegradation and biodegradable polymers: A review. *Polish Journal of Environmental Studies, 19*(2), 255–266.
10. Van, D. O. M., Molenveld, K., Van, D. Z. M., & Bos, H., (2017). *Bio-Based and Biodegradable Plastics: Facts and Figures: Focus on Food Packaging in the Netherlands.* Wageningen Food & Biobased Research.
11. Kunioka, M., (2013). Measurement methods of biobased carbon content for biomass-based chemicals and plastics. *Radioisotopes (Tokyo), 62*(12), 901–925.
12. Mohanty, A. K., Vivekanandhan, S., Pin, J. M., & Misra, M., (2018). Composites from renewable and sustainable resources: Challenges and innovations. *Science, 362*(6414), 536–542.
13. Seadon, J. K., (2010). Sustainable waste management systems. *Journal of Cleaner Production, 18*(16/17), 1639–1651.
14. Kulkarni, V. S., Butte, K. D., & Rathod, S. S., (2012). Natural polymers: A comprehensive review. *International Journal of Research in Pharmaceutical and Biomedical Sciences, 3*(4), 1597–1613.
15. Paul, S., Jayan, A., Sasikumar, C. S., & Cherian, S. M., (2014). Extraction and purification of chitosan from chitin isolated from sea prawn *Fenneropenaeus indicus. Extraction, 7*(4).
16. Rinaudo, M., (2006). Chitin and chitosan: Properties and applications. *Progress in Polymer Science, 31*(7), 603–632.
17. Moura, D., Mano, J. F., Paiva, M. C., & Alves, N. M., (2016). Chitosan nanocomposites based on distinct inorganic fillers for biomedical applications. *Science and Technology of Advanced Materials, 17*(1), 626–643.
18. D'Angelo, G., Elhussieny, A., Faisal, M., Fahim, I., & Everitt, N., (2018). Mechanical behavior optimization of chitosan extracted from shrimp shells as a sustainable material for shopping bags. *Journal of Functional Biomaterials, 9*(2), 37.
19. Daniels, C. A., (1989). *Polymers: Structure and Properties.* CRC Press.
20. Al Marzouqi, M. H., Abdulkarim, M. A., Marzouk, S. A., El-Naas, M. H., & Hasanain, H. M., (2005). Facilitated transport of $CO_2$ through immobilized liquid membrane. *Industrial and Engineering Chemistry Research, 44*(24), 9273–9278.
21. Castillo, L. A., Farenzena, S., Pintos, E., Rodríguez, M. S., Villar, M. A., García, M. A., et al., (2017). Active films based on thermoplastic corn starch and chitosan oligomer for food packaging applications. *Food Packaging and Shelf Life, 14,* 128–136.
22. Fahim, I., Chbib, H., & Mahmoud, H. M., (2019). The synthesis, production and economic feasibility of manufacturing PLA from agricultural waste. *Sustainable Chemistry and Pharmacy, 12,* 100142.
23. Harrington, R., (2012). *Project Using Egg Shell to Make Plastic Packaging.*
24. Faisal, M., Elhussieny, A., Ali, K., Samy, I., & Everitt, N., (2018). Extraction of degradable biopolymer materials from shrimp shell wastes by two different methods. *IOP Conference Series: Materials Science and Engineering.* IOP Publishing.
25. Morais, J. P. S., De Freitas, R. M., Nascimento, L. D., Do Nascimento, D. M., & Cassales, A. R., (2013). Extraction and characterization of nanocellulose structures from raw cotton linter. *Carbohydrate Polymers, 91*(1), 229–235.
26. Fahim, I., Aboulkhair, N., & Everitt, N., (2018). Nanoindentation investigation on chitosan thin films with different types of nanofillers. *J. Mater. Sci. Res., 7*(11).

27. Ummartyotin, S., Pisitsak, P., & Pechyen, C., (2016). Eggshell and bacterial cellulose composite membrane as absorbent material in active packaging. *International Journal of Polymer Science*.

28. Celebi, H., & Kurt, A., (2015). Effects of processing on the properties of chitosan/cellulose nanocrystal films. *Carbohydrate Polymers, 133*, 284–293.

29. Grząbka-Zasadzińska, A., Amietszajew, T., & Borysiak, S., (2017). Thermal and mechanical properties of chitosan nanocomposites with cellulose modified in ionic liquids. *Journal of Thermal Analysis and Calorimetry, 130*(1), 143–154.

30. Ofem, M., Anyandi, A., & Ene, E., (2017). Properties of chitin reinforce composites: A review. *Nigerian Journal of Technology, 36*(1), 57–71.

# CHAPTER 3

# Designing and Synthesis of Green Polymeric Nanomaterials for Pharmaceutical Applications

ALAA A. A. ALJABALI,[1] MAZHAR S. AL ZOUBI,[2]
KHALID M. AL-BATANYEH,[3] ALAA ALQUDAH,[1]
MOHAMMAD A. OBEID,[1] PARTEEK PRASHER,[4] VIJAY MISHRA,[5]
GAURAV GUPTA,[6] POONAM NEGI,[7] DEEPAK N. KAPOOR,[7]
HARISH DUREJA,[8] SAURABH SATIJA,[5] DINESH KUMAR CHELLAPPAN,[9]
KAMAL DUA,[10] and MURTAZA M. TAMBUWALA[11]

[1]*Department of Pharmaceutical Science, Faculty of Pharmacy, Yarmouk University, Irbid, Jordan*

[2]*Department of Basic Medical Studies, Yarmouk University, Irbid, Jordan*

[3]*Department of Biological Sciences, Yarmouk University, Irbid, Jordan*

[4]*Department of Chemistry, University of Petroleum and Energy Studies, Dehradun – 248007, India*

[5]*School of Pharmaceutical Sciences, Lovely Professional University, Phagwara, Punjab – 144411, India*

[6]*School of Pharmacy, Suresh Gyan Vihar University, Jagatpura, Jaipur – 302017, India*

[7]*School of Pharmaceutical Sciences, Shoolini University of Biotechnology and Management Sciences, Solan – 173229, India*

[8]*Department of Pharmaceutical Sciences, Maharshi Dayanand University, Rohtak – 124001, India*

[9]*Department of Life Sciences, School of Pharmacy, International Medical University, Bukit Jalil, Kuala Lumpur – 57000, Malaysia*

[10]*Discipline of Pharmacy, Graduate School of Health, University of Technology, Sydney, NSW – 2007, Australia*

[11]*SAAD Center for Pharmacy and Diabetes, School of Pharmacy and Pharmaceutical Science, Ulster University, Coleraine, UK*

## ABSTRACT

Nanotechnology provides areas that vary from conventional chemistry innovations to medical and climate technologies with productive applications. In practice, NPs have been synthesized by physical and chemical processes, including hydrothermal pyrolysis, spray pyrolysis, sonochemical, sol-gel, coprecipitation, and so on, using different chemical agents to minimize and maintain the harsh conditions of different chemicals to control the properties of the generated nanomaterials. NPs have been used as toxic agents. Biological synthesis is emerging as a green and safe method for synthesizing metal/metal oxide NPs with precursor materials from plants and microbes. Green synthesis of nanomaterials has emerged as an eco-friendly and alternative approach for the synthesis of novel nanomaterials with great potential in medical and pharmaceutical applications. The nanomaterials generated from biomolecules, plant extract, algae, and microorganisms have been given considerable appreciation. It is believed the phytochemicals, alkaloids, flavonoids, and sugar compounds content to act as reducing and stabilization agents to prevent the agglomeration of the nanoparticles.

## 3.1  INTRODUCTION

Nanomaterials have extraordinary physical and chemical properties and are essential in the development of revolutionary and effective drugs, sensors, catalytic converters, and molecular imaging. Three primary methods can achieve nanomaterial synthesis: physical method (Electron beam lithography, ion implementation, mechanical grinding, vacuum sputtering), chemical methods (Coprecipitation method, Chemical reduction of metal salts, pyrolysis, phytochemical method, Sol-gel processes), and biological method (Plant extract, microorganisms, algae, biomolecules, and enzymes).

Compared to conventional chemical synthesis, green synthesis of NPs can be an effective alternative. Green synthesis of nanoparticles has evolved over the past two decades to generate different compositions of nanomaterials from different biological sources like bacteria fungi and plants. Typically, green synthesis refers to the eco-friendly approach to generate nanomaterials that are biodegradable by biocompatible by using plant extract as reducing and capping agents to prevent particle agglomeration.

This approach for nanomaterial generation is implemented to minimize the generated waste reaction by-product but is mainly associated with nanomaterial synthesis. Using plant extract relies on mild reaction conditions to generate nontoxic precursors for various applications [1–3]. Green synthesis of nanomaterials is straightforward, cost-effective, very reproducible, generates stable material. However, this approach, due to its slow synthesis, can only generate a minimal number of sizes and shapes that are amenable for surface modifications. Green synthesis does not require high pressure, a large amount of energy, elevated reaction temperatures, or toxic chemicals. Besides, Nanomaterials from green synthesis can be scaled up for large production easily, and it relies on the use of plant extracts as are reducing and capping agents to generate various types of nanomaterials by using plant extracts chemical content as reducing agent after reaction desired metallic salts.

There are few essential reducing agents (glucose, starch, amine, certain amino acids such as tyrosine), which can be used by simple chemical processes, with less costly wastewater disposal and less capital investment to produce nanoparticles.

Nanoparticles' green synthesis is affected by the incubation / reactive period, which significantly affects nanoparticles' shape, size, and yield. The period of incubation/reaction time is necessary to complete the reaction medium to obtain the best-synthesized nanoparticles and stability.

### 3.1.1   SYNTHESIS OF NANOPARTICLES

Green synthesis of nanomaterials is driven by microorganisms (fungi, bacteria, algae, and yeast), biomolecules (enzymes), plant extract. Green synthesis holds significant advantages as it reduces the risk of contamination and the expensive lab equipment necessary for the synthesis. In this framework, the present chapter includes selected studies highlighting the advancement in green synthesis of nanomaterials and their related applications. Figure 3.1 summarizes different approaches for the synthesis of nanomaterials generated from using different biomolecules.

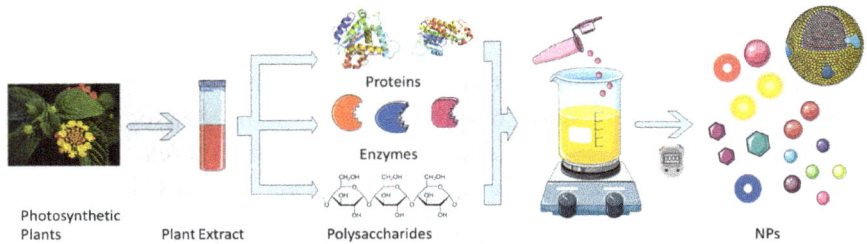

**FIGURE 3.1**    Schematic illustration of the synthesis of nanoparticles from photosynthetic plants containing polysaccharides, proteins, and enzymes. Upon mixing the plant extract with the desired metallic solution, nanoparticles will be generated for various applications.

### 3.1.2    MICROORGANISM-MEDIATED TECHNIQUE

Thanks to their defense mechanism, nanoparticles are synthesized through a microbe. The exposure of microorganisms to reactive ions in their environment induced by bacterial cells is essential for their production of nanoparticles. The high concentration of ions for bacterial cells is usually harmful. Therefore, the cellular machinery tends to prevent cell death and transform reactive ions into nanoparticles. That is to suggest the corresponding nanoparticles. This bacterial product is used for nanoparticle biosynthesis. Cell damage can occur when nanoparticles are formed at a high level.

Several microorganisms can synthesize both extra and intracellular nanoparticles. The composite community of bacteria associated with various biogeochemical processes usually removes metallic salts to their ionic state by specific enzymatic behaviors (e.g., nitrate reductase found in the nitrogen cycle-built bacteria). Extracellular synthesis is carried out during enzymatic operation, where the intracellular synthesis of nanoparticles utilizes bacteria through macrophages and reduces to a nano form, which is further excreted or processed for use in vacuoles (Figure 3.2).

### 3.1.3    PLANT-MEDIATED TECHNIQUES

Plant extracts offer an alternative approach for novel nanomaterials synthesis by using plant extract or parts of the plant as a reducing and capping agent. Photosynthetic plants have a complex biological network of metabolites and enzymes, together acting to keep cellular components from having oxidative damaging effects. Recent studies suggest that the plant extracts produce biomolecules that may serve as a metal reducer to produce metal cations, including polyphenols, flavonoids, ascorbic acid, sterols, triterpenes, alkaloids, alcoholic compounds, saponins, β-Phenyletherylamines, polysaccharides, glucose, fructose, vitamins, proteins, and enzymes [4]. Glucose and ascorbate are also likely to reduce silver and gold ions to nanoparticles at high temperatures [2, 5–7]. Within plant leaf extracts, protein, enzymes, phenolics, and other chemical compounds may reduce silver salts and exquisitely resist the agglomeration of the nanoparticles created [8]. Terpenoids, polyphenols, carbohydrates, alkaloids, phenolic acids, and proteins have been reported to have a vital role in the reduction of metal ions, resulting in nanoparticle formation [9]. Figure 3.3 shows an illustration of nanoparticle synthesis using photosynthetic plants.

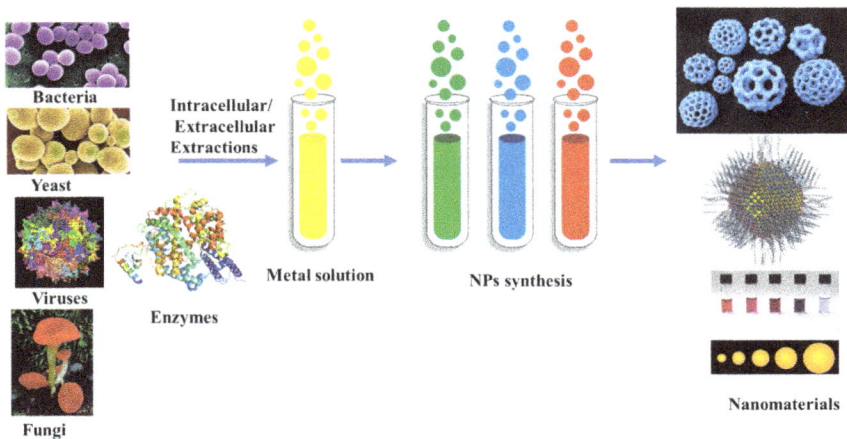

**FIGURE 3.2** Schematic representation of microorganism mediated synthesis. Cellular extracts from bacterial, viral, fungal, or yeast will act as capping and reducing agents to generate the desired NPs with different morphologies and applications.

Flavonoids contain different functional groups that allow metal ions to be reduced. Because of the tautomeric transitions of flavonoids, the reactive hydrogen atom is produced by the transition of enol into the keto form. This is done by reducing metal ions to metal nanoparticles. Enol-to-keto conversion is a critical factor in the production of green NPs in sweet basil (*Ocimum basilicum*) extracts.

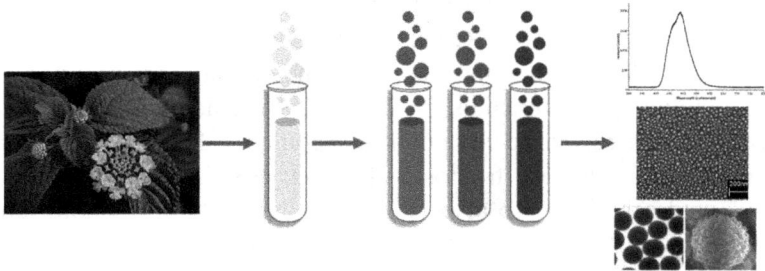

**FIGURE 3.3**    Green synthesis of metallic nanoparticles using plant extract as a capping and reducing agent to generate different types of NPs.

AuNPs are becoming more prevalent using plant extract because of the powerful and the simple reduction of the desired metallic nanoparticles by plant sap. This approach is a straightforward, single-step approach, which is very desirable to scale-up to produce large quantities, on a low coast, effectively, and rapid step. AuNPs have been synthesized from any plant extracts such as *Cucurbita pepo*, *Malva Crispa*, and *Ziziphus* to generate AuNPs with a size range between 20–50 nm [4, 10].

Tea extracts have been used to generate zero-valent iron oxide NPs. It is believed that phenolic compounds acted as a reducing agent to generate FeO NPs [11]. Such particles were used as magnetic biosensors for the detection of various pathogens and the detection of anionic dyes [12].

Two oxidation states can exist in cerium: $Ce^{3+}$ and $Ce^{4+}$. Cerium dioxide ($CeO_2$) can, thus, have two different forms on the nanoscale in comparison to the bulk material: $CeO_2$ ($Ce^{4+}$) or $Ce_2O_3$ ($Ce^{3+}$). $CeO_2$ has a cubic fluorite lattice with both $Ce^{3+}$ and $Ce^{4+}$ coexist on the surface of NPs. The presence of $Ce^{3+}$ leads to localized sites of oxygen defects, which, in turn, act as catalytic reaction sites [13]. $CeO_2$ has an essential role in scavenging reactive oxygen and nitrogen. Therefore, $CeO_2$ is very effective against chronic oxidative stress and inflammation [14]. $CeO_2$ NPs cannot penetrate cells that are both bacterial and algal. Noninternalized $CeO_2$ NPs tend to have toxic effects precisely once bound to algae and bacterial cell walls. $CeO_2$ NPs have been reported as an effective inhibitor toward against gram-negative and gram-positive bacteria. The generated particles through the green synthesis route were 20 nm in diameter, with its antibacterial properties arises from the surface $Ce^{3+}$ [15]. Besides, $CeO_2$ NPs properties of removing ROS have been shown to affect the signal transduction pathway responsible for the neural death and neuroprotection makes $CeO_2$ NPs ideal for Alzheimer's disease (AD) ischemic stroke, Parkinson's disease, trauma, and aging [16]. Another unique property of $CeO_2$ NPs is their capabilities to induce angiogenesis *in vivo* by modulating the Intracellular oxygen condition and stabilizing endogenous hypoxia factor 1α, which affects gene expression [17, 18].

*Gloriosa superba* leaf exhibits impressive antimicrobial characteristics as a result of $CeO_2$ NPs synthesized from the leaf extract to generate spherical particles of 5 nm in diameter [19, 20]. *Acalypha indica* was also utilized for the synthesis of $CeO_2$ NPs with spherical geometries and 36 nm in diameter for potential antimicrobial use [15]. Furthermore, *Aloe vera* was used to generate spherical $CeO_2$ with 63.6 nm in diameter [15]. It has been reported that the green synthesis of $CeO_2$ has many advantages in comparison to the chemical approach: (a) capability of generating spherical NPs with potential in reducing cytotoxicity, (b) the ability to generate stable, water-soluble, and highly fluorescent NPs. However, some of the disadvantages have been reported as well, such as: (i) it is challenging to generate nonuniform NPs geometries leading to particle aggregation, (ii) complicated to control the size range between 5–63.6 nm [19].

### 3.1.4   ENZYMES-MEDIATED TECHNIQUES

Extracellular microbial enzymes play an essential role in reducing salt ions to generate nanomaterial. Published research suggests that enzymatic cofactors, including adenine dinucleotide nicotinamide (NADH) and reduced types of phosphorous dinucleotide adenine nicotinamide (NADPH), also perform vital roles as a reducing agent through the electron transfer mechanism [21, 22]. This mechanism was utilized to generate gold nanoparticles (AuNPs) via electron transfer from NADH by NADH-reliant reductase enzymes present in *R. capsulata*. $Au^{3+}$ ions accept electrons from NADH to generate $Au^0$, subsequently generating AuNPs [23]. Acetyl xylan esterase, and cellobiohydrolase D, glucosidase, and β-glucosidase are some enzymes that are produced extracellularly by several fungi-species [24]. The nitrate reductase, which is secreted by fungi, was used for the generation of AgNPs, as shown in Figure 3.4 [25, 26]. *Fusarium oxysporum* extracellular reductase enzyme was utilized to the generated reduction of $Au^{3+}$ and $Ag^{1+}$ to Au-Ag alloy NPs [27, 28]. Furthermore, *F. oxysporum* was utilized for the extracellular synthesis of semiconductor CdS NPs [29].

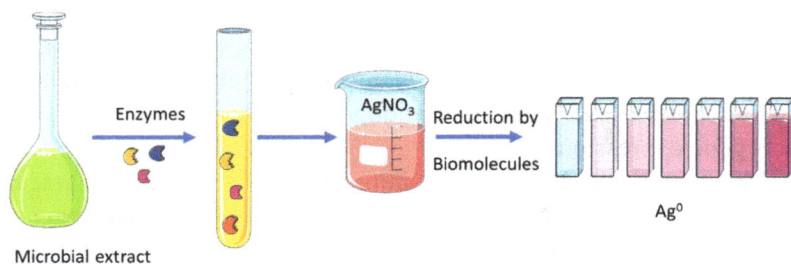

**FIGURE 3.4** Schematic illustration of the biogenic synthesis of, for example, AgNPs from extracted microbial enzymes. Upon the addition of the microbial extract to the desired metallic solution, NPs will be generated. In this example, Ag cations will be reduced to the metallic form $Ag^0$.

### 3.1.5  VITAMINS-MEDIATED TECHNIQUES

One of the unique approaches in the green synthesis of nanomaterials is the use of vitamins as a reducing agent. In particular, the use of vitamin B2 as a reducing agent to generate nanowires and nanorods [30]. Furthermore, ascorbic acid (vitamin C) and chitosan were utilized as capping and reducing agent to generate AuNPs and AgNPs [31, 32]. Antioxidants were also used for the generation of AgNPs [33]. Besides, vitamin E was used in a one-step approach to generate Langmuir monolayers with vitamin E, which reduces the silver cations to generate the metallic monolayer [34]. The schematic illustration that summarizes the process is depicted in Figure 3.5.

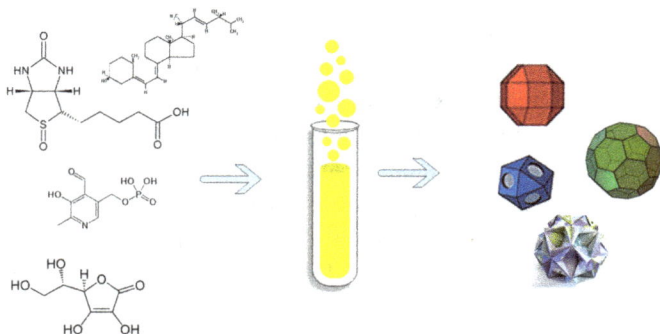

**FIGURE 3.5** Schematic illustration of the biogenic synthesis of, for example, AgNPs from extracted microbial enzymes.

## 3.2 MECHANISM OF GREEN SYNTHESIS

Plant extract contains various molecules from polyphenols, phytochemicals, flavonoids, alkaloids, phenols, tannins, saponins, etc. The presence of flavonoids and phenols within a normal plant cell is essential as an antioxidant and its ability to scavenging free radicals. However, the detailed mechanism of NPs synthesis is still not yet precise. However, the proposed mechanism of green synthesis of nanomaterials from plant extract involves three phases: (1) nucleation (activation) phase (2) crystal growth phase (3) crystallization and process termination phase. Salt ions reduction occurs during the activation phase. This will initiate the nucleation (self-organization) of the reduced salt ions of the desired materials. The second phase involves a further reduction of the salt ions and the growth of the metallic nucleus with an increase in the reaction thermodynamics of the formed NPs. In the third phase, the shape and the crystallinity of the desired materials are achieved, and the generated NPs are stabilized with the biomolecules and enzymes. However, many factors are influencing the synthesis of nanomaterials. The published work suggests the presence of biomolecules that act as reducing/capping agents. Some other factors that influence the NPs synthesis include temperature, pH, concentration extracts, and the desired particle size. The generated size depends on the concentration of the polyphenols [35], reaction pH (acidic pH leads to agglomeration over the nucleation, basic pH leads to particle instability), NPs size, and shape.

Furthermore, the reaction temperature plays a vital role in nanomaterials generation as higher temperatures (above ambient temperature) lead to faster nanoparticle growth leading to crystal defect formation affecting the crystal quality. In addition, nucleation time is essential to control the size and the particle distribution, and minimal nucleation time leads to overall control on the particle size and distribution. Furthermore, green synthesis of nanomaterials requires optimization of reaction times, mixing ratio of plant extract to metal salts, temperature, and pH. The majority of the described nanomaterials discussed in this section are reported in Table 3.1.

## 3.3 GREEN SYNTHESIS OF AGNPS BY MICROBES

The application of AgNPs in molecular medicine, diagnostic probes, bioconjugation, nano-therapeutics, and next-generation antibiotics,

**TABLE 3.1** Summarizes the Different Approaches for the Synthesis of Nanomaterials and Their Sizes, Characterization, and Geometrical Arrangement

| Organism/Plant | Constitution Chem./Bio | NPs Size Shape | Characterization | References |
|---|---|---|---|---|
| *Ziziphus ziziphus (leaves)* | Leaf extract | 40–50 nm (spherical) | UV-vis, HRTEM, FTIR, DLS, XRD, EDS, TGA, ζ potential | [10] |
| *Acacia nilotica (pod)* | Gallic acid, epicatechin | 20–30 nm (distorted spherical) | UV-vis, HRTEM, FTIR, DLS, XRD, EDS, ζ potential | [32] |
| *Emblica officinalis* | Plant extract | 22 nm spherical FeO | FTIR, DLS, XRD, ζ potential | [46] |
| *Eucalyptus sp.* | Plant extract | 20–80 nm spherical FeO | FTIR, DLS, XRD, TEM, ζ potential | [47] |
| *Salvia officinalis* | Plant extract | 5–25 nm spherical FeO | TEM, DLS | [12] |
| *Quercus petraea, Morus alba, Prunus cerasus* | Plant extract | 10–30 nm spherical FeO | DLS, XRD, TEM, ζ potential | [48] |
| **Fungi and Algae Species** | | | | |
| *Aspergillus niger* | Fungi extract | 53–69 nm spherical ZnO NPs | TEM, FTIR, DLS, XRD, EDS, TGA, ζ potential | [49] |
| *Duddingtonia flagrans* | Fungi extract | 30–60 nm spherical AgNPs | UV-Vis, TGA, ζ potential | [50] |
| *Trametes trogii* | Fungi extract | 40–100 nm spherical, core-shell ellipsoidal AgNPs | TEM, FTIR, DLS, XRD, EDS, | [51] |
| *Chlamydomonas reinhardtii* | Fungi extract | 6 nm spherical AgNPs | EDS, TGA, ζ potential | [22] |

**TABLE 3.1** (Continued)

| Organism/Plant | Constitution Chem./Bio | NPs Size Shape | Characterization | References |
|---|---|---|---|---|
| Penicillium polonicum | Fungi extract | 10–15 nm spherical AgNPs | TEM, FTIR, DLS, XRD, EDS | [52] |
| Candida glabrata | Fungi extract | 2–15 nm spherical AgNPs | EDS, TGA, ζ potential | [53] |
| Aspergillus terreus | Fungi extract | 16–57 nm spherical AgNPs | TEM, EDS, TGA, ζ potential | [54] |
| Fusarium oxysporum | Fungi extract | 21.3–37 nm spherical AgNPs | TEM, FTIR, DLS, XRD, EDS | [55] |
| Microbes Mediated Synthesis | | | | |
| Escherichia coli | Gram-negative | 2–3.2 nm (spherical CdTe NPs) at 37°C | FTIR, DLS, XRD, EDS, | [56] |
| Escherichia coli | Gram-negative | 20–30 nm (Hexagonal, Triangle AuNPs) at 37°C | FTIR, DLS, XRD, ζ potential | [57] |
| Pseudomonas aeruginosa | Gram-negative | 15–30 nm AuNPs at 37°C | UV-vis, HRTEM, FTIR, DLS, XRD, EDS, TGA, ζ potential | [58] |
| Shewanella oneidensis | Facultative Species | 12 nm spherical AuNPs at 30°C | UV-vis, HRTEM, FTIR, DLS, XRD, EDS, TGA, ζ potential | [59] |
| Desulfovibrio desulfuricans | Gram-Negative | 50 nm spherical Pd NPs | UV-vis, HRTEM, FTIR, DLS, XRD, EDS, TGA, | [60] |
| Bacillus licheniformis | Gram-Positive | 50 nm AgNPs spherical at 37°C | UV-vis, HRTEM, FTIR, DLS, EDS, TGA, ζ potential | [61] |

**TABLE 3.1** *(Continued)*

| Organism/Plant | Constitution Chem./Bio | NPs Size Shape | Characterization | References |
|---|---|---|---|---|
| *Ureibacillus thermo sphaericus* | Gram-Positive | 50–70 nm AuNPs spherical at 60–80°C | UV-vis, TEM, FTIR, DLS, XRD, EDS, TGA, ζ potential | [62] |
| *Rhodopseudomonas capsulate* | Phototrophic | 10–20 nm spherical AuNPs at 30°C | UV-vis, TEM, FTIR, DLS, XRD, EDS, TGA, ζ potential | [63] |
| Enzymes (Intercellular) | | | | |
| *Shewanella algae* | Gram-Negative | 5 nm Pt NPs at 25°C | TEM, FTIR, DLS, XRD, EDS, TGA, ζ potential | [64] |
| *Enterobacter species* | Gram Negative-Bacilli | 2–5 nm Hg spherical NPs at 30°C | TEM, FTIR, DLS, XRD, EDS, TGA, ζ potential | [65] |
| *Rhodococcus species* | Actinobacteria | 8–12 nm spherical AuNPs at ambient temperature | TEM, FTIR, DLS, XRD, EDS, TGA, ζ potential | [66] |
| *Brevibacterium casei* | Actinomycetales bacteria | 10–50 nm spherical AuNPs and AgNPs at 37°C | EDS, TGA, ζ potential | [67] |
| *Escherichia coli* | Gram-negative Bacteria | 2–3.2 nm spherical CdTe NPs | TEM, FTIR, DLS, XRD, EDS, TGA, ζ potential | [56] |
| *Escherichia coli* | Gram-negative Bacteria | 20–30 nm hexagonal and Triangles AuNPs | EDS, TGA, ζ potential | [68] |

necessitates their synthesis by green routes to ensure physiological benevolence [26]. Microbes such as bacteria, fungi, and algae mediate the intracellular and extracellular green synthesis of AgNPs by biosorption of the ionic silver and converting it into the metallic form [36]. The microbial biomass possesses biomacromolecules, such as enzymes, cofactors, peptidoglycans, exopolysaccharides, glucans, hyaluronic acid, xylans, chitosan, fucoidan, chitin, and mannans [28]. These biomolecules are enriched with diverse functional head groups such as –COOH, -SH, -NH$_2$, -S-, -OH, and CONH$_2$, serving as the sorption sites for ionic silver and prompt its reduction to stabilized AgNPs [37, 38]. The microbial enzymes such as nitrate reductase and lactate dehydrogenase reportedly mediate the intracellular bio-reduction of Ag$^+$ ions to AgNPs in the presence of cofactors such as NADPH, and mitochondrial electron shuttle, with pH being the deciding factor [39]. Similarly, the extracellular green synthesis of AgNPs occurs in the presence of microbial supernatant containing the complex biomolecules and biopolymers. Varying the physicochemical conditions such as temperature, pH, the concentration of the target ions, and biosorbent helps in maneuvering the morphology of the resulting AgNPs [40]. Except for *Trichoderma viride*, the rate of AgNPs synthesis and the particle size mainly enhances at the temperature higher than 40°C due to the transfer of an electron from free amino acids present in the microbial biomass to the Ag$^+$ ions [41]. However, the temperatures >80°C onsets the denaturation of peptides participating as nanoparticle capping agents, thereby disturbing the nucleation of Ag$^+$ ions leading to their aggregation and increase in size [42]. Similarly, the optimum synthesis of AgNPs occurs at a neutral pH because both acidic and basic pH results in a diminished biosorption of Ag$^+$ ions to the microbial biomass, adversely affecting their bioreduction to AgNPs [43]. However, in some microbial strains, the deprotonation of the Ag$^+$ ion binding sites at higher pH enhances the rate of biosorption, but the bioreduction does not necessarily enhance due to competitive binding between the protons and Ag$^+$ ions for the available sites [44]. The concentration of microbial biomass and its contact time with the Ag$^+$ ion serves as another vital parameter for guiding biosorption of silver ions and their subsequent bio-reduction to AgNPs [45]. Principally, the electrostatic interactions between the Ag$^+$ ions and microbial biomass enhance at higher concentrations of the latter resulting in agglomerates, whereas conversely, the specific biosorption enhances at the lower microbial biomass concentration [36]. Similarly, the high initial concentration of the $Ag^+$ ions only enhances their rate of biosorption on microbial biomass as many metal ions compete for the limited binding sites on biomass. Table 3.1 presents recent reports on the green synthesis of AgNPs by microbes.

## 3.4  CONCLUSIONS

This chapter addressed the processes and classification of different nanomaterials and the challenges involved in their planning. It is evident from the discussions above list, mainly due to its inherent properties, the thickness, the full surface area, and the formulations crystallize, form, and many more, that the application of nanomaterials from nanocellulose and metal oxides, carbonated, and clay minerals are essential globally. The use of toxic and costly chemicals, production of secondary waste, high-energy consumption, and low output, respectively, constitute major disadvantages of chemical synthesis and a combination of physical and chemical synthesis. On the contrary, green plant extract NP synthesis was identified as a potential upscaling technique when plant-based materials were usable. Different methods were explored, which focused on the advancement of manufacturing and future potential scale-up.

## KEYWORDS

- Alzheimer's disease
- green synthesis
- nanomaterials
- nanoscience
- pharmaceutical applications
- plant-mediated nanomaterial synthesis

## REFERENCES

1.  Al-Trad, B., et al., (2017). Inhibitory effect of thymoquinone on testosterone-induced benign prostatic hyperplasia in Wistar rats. *Phytother Res., 31*(12), 1910–1915.

2. Al-Trad, B., et al., (2019). Effect of gold nanoparticles treatment on the testosterone-induced benign prostatic hyperplasia in rats. *Int. J. Nanomedicine, 14*, 3145–3154.

3. Aljabali, A. A. A., et al., (2020). Albumin nano-encapsulation of piceatannol enhances its anticancer potential in colon cancer via downregulation of nuclear p65 and HIF-1alpha. *Cancers (Basel), 12*(1).

4. Lu, Y., & Foo, L. Y., (2002). Polyphenolics of salvia: A review. *Phytochemistry, 59*(2), 117–140.

5. Prasad, R., (2014). Synthesis of silver nanoparticles in photosynthetic plants. *Journal of Nanoparticles, 2014*.

6. Aljabali, A. A. A., et al., (2019). Gold-coated plant virus as computed tomography imaging contrast agent. *Beilstein. J. Nanotechnol., 10*, 1983–1993.

7. Alomari, G., et al., (2020). Gold nanoparticles attenuate albuminuria by inhibiting podocyte injury in a rat model of diabetic nephropathy. *Drug Deliv. Transl. Res., 10*(1), 216–226.

8. Saxena, A., et al., (2012). Green synthesis of silver nanoparticles using aqueous solution of *Ficus benghalensis* leaf extract and characterization of their antibacterial activity. *Materials Letters, 67*(1), 91–94.

9. Shankar, S. S., et al., (2004). Rapid synthesis of Au, Ag, and bimetallic Au core–Ag shell nanoparticles using neem (*Azadirachta indica*) leaf broth. *Journal of Colloid and Interface Science, 275*(2), 496–502.

10. Aljabali, A. A. A., et al., (2018). Synthesis of gold nanoparticles using leaf extract of *Ziziphus zizyphus* and their antimicrobial activity. *Nanomaterials (Basel), 8*(3).

11. Malik, P., et al., (2014). Green chemistry based benign routes for nanoparticle synthesis. *Journal of Nanoparticles, 2014*, 14.

12. Wang, Z., Fang, C., & Mallavarapu, M., (2015). Characterization of iron-polyphenol complex nanoparticles synthesized by sage (*Salvia officinalis*) leaves. *Environmental Technology and Innovation, 4*, 92–97.

13. Das, S., et al., (2013). Cerium oxide nanoparticles: Applications and prospects in nanomedicine. *Nanomedicine (Lond.), 8*(9), 1483–1508.

14. Celardo, I., et al., (2011). Pharmacological potential of cerium oxide nanoparticles. *Nanoscale, 3*(4), 1411–1420.

15. Kannan, S., & Sundrarajan, M., (2014). A green approach for the synthesis of a cerium oxide nanoparticle: Characterization and antibacterial activity. *International Journal of Nanoscience, 13*(03), 1450018.

16. Uttara, B., et al., (2009). Oxidative stress and neurodegenerative diseases: A review of upstream and downstream antioxidant therapeutic options. *Curr. Neuropharmacol., 7*(1), 65–74.

17. Das, S., et al., (2012). The induction of angiogenesis by cerium oxide nanoparticles through the modulation of oxygen in intracellular environments. *Biomaterials, 33*(31), 7746–7755.

18. Fitzpatrick, S. F., et al., (2011). An intact canonical NF-κB pathway is required for inflammatory gene expression in response to hypoxia. *The Journal of Immunology, 186*(2), 1091–1096.

19. Charbgoo, F., Ahmad, M. B., & Darroudi, M., (2017). Cerium oxide nanoparticles: Green synthesis and biological applications. *Int. J. Nanomedicine, 12*, 1401–1413.

20. Fang, X., & Song, H., (2019). Synthesis of cerium oxide nanoparticles loaded on chitosan for enhanced auto-catalytic regenerative ability and biocompatibility for the spinal cord injury repair. *J. Photochem. Photobiol. B, 191*, 83–87.

21. Kumari, R., Singh, J. S., & Singh, D. P., (2017). Biogenic synthesis and spatial distribution of silver nanoparticles in the legume mungbean plant (*Vigna radiata* L.). *Plant Physiol. Biochem., 110*, 158–166.

22. Rahman, A., et al., (2019). A mechanistic view of the light-induced synthesis of silver nanoparticles using extracellular polymeric substances of *Chlamydomonas reinhardtii*. *Molecules, 24*(19).

23. Bharde, A., et al., (2007). Bacterial enzyme mediated biosynthesis of gold nanoparticles. *J. Nanosci. Nanotechnol., 7*(12), 4369–4377.

24. Ovais, M., et al., (2018). Role of plant phytochemicals and microbial enzymes in biosynthesis of metallic nanoparticles. *Appl. Microbiol. Biotechnol., 102*(16), 6799–6814.

25. Anil, K. S., et al., (2007). Nitrate reductase-mediated synthesis of silver nanoparticles from $AgNO_3$. *Biotechnol. Lett., 29*(3), 439–445.

26. Abdelghany, T. M., et al., (2018). Recent advances in green synthesis of silver nanoparticles and their applications: About future directions: A review. *Bio. Nano Science, 8*(1), 5–16.

27. Senapati, S., et al., (2005). Extracellular biosynthesis of bimetallic Au-Ag alloy nanoparticles. *Small, 1*(5), 517–520.

28. Ahmad, S., et al., (2019). Green nanotechnology: A review on green synthesis of silver nanoparticles: An ecofriendly approach. *Int. J. Nanomedicine, 14*, 5087–5107.

29. Xu, J., et al., (2019). Extracellular biosynthesis of biocompatible CdSe quantum dots. *IET Nanobiotechnol., 13*(9), 962–966.

30. Nadagouda, M. N., & Varma, R. S., (2006). Green and controlled synthesis of gold and platinum nanomaterials using vitamin B2: Density-assisted self-assembly of nanospheres, wires and rods. *Green Chemistry, 8*(6), 516–518.

31. Arunachalam, K. D., Annamalai, S. K., & Hari, S., (2013). One-step green synthesis and characterization of leaf extract-mediated biocompatible silver and gold nanoparticles from *Memecylon umbellatum*. *Int. J. Nanomedicine, 8*, 1307–1315.

32. Arya, A., et al., (2018). Biogenic synthesis of copper and silver nanoparticles using green alga *Botryococcus braunii* and its antimicrobial activity. *Bioinorg. Chem. Appl., 7879403*.

33. Ahmad, N., et al., (2011). Biosynthesis of silver nanoparticles from *Desmodium triflorum*: A novel approach towards weed utilization. *Biotechnol. Res. Int., 2011*, 454090.

34. Zhang, L., et al., (2006). One-step synthesis of monodisperse silver nanoparticles beneath vitamin E Langmuir monolayers. *J. Phys. Chem. B., 110*(13), 6615–6620.

35. Goncalves, A. C., et al., (2018). Antioxidant status, antidiabetic properties and effects on caco-2 cells of colored and non-colored enriched extracts of sweet cherry fruits. *Nutrients, 10*(11).

36. Parashar, U. K., et al., (2011). Study of mechanism of enhanced antibacterial activity by green synthesis of silver nanoparticles. *Nanotechnology, 22*(41), 415104.

37. Mabey, T., et al., (2019). Bacteria and nanosilver: The quest for optimal production. *Crit. Rev. Biotechnol., 39*(2), 272–287.

38. Rahman, A., Kumar, S., & Nawaz, T., (2020). Chapter 17: Biosynthesis of nanomaterials using algae. In: Yousuf, A., (ed.), *Microalgae Cultivation for Biofuels Production* (pp. 265–279). Academic Press.

39. Soshnikova, V., et al., (2018). Cardamom fruits as a green resource for facile synthesis of gold and silver nanoparticles and their biological applications. *Artif. Cells Nanomed. Biotechnol., 46*(1), 108–117.

40. Rao, T. N., et al., (2019). Green synthesis and structural classification of *Acacia nilotica* mediated-silver doped titanium oxide (Ag/TiO$_2$) spherical nanoparticles: Assessment of its antimicrobial and anticancer activity. *Saudi J. Biol. Sci., 26*(7), 1385–1391.

41. Zhang, Z., et al., (2019). Green synthesis of silver nanoparticles from *Alpinia officinarum* mitigates cisplatin-induced nephrotoxicity via down-regulating apoptotic pathway in rats. *Artif. Cells Nanomed. Biotechnol., 47*(1), 3212–3221.

42. Tripathi, D., et al., (2019). Green and cost effective synthesis of silver nanoparticles from endangered medicinal plant *Withania coagulans* and their potential biomedical properties. *Mater. Sci. Eng. C Mater. Biol. Appl., 100*, 152–164.

43. Mallmann, E. J., et al., (2015). Antifungal activity of silver nanoparticles obtained by green synthesis. *Rev. Inst. Med. Trop. Sao. Paulo., 57*(2), 165–167.

44. Francis, S., Koshy, E. P., & Mathew, B., (2018). Green synthesis of *Stereospermum suaveolens* capped silver and gold nanoparticles and assessment of their innate antioxidant, antimicrobial and antiproliferative activities. *Bioprocess Biosyst. Eng., 41*(7), 939–951.

45. Ghaseminezhad, S. M., Hamedi, S., & Shojaosadati, S. A., (2012). Green synthesis of silver nanoparticles by a novel method: Comparative study of their properties. *Carbohydr. Polym., 89*(2), 467–472.

46. Desalegn, B., et al., (2019). Green synthesis of zero valent iron nanoparticle using mango peel extract and surface characterization using XPS and GC-MS. *Heliyon., 5*(5), e01750.

47. Bibi, I., et al., (2019). Green synthesis of iron oxide nanoparticles using pomegranate seeds extract and photocatalytic activity evaluation for the degradation of textile dye. *Journal of Materials Research and Technology, 8(6)*, 6115–6124.

48. Poguberović, S. S., et al., (2016). Removal of As(III) and Cr(VI) from aqueous solutions using "green" zero-valent iron nanoparticles produced by oak, mulberry and cherry leaf extracts. *Ecological Engineering, 90*, 42–49.

49. Kalpana, V. N., et al., (2018). Biosynthesis of zinc oxide nanoparticles using culture filtrates of *Aspergillus niger*: Antimicrobial textiles and dye degradation studies. *Open Nano, 3*, 48–55.

50. Gnanakani, P. E., et al., (2019). *Nannochloropsis* extract-mediated synthesis of biogenic silver nanoparticles, characterization and in vitro assessment of antimicrobial, antioxidant and cytotoxic activities. *Asian Pac. J. Cancer Prev., 20*(8), 2353–2364.

51. Kobashigawa, J. M., et al., (2019). Influence of strong bases on the synthesis of silver nanoparticles (AgNPs) using the ligninolytic fungi *Trametes trogii*. *Saudi J. Biol. Sci., 26*(7), 1331–1337.

52. Neethu, S., et al., (2018). Efficient visible light induced synthesis of silver nanoparticles by *Penicillium polonicum* ARA 10 isolated from *Chetomorpha antennina* and its

antibacterial efficacy against salmonella enterica serovar typhimurium. *J. Photochem. Photobiol. B., 180*, 175–185.

53. Jalal, M., et al., (2018). Biosynthesis of silver nanoparticles from oropharyngeal candida glabrata isolates and their antimicrobial activity against clinical strains of bacteria and fungi. *Nanomaterials (Basel), 8*(8).

54. Valsalam, S., et al., (2019). Rapid biosynthesis and characterization of silver nanoparticles from the leaf extract of *Tropaeolum majus* L. and its enhanced *in-vitro* antibacterial, antifungal, antioxidant and anticancer properties. *J. Photochem. Photobiol. B., 191*, 65–74.

55. Ahmed, A. A., Hamzah, H., & Maaroof, M., (2018). Analyzing formation of silver nanoparticles from the filamentous fungus *Fusarium oxysporum* and their antimicrobial activity. *Turk J. Biol., 42*(1), 54–62.

56. Bao, H., et al., (2010). Extracellular microbial synthesis of biocompatible CdTe quantum dots. *Acta Biomater., 6*(9), 3534–3541.

57. Karthick, V., et al., (2015). Biosynthesis of gold nanoparticles and identification of capping agent using gas chromatography-mass spectrometry and matrix assisted laser desorption ionization-mass spectrometry. *J. Nanosci. Nanotechnol., 15*(6), 4052–4057.

58. Husseiny, M. I., et al., (2007). Biosynthesis of gold nanoparticles using *Pseudomonas aeruginosa. Spectrochim. Acta A Mol. Biomol. Spectrosc., 67*(3/4), 1003–1006.

59. Suresh, A. K., et al., (2011). Biofabrication of discrete spherical gold nanoparticles using the metal-reducing bacterium *Shewanella oneidensis. Acta Biomater., 7*(5), 2148–2152.

60. Lloyd, J. R., Yong, P., & Macaskie, L. E., (1998). Enzymatic recovery of elemental palladium by using sulfate-reducing bacteria. *Appl. Environ. Microbiol., 64*(11), 4607–4609.

61. Kalimuthu, K., et al., (2008). Biosynthesis of silver nanocrystals by *Bacillus licheniformis. Colloids Surf. B Biointerfaces., 65*(1), 150–153.

62. Juibari, M. M., et al., (2011). Intensified biosynthesis of silver nanoparticles using a native extremophilic *Ureibacillus thermosphaericus* strain. *Materials Letters, 65*(6), 1014–1017.

63. He, S., et al., (2007). Biosynthesis of gold nanoparticles using the bacteria *Rhodopseudomonas capsulata. Materials Letters, 61*(18), 3984–3987.

64. Konishi, Y., et al., (2007). Bioreductive deposition of platinum nanoparticles on the bacterium *Shewanella algae. J. Biotechnol., 128*(3), 648–653.

65. Sinha, A., & Khare, S. K., (2011). Mercury bioaccumulation and simultaneous nanoparticle synthesis by *Enterobacter sp.* cells. *Bioresour. Technol., 102*(5), 4281–4284.

66. Markus, J., et al., (2016). Intracellular synthesis of gold nanoparticles with antioxidant activity by probiotic *Lactobacillus kimchicus* DCY51(T) isolated from Korean kimchi. *Enzyme Microb. Technol., 95*, 85–93.

67. Kalishwaralal, K., et al., (2010). Biosynthesis of silver and gold nanoparticles using *Brevibacterium casei. Colloids and Surfaces B: Biointerfaces., 77*(2), 257–262.

68. Djohan, Y., et al., (2019). Molecular chaperone prefoldin-assisted biosynthesis of gold nanoparticles with improved size distribution and dispersion. *Biomater. Sci., 7*(5), 1801–1804.

# CHAPTER 4

# Natural Green Biopolymers (Chitosan and Collagen) Extraction, Characteristics, and Biomedical Applications

APARNA TIRUMALASETTI,[1] KESANA SURENDRA BABU,[2]
MANNAM KRISHNAMURTHY,[2,3] MURTHY CHAVALI,[2,4] and
ENAMALA MANOJ KUMAR[5]

[1]Department of Chemistry, International Institute of Information
Technology (IIIT), Nuzvid Campus, Rajiv Gandhi University of
Knowledge Technologies, Nuzvid (RGUKTN)-AP, Mylavaram Road,
Nuzvid – 521202, Krishna District, Andhra Pradesh, India

[2]Department of Chemistry (PG Studies), Shree Velagapudi Rama
Krishna Memorial College, Nagaram – 522268, Guntur District,
Andhra Pradesh, India

[3]Varsity Education Management Limited, Ayyappa Society Main Road,
Hyderabad – 500081, Telangana, India

[4]NTRC-MCETRC and Aarshanano Composite Technologies Pvt. Ltd.,
Guntur District – 522201 Andhra Pradesh, India

[5]Bioserve Biotechnologies (India) Private Ltd., Hyderabad, A Reprocell
Company, 3-1-135/1A, CNR Complex, Genome Valley Main Road,
R.R. District, Mallapur, Hyderabad – 500076, Telangana, India

## ABSTRACT

The intention of this chapter was to summarize the extraction, characteristics, and biomedical applications of natural green biopolymers,

chitosan, and collagen from aquatic animals. Over the decades, there has been strong ever-increasing attention in using numerous forms of chitosan and collagen for various biomedical applications. Chitosan is a natural, polycationic, linear polysaccharide resultant from chitin, and collagen is an elongated fibrillar structure having a repeating motif Gly-X-Y, where X and Y can be any amino acids, but mostly are proline and hydroxyproline. Chitosan has several impressive biological characteristics resulting from chitin; chitosan is an exceptional biopolymer that parades outstanding properties, alongside biocompatibility and biodegradability, anti-bacterial properties, and cytocompatibility. Many researchers have concentrated on these biopolymers as an impending source of bioactive materials in the past 25-year sowing to their non-toxic, biocompatible, and are biodegradable. The understanding of the production processes of chitosan and collagen and the confirmation of these biomaterials are crucial for promoting theoretical and practical availability. These biopolymers can be easily processed into gels, sponges, membranes, beads, and scaffold forms for various applications in the biomedical field.

This chapter presents the detailed picture of selective biomedical applications of natural green biopolymers, chitosan, and collagen to human health. The main focus of this chapter is to address the biomedical applications of chitosan and collagen towards the generation of fibrous scaffolds for tissue engineering (bone tissue, cartilage tissue, skin tissue, and neural tissue with respect to chitosan and collagen scaffolds, their enzyme immobilization via chitosan and collagen matrices and matrix drug delivery mechanisms via chitosan and collagen matrices.

## 4.1 INTRODUCTION

Biopolymers are high-molecular-weight (MW) compounds fabricated by interlinking, perennial elementary building blocks called monomers produced by living organisms [1]. Biopolymers can be either naturally formed or can be produced from renewable resources such as macromolecules of the plant, animal, or even microbial origin [2]. Biological macromolecules include carbohydrates (starch, chitin, cellulose, pectin, lignin, etc.), proteins (collagen, gelatin, casein, whey, silk, gluten, wool, etc.), lipids (oil and fats), polyesters formed by microorganisms through fermentation such as (polyhydroxyalkanoate (PHA), poly(4-hydroxybutyrate)

(PHB), poly-hydroxyvalerate (PHV), poly(lactic acid) (PLA)) [3], and various polymers like natural rubbers, other composites, etc. [4].

## 4.1.1 CLASSIFICATION OF BIOPOLYMERS

Polymers are noticeable practically in nearly every feature of current life ranging from common synthetic materials such as polystyrene (PS) to naturally available biopolymers and DNA to proteins-fundamental to biological function and structure. Natural macromolecules are critical to daily life; they arise from renewable biomass, originated from the organic macromolecular matter of plants, animals, and microbes. Natural polymers are distinct materials extensively occur in nature or are usually obtained from plants or animals. Proteins and nucleic acids, natural rubber, cellulose, silk, and wool are a few examples of natural polymers. The natural polymers market is obsessed with an increasing mandate towards therapeutic, pharmacological, and health applications. These are also employed in adhesives, food packaging, beverage, paint, and inks industries, specifically in cosmetics and toiletries.

Going green, going natural is the order of the day; coming to polymers, green and natural are different. On the other hand, green polymers are created under green (or sustainable) chemistry rules, a word that was coined in the early 1990s. The main task of expending natural polymers or emerging novel biomaterials lies with coordinating the multifarious interaction between chemical, biological, physical sciences, and engineering/technology and also in understanding their correct mode of action.

In general, biopolymers are aliphatic polyesters, which are categorized into two groups, natural and synthetic polymers; in spite of their origin, both groups are widely used for biomedical applications centered on specific properties and possibilities of developing the final products [5]. Natural biopolymers are produced from living organisms as structural components of tissues, which include mainly proteins and polysaccharides. Collagen is considered the oldest and most popular among proteins, followed by fibrinogen and elastin as biopolymers. Similarly, polysaccharides like cellulose, hyaluronate, chitosan, and heparin are also extensively used as biopolymers for various applications [6].

Synthetic polymers are further divided into biodegradable and non-biodegradable polymers based on the mode of degradation/susceptible to the active biological environment [7]. Both the groups are commercially viable due to their specific applications; non-degradable synthetic polymers are used in various surgeries, i.e., plastic surgeries, reconstructive procedures, vascular or trauma treatment [8]. Silicones, polyethylene (PE), polypropylene (PP), polyamide (PA), polyurethane (PU), polymethacrylates (PMA), polytetrafluoroethylene (PTFE), polycarbonates (PC), acrylic resins, and polyvinyl chloride (PVC) are the popularly used non-degradable synthetic polymers [9, 10]. Similarly, polylactide (PLA), polyglycolide (PGA) and its copolymers with lactides, polycaprolactone (PCL), polydioxanone (PDS), polyhydroxybutyrate (PHB), polypropylene fumigates (PPF), polyorthoesters, polyesteramides, and polyanhydrides comes under the category of biodegradable polymers and have enormous usages in the areas of tissue engineering, orthopedics, drug delivery and short-term implants [11].

In spite of the various advantages of synthetic or fermented polymers, biopolymers are environment-friendly resins because they are biodegradable, and the biomass, especially plants, which act as the raw materials, participate in the carbon cycle and help in carbon fixation through photosynthesis [12].

On the other hand, they acted as alternatives for fossil fuel-based polymers and preferred due to their biodegradable nature upon exposure to certain enzymes or bacteria present in the soil, compost, or marine sediment. Compared to the degradation of fossil fuel-based polymers, biopolymers reduce the emission of $CO_2$ with conventional incineration [13]. In consideration of global warming and other major environmental issues, much attention is given to biopolymers in spite of the problems like low softening temperatures (Tm) and lacking uniform mechanical strength [14]. Moreover, molecules of carbohydrate and proteinaceous in nature are very popular because of their diversity in number, type, distribution, and bonding of the monomer units. Due to their gigantic molecular structure and their capability to self-assemble makes these biopolymers suitable to build systems for biomedical applications. Therefore, this chapter highlights the structure, function, properties, extraction, characterization, and biomedical applications of chitosan (polysaccharide) and collagen (protein).

## 4.1.1.1 CHITOSAN

A deacetylated form of chitin consisting of β-the (1→4)-linked 2-acet-amido-2-deoxy-D-glucopyranose and 2-amino-2-deoxy-D-glucopyranose units called chitosan. Chitin and chitosan are natural polysaccharides conforming to the 2nd most plentiful polysaccharide (to cellulose), after cellulose. Chitin is a usual constituent of the exoskeleton in several water-dwelling organisms, land-dwelling organisms, and few microorganisms [15]. Generally, chitosan is commercially obtained from crustaceans and mollusks via the chemical process (conc. alkali solutions at high tempera-tures) or enzymatic method (acetyl xylan esterase or deacetylase chitin) [16].

1. **Structure of Chitosan:** Chitosan (poly-β-1,4-glucosamine) is a modified, linear naturally occurring helical polysaccharide macro-molecule, an amino polysaccharide, obtained from crustaceans and insects. Equally, chitin and chitosan have few extraordinary biological properties such as hydrophilicity, bioresorbable degra-dation products, biocompatibility, cellular binding capability, and wound healing accounting for their extensive applications in food, biomedical, cosmetic, and pharmaceutical industries.

   The chitosan structure is similar to cellulose but comparatively owing to chitin inertness, and less attention was given. So under-standing its properties is very important to make it viable for various applications, which begin with the structure and degree of deacetylation (DD). The key variance between chitin and chitosan lies within the structural arrangement of its monomer units. Chitin is a hetero-polymer of N-acetyl-d-glucosamine (GlcNAc) and d-glucosamine (GluN) units linked with β-(1-4) glycosidic bonds; in this linear chain, GlcNAc units are more predominant. On the other hand, chitosan consists of pyranose cycles of β-(1,4)-2-amino-2-deoxy-β-d-glucose (GluN) linked with a glycosidic bond [17]; during the deacetylation process, an arbitrary dispersal of acetylated, deacetylated units alongside chitosan chains are formed. The degree of deacetylation and polymerization (DP) is responsible for the size and MW of the molecule; usually, 40% to 98% of DD leads to an MW range from $5 \times 10^4$ to $2 \times 10^6$ Da [18]. Chitosan has a pKa of ~6.3; decreasing pH makes it is positively charged and water-soluble, similarly increasing pH makes it is negatively charged and hydrophobic [19]. By properly understanding and applying the pH, various types, such as powder, paste, film, and fiber can be produced for various biomedical applications [20]. Much attention was particularly laid on biomedical materials based on chitosan because of its exceptional properties such as renewable, non-toxic, biodegradability, biocompatibility, antibacterial properties, and excellent wound healing properties because of its ability to stimulate hemostasis and tissue regeneration [21]. Despite these advantages, its real-world use was largely restricted due to its meager solubility at pH 7, also for its reduced workability, little antioxidant activity, etc. See Figure 4.1 for the structures of (a) chitin and chitosan, and (b) collagen.

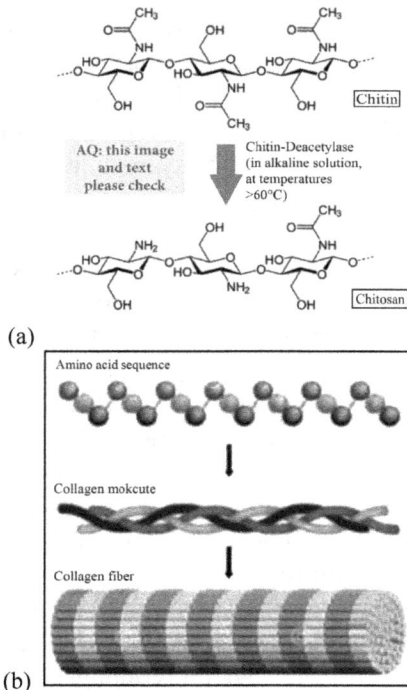

(a)

(b)

**FIGURE 4.1**    Structure of (a) chitin and chitosan, (b) collagen.

2. **Extraction of Chitosan**: The significant sources of chitosan are crab and shrimp shells, such as *Callinectes sapidus* [22] and *Chionoecetes opilio* (snow crab sps., also known as opilio crab

or opies crab) [23]; and *Pandalus borealis, Crangon crangon* (important species of caridean shrimp); *Penaeus merguiensis, Penaeus indicus, Penaeus penicillatus,* and *Penaeus monodon* (Indian shrimps) [24]. Generally, crustacean shell contains $CaCO_3$ and $Ca_3(PO_4)_2$ (34–46%), protein (25–35%) and chitin (28–29%). Chitin is a hydrophobic molecule, but after deacetylation, it yields chitosan; this conversion can be achieved by chemical, microbiological, and enzymatic methods. The chemical method of chitosan extraction includes de-mineralization, deproteiniza-tion, and deacetylation using either strong acids or strong alkalis. Demineralization process is done by adding 1.5N HCl at RT for 1 hour followed by de-deproteinization (0.5% NaOH at 100°C for 30 min.) primarily to deteriorate the protein tertiary structure in shells. It was then frequented till decolorization with 3% NaOH at 100°C for 30 min to get chitin slurry followed by deacetylation via treating with 40% aqueous NaOH at 95°C for 1.5 hours followed by washing and then dried. The duration of the deacetylation process may vary from 45 hr, 55 hr, 65 hr, and 72 hr; similarly, instead of NaOH, potassium permanganate oxalic acid is also used for decolorization. An illustration for the extraction of Chitosan is shown in Figure 4.2.

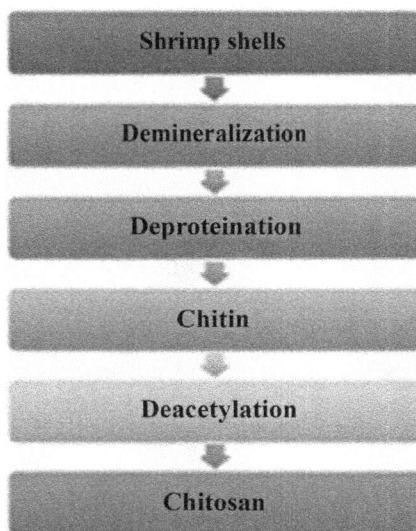

**FIGURE 4.2** Extraction of chitosan.

Bacteria like *Lactobacillus plantarum* [25]; *Serratia marcescens* [26] are used for the deacetylation of chitin [27]. Usually, sterilized shrimp shell powder is used to inoculate seed culture and left for batch fermentation at 30°C and 180 rpm for 7 days, and raw chitin acquired is cured with HCl followed by NaOH (~2 hours) respectively at RT and washed. The cleansed chitin is treated with 56% NaOH for 4 hours in a water bath under steaming conditions (95°C), trailed by washing and drying. In this process, chitosan can be extracted with 83% DD. Similarly, in the enzymatic method, shell waste after thoroughly washed, cooked with double distilled water at a ratio of 1:2 (w/v) for 30 min at 90°C, and enzymes like bromelain and alcalase are used for deproteinization experiments in the ratio of 1:3. Demineralization is done out in HCl solution (1.5 M) in 1:10 (w/v ratio) for 6 h at 50°C while stirring constantly, and deacetylation is done by treating with NaOH in a similar ratio at 140°C for 4 h; thus, obtained filtrate was filtered, washed with deionized water, and dried overnight at 50°C to obtain crude chitosan. The enzymatic method can also be performed using papain, tryptase, and pepsase, but it has shortcomings like the high cost of enzymes and low extraction [28]. Chitosan extracted by any of the aforementioned methods, due to its biocompatibility, mucoadhesion, high charge density, adaptability, hemostatic activity, film-forming, coagulating ability, and wound-healing properties, has attracted much attention for biomedical applications.

## 4.1.1.2 COLLAGEN

Collagen was used by Egyptians (as an adhesive) some 4,500 years ago, and by Native Americans (in bows) some 1,600 years ago [29]. Collagen is an extensively found animal protein with nearly 25% of protein mass, which is a key source of tissue strength [30]. A characteristic collagen molecule consists of three intertwined chains polymerized together to forms a helical structure with varying lengths, thickness, and inter-weaving patterns depending on the species and organs [31]. Collagen typically consists of 35% glycine (Gly), 21% proline-Pro, and hydroxyproline-Hyp. The amino acid sequence in collagen is usually a repetitive tripeptide unit (Gly-X-Y), where X is frequently Pro, and Y is Hyp [32]. The high glycine content of collagen has a significant role regarding the stabilization of the collagen helix tolerating the close link between the collagen fibers, facilitates intermolecular cross-links through hydrogen bonding [33]. Because glycine (Gly) is the tiniest amino acid without any side chain (R), it plays an exclusive role in fibrous structural proteins. Moreover, it has an important part in recognition of phenotype cell, cell adhesion, tissue regulation; non-proline-rich segments of collagen have cell regulatory roles [34].

1. **Structure of Collagen:** There are almost 29 diverse types of collagen differing in their construction, location, purpose, and additional characteristics. They are categorized based on their structure into fibrous (*striatum*), non-fibrous (*network forming*), micro-fibrillar (*filamentous*), and those associated with fibrils [35]. However, the predominant form for biomaterial application, type-I collagen, which is known as "rope-forming" collagen and can be found in skin, tendons, and bone [36] consisting of three polypeptide chains, of which two are identical ($\alpha 1$ (I) and $\alpha 2$ (I) chains), but their composition of amino acids vary. Type-II collagen occurs only in cartilage tissue, and it was thought that the $\alpha 1$ (II) subunit is similar to the $\alpha 1$ (I) subunit. Other types of collagen only exist in small aliquots, mainly in explicit organs such as the basement membranes, cornea, lung tissue, heart muscle, and intestinal mucosa [37]. Collagen is intensely reliant on age; in the early stages of life, skin contains up to 50%, and during the aging process, it gets reduced to 5–10%.

2. **Extraction of Collagen:** Collagen is generally formed by chemical hydrolysis and enzymatic hydrolysis [38]. Chemical hydrolysis is a common procedure, but enzymatic hydrolysis is more promising when compared to the yield of products with improved functionality and reduces the processing time [33] but extremely costly. To extract collagen, pre-treatment is essential to eliminate plentiful covalent intra and intermolecular cross-links, either by using an acid or alkaline process, that differs agreeing to the origin of the raw material, also removes non-collagenous substances and higher yields are obtained with pre-treatment. The utmost frequently used extraction methods are based on the collagen solubility in neutral saline, acidic solutions, and acidic solutions with added enzymes [39]. However, a widely accepted and effective method for collagen extraction is treating the tissue with 0.05 to 0.1 M

NaOH at 5–20°C based on the structural modifications [40]. An illustration for the extraction of Collagen is shown in Figure 4.3.

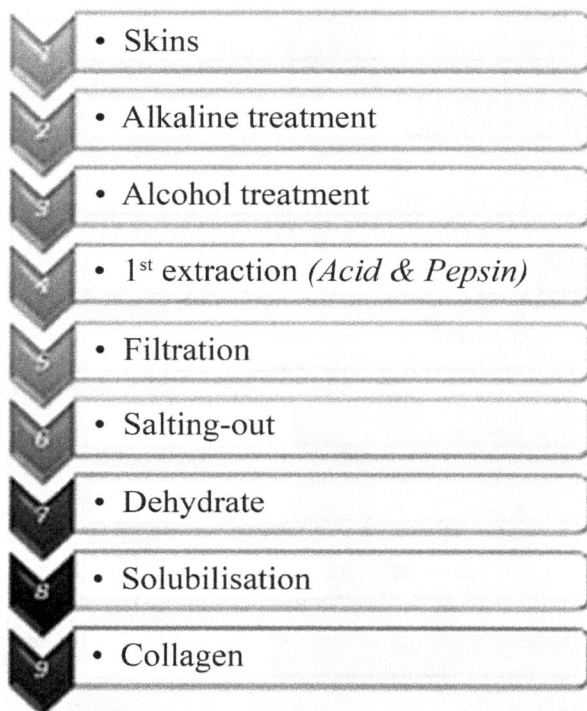

1. • Skins
2. • Alkaline treatment
3. • Alcohol treatment
4. • 1ˢᵗ extraction *(Acid & Pepsin)*
5. • Filtration
6. • Salting-out
7. • Dehydrate
8. • Solubilisation
9. • Collagen

**FIGURE 4.3**   Extraction of collagen.

In extracting collagen, saline solutions (pH-7) such as NaCl, Tris-HCl (Tris (hydroxyl methyl) amino-methane HCl), phosphates or citrates [41] were used. Even though the process is cost-effective, it has a lot of limitations, and these were rectified in the acid hydrolysis method using carboxylic acids (organic), for example, acetic acid, citric acid, and lactic acid [42, 43]. Acetic acid is capable of solubilizing non-crosslinked and interstrand cross-links of collagen, leading to a higher solubility of collagen during the extraction process [40]. For the extraction of acid-soluble collagen: pre-treated material was added to the acid solution, typically 0.5 M acetic acid, and maintained at 4°C under constant stirring for 24 to 72 hours, depending on the raw material [44]. On the other hand, collagen can be extracted by enzymatic hydrolysis; the insoluble raw material (in acetic acid) was used to extract pepsin-solubilized collagen (PSC) with 0.15% (w/v) pepsin in 0.015 M HCl for 48 hours and filtered. The filtrate was then subjected to precipitation and dialysis under the same conditions to obtain acid-soluble collagen.

### 4.1.2 INFORMATION BASED ON PUBLICATIONS

Publications wise we have collected information on chitosan and collagen with respect to biomedical applications. Data we recollected from 1996 to 2020 (Jan. 2020) via ScienceDirect (https://www.sciencedirect.com/). A maximum number of publications (all types) were observed for collagen-based biomedical applications (40,982) compared to that of chitosan (20,856) as on today. Of which increased number of publications for collagen seen from the year 2005 compared to that of chitosan (2012). Statistical data was presented in Figures 4.4(a) and 4.4(b).

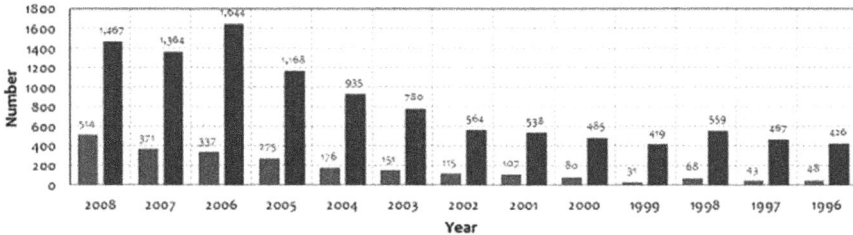

(a)

■ Chitosan/Biomedical    ■ Collagen/Biomedical

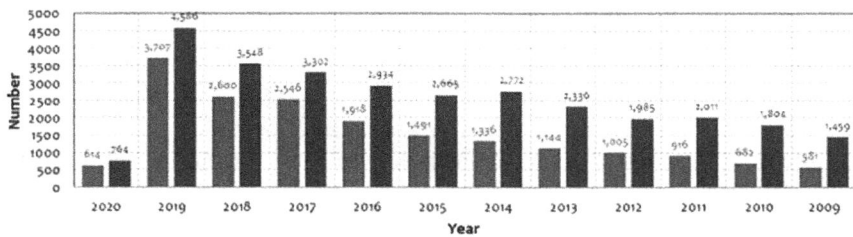

(b)

■ Chitosan/Biomedical    ■ Collagen/Biomedical

**FIGURE 4.4** Statistical data illustrating the number of publications (all types) for chitosan and collagen-based biomedical applications, (a) 1996–2008, (b) 2009–2020.

Data collected from 1996 to 2020 (Jan. 2020) via ScienceDirect was further segregated based on the type of publication, say for example review, mini-reviews, editorials, etc. Statistical data based on article types for chitosan and collagen with reference to biomedical applications are presented in Figures 4.5(a) and 4.5(b).

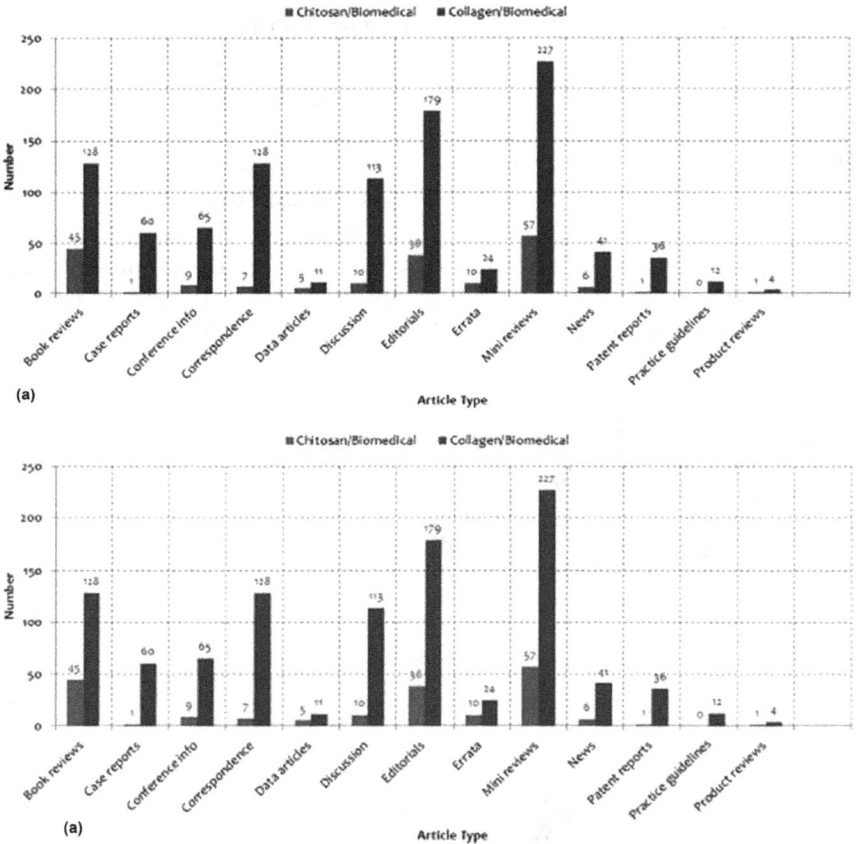

(a)

(a)

**FIGURE 4.5** Statistical data based on article types for chitosan and collagen with reference to biomedical applications.

Data were further segregated based on journal titles for chitosan and collagen with reference to biomedical applications. Details were illustrated in Figure 4.6(a) for chitosan and biomedical applications and Figure 4.6(b) for collagen and biomedical applications.

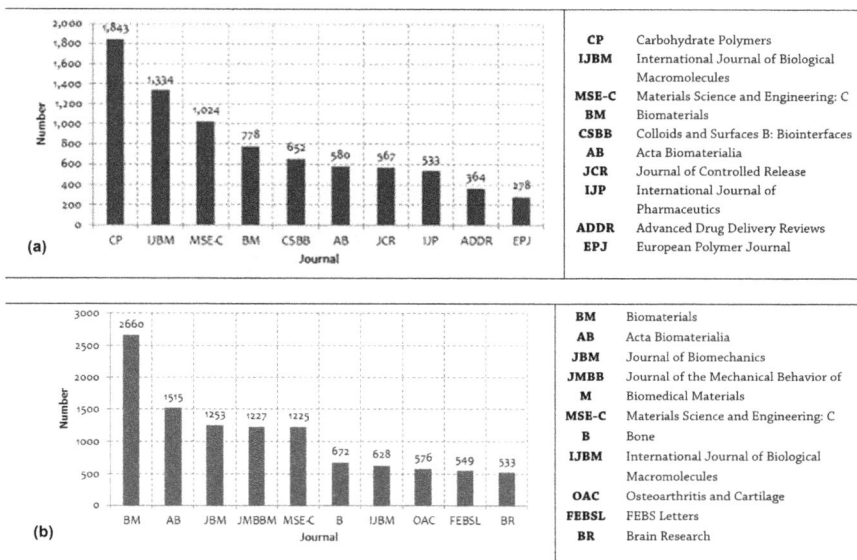

| CP | Carbohydrate Polymers |
| IJBM | International Journal of Biological Macromolecules |
| MSE-C | Materials Science and Engineering: C |
| BM | Biomaterials |
| CSBB | Colloids and Surfaces B: Biointerfaces |
| AB | Acta Biomaterialia |
| JCR | Journal of Controlled Release |
| IJP | International Journal of Pharmaceutics |
| ADDR | Advanced Drug Delivery Reviews |
| EPJ | European Polymer Journal |

| BM | Biomaterials |
| AB | Acta Biomaterialia |
| JBM | Journal of Biomechanics |
| JMBB | Journal of the Mechanical Behavior of Biomedical Materials |
| M | Biomedical Materials |
| MSE-C | Materials Science and Engineering: C |
| B | Bone |
| IJBM | International Journal of Biological Macromolecules |
| OAC | Osteoarthritis and Cartilage |
| FEBSL | FEBS Letters |
| BR | Brain Research |

**FIGURE 4.6** (a) Journal titles for chitosan and biomedical applications, (b) Journal titles for collagen and biomedical applications.
[*Abbreviations:* CP: Carbohydrate Polymers; IJBM: International Journal of Biological Macromolecules; MSE-C: Materials Science and Engineering-C; BM: Biomaterials; CSBB: Colloids and Surfaces B: Biointerfaces; AB: *Acta biomaterialia*; JCR: Journal of Controlled Release; IJP: International Journal of Pharmaceutics; ADDR: Advanced Drug Delivery Reviews; EPJ: European Polymer Journal; JBM: Journal of Biomechanics; JMBBM: Journal of the Mechanical Behavior of Biomedical Materials; B: Bone; OAC: Osteoarthritis and Cartilage; FEBSL: FEBS Letters; BR: Brain Research].

## 4.2 APPLICATIONS OF CHITOSAN AND COLLAGEN

Chitosan has great potential in diverse fields has long been familiar. Its chemical characteristics provide chitosan with an exceptional set of practical properties. These properties have led to its increased utility in precise applications such as controlled release coatings, gene delivery, antibacterial coatings, nanofiltration, anti-biofouling coatings, microcapsules, drug delivery hydrogel, and tissue engineering scaffolds. For biomedical applications, chitosan derived from the non-animal origin is preferred towards in vivo testing. Chitosan was also used in diverse fields, including medicine, food, biomedical, waste management, and agricultural applications. Chitosan possesses properties like antibacterial, and antifungal and was extensively studied for antimicrobial properties (as a potential natural agent) in agricultural, pharmaceutical, cosmetic, and food industries. Chitosan has many other beneficial properties; it is a non-toxic, antibacterial, and environmentally friendly with no acidic degradation products; although common applications range from water treatment to chromatography, cosmetics, textile treatment, textiles, photographic papers, biomedical devices, tissue engineering and wound healing (regeneration), hemodialysis membranes and implant coatings for the controlled release in gene or drug delivery, major applications are in the development of edible films, PU paint, and biopesticides. Therapeutic applications for chitosan have been proposed due to their properties such as antioxidant activity, antibacterial, trapping triglyceride, and hypoglycemic effects towards prevention, treatment, and management of long-lasting ailments.

A natural polymer matrix, collagen is extremely conserved through species. Inside the mammalian body, it is comprising 1/3rd of all the protein mass in tissues, as a predominant extracellular matrix (ECM) component. Collagen is an extracellular protein and is the most abundant material as a building block for skin, tendons, and bones. There are 27 known types of Collagens mainly have a structural role to play. The protein configuration significantly affects its role in tissue architecture. Collagen types contain diverse proteins which assist distinct purposes within the body. Collagen type-I plays an imperative role in maximum matrix rich tissues, but there are plentiful other protein components that are perilous to the exclusive architecture of tissues.

### 4.2.1 BIOMEDICAL APPLICATIONS

Tissues and organs highly organized hierarchical, nanosize fibrous structures, which include skin, collagen, cartilage, dentin, and bone, in one way or another, have some sort of structural resemblance. Thus, research on biomedical applications has concentrated on the:

1. Fibrous scaffolds generation for tissue engineering;
2. Enzyme immobilization;
3. The mechanism in drug delivery [45].

## 4.2.1.1 *GENERATION OF FIBROUS SCAFFOLDS FOR TISSUE ENGINEERING*

Tissue engineering is an essential practice to substitute the damaged tissues/ organs and a perfect replacement for autografts or allografts because of the restrictions such as the transmission of diseases, pain (graft site), morbidity (donor site) and cost. The achievement of tissue engineering lies in the selection of proper cells for tissue/organ replacement, appropriate biomaterials with optimum physio- and biochemical properties.

Amongst the numerous natural and synthetic polymers, chitosan, and collagen have shown extraordinary promise in the biomedical field because of their exclusive nature and ability to offer the target cells with a native environment by mimicking the ECM. In this chapter, we are concentrating on the exact applications of chitosan and collagen scaffolds in bone, cartilage, skin, and neural regeneration.

1. **Bone Tissue Engineering (BTE):** All over the world, the transplant crisis is a key concern in the healthcare industry, lack of donors, persons on transplant waiting list is growing annually. Presently, it is considered as one of the most abused fields in the regenerative medicine was tissue engineering which wishes to combine engineering concepts with biological facts by using the human body's potential to repair or create fresh tissues. Collagen-I is a vital component of the bone matrix, its structure has a crucial role to play in mineralization process. Bone is a firm, very greatly specialized, strong, ordered, and with dense connective tissue in a human body composed of cells, organic (collagen, growth factors, and other non-collagenous proteins) and inorganic matrix (hydroxyapatite (HA)) [46]. The bone tissue is the utmost complex composite organ of the human body mainly composed of components (3): HA, represents ~70% from the total mineral phase, collagen-I-nearly 20%, water-8% and additional constituents such as Mg, proteins (non-collagenous) (usually function as growth factors, promoting bone formation), lipids, etc. BTE is a regeneration of natural human bone through artificial means, which requires a scaffold matrix with or without cells and biological cues for an effective outcome.

In BTE, scientists say, the current challenges in terms of medical issues and the economic impact of the available treatments are the two main aspects to be considered in the future. The need for bone tissue treatments is becoming clear. Bone tissue ailments are affecting nearly 76 M in the USA, Europe, and Japan. During the past 20–30 years, the USA spent more than 20 Bn US$ on treatments based on bone trauma. Further, more than 300000–350000 spinal fusions were conducted only in the year 2005.

Scaffolds are the chief tools used in tissue engineering, a synthetic ECM categorized by a specific shape providing mechanical sustenance for the new tissue formation. At present, several technologies are used in order to generate scaffolds with specific requirements. A recent novel methodology in the field is 3D printing process-rapid prototyping (RP) can overwhelm the weaknesses reported by the conventional methods. Scaffold requirements for BTE and various types of manufacturing methods were listed in Figure 4.7.

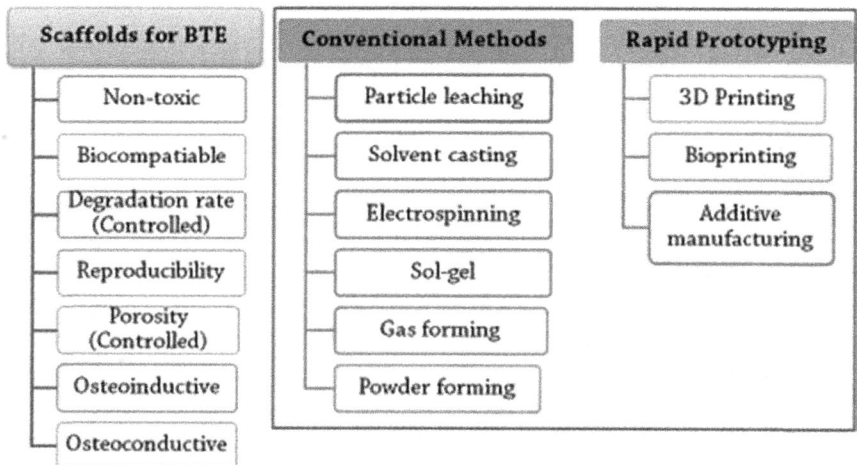

**FIGURE 4.7** Bone tissue-engineering (a) requirements for scaffolds; (b) types of manufacturing methods both conventional methods/rapid prototyping.

i. **Chitosan Scaffold:** Chitosan is a natural biomaterial used for developing scaffold matrix due to certain rewards such as biodegradability, simple processing methods, biocompatibility, flexibility, and porosity [47]; however, it is weak and unstable mechanically. Hence, chitosan polymeric blends progressed as an alternative to augment the mechanical strength and serve as osteoconductive matrices. Saad et al. [48] established chitosan-HA hybrid scaffold, a challenging approach has been adapted to reconstruct and restore the functionality of the impaired tissue. This combination enhanced the hard tissue regeneration; scaffold showed (within 30 days of implantation) complete in-vivo biodegradation. Similarly, Ming et al. [49] reported the addition of raloxifene in chitosan scaffold which has estrogenic actions on the bone; this combination has significantly enhanced cell proliferation, higher mineralization capacity and showed high alkaline phosphatase (ALP) activity designates the bone regeneration capability of MC3T3-E1 cells after 15 days of exposure.

With the advancement of nanotechnology and its application in tissue culture has also revolutionized the utilization of chitosan in tissue culture. Because nanotechnology includes manipulation of structures within a size range of 1 to 100 nm at least in one dimension and displays new properties and functionalities different from their bulk counterparts. The small-size tailored surface, enhanced solubility, multi-functionality, and tissue adhesion properties of chitosan-based nanomaterials have produced a vast influence in the biomedical area [50]. Tan et al. [51] demonstrated the promotion of osteoblast propagation and osteogenic differentiation of MSCs while plummeting osteoclastogenesis through free chitosan nanoparticles.

Besides the above properties, piezoelectricity, and extraordinary mechanical strength are the two vital characteristics of bone tissue, these characters were achieved by composite scaffolds comprised of functionalized multi-walled carbon nanotubes (f-MWCNT), medium MW chitosan, and β-Glycerophosphate. f-MWCNT content was between 0.1 w/v% and 0.5 w/v% are the most appropriate compositions in BTE with no significant cytotoxicity and improved electrical conductivity [52]. The introduction of nanoparticles with magnetic properties into chitosan scaffold through reverse co-precipitation method has been showing promising results [53].

ii.  **Collagen Scaffold:** Collagen is extracted from animal sources such as porcine, bovine skin, rat-tail, and fish for biomedical applications. Nonetheless, pure collagen cannot be directly used as a material for the bone substitute, due to its meager mechanical strength. Hence, much attention was concentrated on composite scaffolds of collagen with hydroxyapatite (HA) or calcium phosphates (CaP) such as beta-tricalcium phosphate ($\beta$-TCP) and biphasic calcium phosphate (BCP), etc., [54]. Moreover, Yu et al. [174] reported that the Type-I collagen presented in collagen-HA scaffolds is readily degraded by enzymes (collagenases) secreted by the surrounding cells, supports the differentiation of progenitor cells into bone-forming osteoblasts. This facilitated the engineering of the bi-component system (CH-HA) and is currently drawing many researchers attention because of their enhanced properties compared with CH (mono).

Ning et al. [55] has engineered porous collagen-hydroxyapatite scaffolds loaded with mesenchymal stem cells for bone regeneration. Similarly, induced pluripotent stem (iPS) cell-derived mesenchymal stem cells were cultured on collagen and HAP scaffolds which enhanced the osteogenic differentiation at *in vitro* and *in vivo* experiments also. Rahmatullah et al. [56] reported the advantage of incorporating hydroxyapatite mesoporous microspheres into collagen scaffolds. The compressive modulus of the composite scaffold at low and high strain values was improved by 1.7 and 2.8 times and cell proliferation rate up to 3 folds by this combination. McDaniel et al. [175] reported the utilization of $\beta$-TCP combined with collagen as a substitute to autografts and successfully implanted in rabbit segmental bone defects and found new bone formation. Instead of these chemicals agents, natural therapeutic molecules such as ginseng compound, K was merged into the composite fish collagen scaffold, which was found to be biocompatible, optimal pore size, adequate swelling, biodegradable, moderate mineralization and sustained the growth of MG-63 cells. Supaporn et al. [57] reported an interesting combination of collagen with decellularized pulp/fibronectin for BTE in alveolar bone resorption and observed predominant biofunctionalities. Chetana et al. [58] has mimicked the formation of vertebrate bone via the efficacious formation of collagen-polycatecholamines-$CaCO_3$ composite structures, resulting significant enhancement in mechanical properties of collagen and biological studies with human fetal osteoblastic (hFob) displayed augmented cell proliferation and osteogenic differentiation.

Thalita et al. [59] have developed and characterized, 3D biocomposite scaffolds using type-I collagen, mineral trioxide aggregate (MTA) and multiwalled carbon nanotubes (MWCNT) for bone tissue regeneration. MC3T3-E1 osteoblasts have successfully migrated into scaffolds and caused a surge in mineralization of scaffolds. Biomimetic collagen scaffolds are also capable of hosting osteoprogenitor cells (MC3T3-E1) and governing kinetic release profile of the encapsulated pro-osteogenic factor (BMP2) without weakening bioactivity over 3 weeks. Gayathri et al. [60] reported that this model offers not only an osteoinductive environment for osteoprogenitor cells to differentiate but also an appropriate biomechanical and biochemical environment to act as a reservoir for osteogenic factors with controlled release profile.

2.  **Cartilage Tissue Engineering:** Cartilage is a firm tissue but is softer and much more flexible than bone, also a key structural component of the body [61]. A connective tissue found in many areas of the body including proliferation, differentiation between the vertebrae in the spine, bronchial tubes or airways, ears, and nose [62]. Cartilage tissue engineering target at generating totally healed, functional, and scarless tissue regeneration by exploiting numerous biodegradable scaffolds seeded with stem cells, growth factors, and serum. In general, chondrocytes have the capability to grow again via articular cartilage, utilization of induced bone marrow stems cells, and adipose-derived stem cells (ADSCs) are the more potential source [63]. These cells can be dedifferentiated by exposing to growth factors such as insulin growth factor-I, transforming growth factor $\beta$ (TGF-$\beta$), and bone morphogenic proteins. Scaffolds derived from natural polymers such as alginate, fibrin, chitosan, and silk have shown to have increased biocompatibility, cell adherence and chondrogenic differentiation of stem cells due to their structural resemblance to ECM [64].

i.  **Chitosan Scaffold:** Glycosaminoglycans (GAGs) provide a stimulating environment in cartilage regeneration and chitosan having similar structure stimulates chondrogenesis. Chitosan/gelatin hybrid scaffold was combined with ADSCs to fabricate dynamically in vitro. ADSCs grew well in chitosan/gelatin hybrid scaffold and were suitable for tissue engineering applications in cartilage regeneration [65]. Similarly, Park et al. [176] altered chitosan-using hydroxyapatite and encapsulated with chondrocytes and experimentally proved significant cell proliferation, cell differentiation but with a reduced degradation rate. If required the growth of chondrocytes can be improved by TGF-β which were incorporated into chitosan scaffold [66]. Injectable hydrogels of chitosan composites was another advanced method of creating artificial ECM for regenerating cartilage; this approach has shown remarkable effects for of resemblance with the ECM of native tissue.

ii. **Collagen Scaffold:** Regular cartilage was encompassing minor percentage of chondrocytes, an ECM, and water with dissolved electrolytes [67]. The ECM, on the other hand, comprises water, collagen, and proteoglycans. The exclusive physical and mechanical properties of cartilage ECM are due to the abundance of type-I, II, and IX collagen scattered throughout the matrix [68]. The fluctuating amounts and types of collagen, proteoglycan, and chondrocytes give rise to the three different types of cartilage, hyaline, elastic, and fibrocartilage present in the human body [67]. Therefore, collagen is an integral part of the cartilage ECM and considered as an important constituent in cartilage tissue engineering. Collagen-glycosaminoglycan scaffold was used for differentiation of rat MSCs in vitro. In addition, the collagen-HyA (CHyA) scaffolds displayed larger levels of MSC infiltration with noteworthy acceleration of gene expression (SOX-9), collagen type-II and cartilage matrix production [69], which makes this scaffold as an appropriate matrix for encouraging cartilage tissue repair. Birgit et al. [70] reported the role of cross-linkers in increasing the stability of porous collagen extracted from jellyfish *(Rhopilema esculentum)* and subsequent engineering of the scaffold by freeze-drying. This scaffold has up-regulated chondrogenic marker (SOX9), collagen II and aggrecan indirect cultures of hMSCs upon chondrogenic stimulation. The structural design of scaffolds also plays a major role in cartilage tissue engineering [71], 3D scaffolds were fabricated with natural type-I collagen and synthetic

PLGA crocheted mesh in three different compositions as thin, semi, and sandwich, respectively. Bovine chondrocytes were cultured in these scaffolds and transplanted subcutaneously into nude mice, all groups showed homogeneous cell distribution, natural chondrocyte morphology, and abundant cartilaginous ECM deposition but varied in the expression of type-II collagen and aggrecan mRNA was advanced in the semi, and sandwich groups could be used for cartilage tissue engineering [72].

3. **Skin Tissue Engineering (STE):** The largest organ of the body is skin, as an outer covering protects from injury, hazards, and invasion. The skin with seven layers of ectodermal tissue and sentries the essential muscles, bones, ligaments, internal organs and has been the genesis of many tissue engineering constructs [73]. Naturally, in a mechanical injury to the skin, the body activates a response called regeneration or wound healing, but during major injuries, the repair mechanisms are not capable of restoring the skin to its original condition [74]. Skin regeneration can be achieved through tissue engineering; the early methodology to skin tissue engineering (STE) is to mimic the natural skin constituents comprising collagen, GAGs, and elastins [75]. A porous scaffold can be fabricated by assembling these natural components, providing support (for an overlying epidermis) as well as an internal architecture capable of permitting angiogenesis [76]. Natural materials such as collagen and chitosan were spun on their own or together with synthetic polymers to produce scaffolds for STE.

i. **Chitosan Scaffold:** Chitosan is known to quicken wound healing, energizing for the migration of polymorphonuclear leukocytes into the wound causing debridement [77]. It has exclusive tissue-adhesive and properties like antimicrobial, that sterilize the wound by releasing bactericidal reactive oxygen species (ROS) escorting phagocytotic activity of the polymorphonuclear leukocytes [78]. Chitosan in amalgamation with collagen forms an outstanding proangiogenic biomaterial, creating a vascularized site towards tissue regeneration [79]. Chitosan scaffold fabricated with poly(caprolactone) showed significant improvement in the hydrophilicity, protein adsorption and cytocompatibility for human cells was considered an excellent system for STE [80]. Chitosan-graft-poly (ε-caprolactone) was developed in various compositions to improve cellular adhesion profiles and stability of the 3D fibrous structure, as probable scaffolds for STE. Chitosan is also blended with poly(3-hydroxybutyrate-co-3-hydroxyvalerate) to fabricate scaffolds for skin engineering. PHBV/chitosan 4:1 (w/w) demonstrated a greater in vitro biocompatibility and an improved ability for cell adhesion and growth against L929 cell line and same has improved the wound healing process in rats [81]. Yunyun et al. [82] developed a facile technique to make the glutaraldehyde (GA) cross-linked collagen/chitosan porous scaffold for STE. This technique produced scaffolds with a smooth surface, controlled size, sufficient swelling ratios (sufficient to guarantee the nutrient source), in vitro degradation, enhanced tensile and compression properties, accelerated cell infiltration and proliferation.

A series of norfloxacin-loaded scaffolds were synthesized in combination with collagen and chitosan for treatment of wounds. Rafael et al. [83] produced a double layer scaffolds using electrospinning technique, where one layer was composed of PCL (for mechanical support), and another layer by chitosan (primary wound dressing). The double-layer scaffolds have a water vapor permeation rate ($\sim730\ \mathrm{g\ m^{-2}\ day^{-1}}$) and a PBS solution uptake capability (up to 369%) attributes to the extraordinary volumetric porosity of these scaffolds (~80%) meeting the necessities for skin lesion dressing applications.

ii.  **Collagen Scaffold:** Collagen is a biological activity protein in the ECM and choice for skin regenerations due to its properties like superior biocompatibility, biodegradability, and low immunogenicity [84]. Collagen acts like an adhesive for cells within the regenerated organs, specifically used as a wound dressing in burns and chronic wounds for decades [85]. Molecular architecture of collagen within the scaffold supports the integration and infiltration of cells, due to precise cellular adhesion and migration [86] but the mechanical properties and tensile strength of pure collagen are one of the limitations, which can be overcome by blending with certain cross-linkers.

Xingang et al. [87] has fabricated collagen-chitosan scaffolds incorporated with poly(l-lactide-co-glycolide) to enhance the mechanical properties as a hybrid dermal substitute for tissue engineering. Collagen scaffold blended with hydroxyethyl cellulose/poly(vinyl) alcohol was considered as an impending substrate for STE owing to slower degradation rate, uneven, and rough surfaces near the final week of incubation in PBS and DMEM solution [88].

Fourier transform infrared (FT-IR) spectroscopy and thermo-gravimetric (TG) results confirmed the surface alteration of PCL/gelatin scaffold by collagen type-I immobilization on the scaffold surface. MTT assay established cell adhesion, viability, and high proliferation rate of L929 mouse fibroblast cells on the collagen type I-modified composite scaffold [89]. To improve the surface feature of scaffold for STE, poly(lactic-co-glycolic acid) (PLGA) hydrolyzed in NaOH (diverse concentrations) was electrospun with collagen. Contact angle measurements, porosimetry, SEM, FTIR spectroscopy, tensile ability, degradation tests, in vitro cell attachment (HDF, HaCat) and cytotoxicity assays have proven the effectiveness of this combination and can be a suitable matrix for skin regeneration [90].

Initially, the collagen was extracted from mammalian source but later to overcome the religious issues and to stop the transmission of contagious diseases; fish collagen was used as an alternative. Huan et al. [91] designed a scaffold with controlled release system for STE using fish collagen/chitosan/chondroitin sulfate scaffolds using the freeze-drying technique. This combinational effect leads to an increase in the protein release, the higher diffusion rate of microspheres incorporated in the scaffolds, sustaining its structural integrity and bioactivity. In vivo evaluation reveal scaffolds/MPs had decent biocompatibility and an ability to encourage fibroblast cell proliferation and STE. Similarly, a hybrid scaffold composed of fish collagen/alginate functionalized by dissimilar mol.wts. of chitooligosaccharides (COSs) with the use of 1-ethyl-3-(3-dimeth-ylaminopropyl) carbodiimide HCl as a cross-linking agent was fabricated. These results indicate that the homogeneous material blending has highly interconnected porous architecture (160–260 µm pore size; 90% porosity), tensile property, retention capacity and in vitro biodegradation behavior assured the FCA/COS scaffolds for STE application [92]. A highly interconnected porous 3D collagen matrix impregnated with bioactive extract was fabricated for efficient wound healing. The dressing substrate possesses the in vitro enzymatic degradability, high swelling capacity, and increase in porosity, antibacterial property and excellent cell adhesion and proliferation against NIH 3T3 fibroblast and human keratinocyte (HaCaT) cell lines equally [93].

4. **Neural Tissue Engineering:** A neuron is an electrically excitable cell which processes and communicates data through electrical and chemical signals. They are the core components of the CNS, and ganglia of PNS. Its regeneration refers to the regrowth or repairs of nervous tissues or cells and can be achieved by a scaffold with good mechanical, electrical, biological properties and compliance match methodically resembling the native ECM [94]. Even though natural polymers (chitosan, collagen, gelatin, and alginate) were used in countless nerve regeneration methodologies, they have certain demerits like surface erosion. Therefore, surface eroding scaffold is likely to provide enhanced contact guidance for nerve regeneration [95].

   i. **Chitosan Scaffold:** Chitosan is an optimal material for scaffolds in the regeneration of damaged peripheral nerves [96]. The same was confirmed by Chuang et al. [97] by culturing rat Schwann cells (RSCs) on porous chitosan scaffolds and observed the higher amount of laminin and collagen secretions. Incorporation of nerve growth factor (NGF) in chitosan/ PVA conjugated scaffolds can act as potential neural tissue engineering matrixes. Because NGF has enhanced the thermodynamic parameters and binding abilities of SKNMC and U373 cell lines. This encouragement is due to the CS/PVA conjugated NGF nanocomposite fibers have a high surface-area-to-volume ratio to support the attachment and proliferation rate of both cell types [98].

   Polymeric scaffolds comprising chitosan, and gelatin with pore geometry of inverted colloidal crystals (ICC) were engineered via self-assembly; cross-linking, infiltration, dehydration, and particle leaching for managing the differentiation of iPS cells toward neurons. Adhesion and proliferation of Schwann cells on the arranged scaffolds was achieved because PAG improved the electrical conductivity and mechanical properties of the matrix [99]. The in vitro Schwann cells culture demonstrated that the silanized scaffolds with 8% APTE (3-aminopropyltriethoxysilane) could facilitate the attachment and proliferation of cells, indicating great potential for the application in peripheral nerve regeneration [100]. A chitosan conduit and silk fibroin (SF) fibers were fabricated as a scaffold and loaded with Schwann cell to bridge a 10 mm rat sciatic nerve gap. The results from morphological and electro-physiological examination showed that regenerative outcomes were comparable to a cellular nerve graft and a lot superior to plain chitosan/SF scaffolds [101]. Guicai et al. [102] established the use of negatively charged heparin and positively charged γ-aminopropyltriethoxysilane (APTE) treatment as a biocompatible modification of lyophilized porous chitosan scaffolds provides an effective modification of surface and displays excessive potential for the application in peripheral nerve regeneration. Incorporating conductive hyaluronic acid doped-poly(3,4-ethylenedioxythiophene) nanoparticles into a chitosan/gelatin matrix for nerve tissue regeneration a novel porous scaffold was developed by Shuping et al., [177] using neuron-like rat phaeochromocytoma (PC12) cells. This combination has augmented the mechanical and electrical properties while decreasing water absorption capacity, the porosity, and in vitro biodegradation of the scaffold.

ii. **Collagen Scaffold:** These are highly suggested for neural tissue reconstitution because they upkeep the elongation of axons past the scaffold and cell growth; vascularization of the engrafted tissue [103]. Moreover, collagen is the key constituent of the ECM which plays a significant role in the regulation of stem cell differentiation, migration, and proliferation during embryogenesis [104]. Molecules such as GAGs, mainly hyaluronan, heparin sulfate, chondroitin sulfate, and integrins are tangled in the control of the nerve cell function and regulation of nervous cell migration [105]. Therefore, the incorporation of these molecules in the collagen scaffold will definitely promote the nerve cell regeneration. Collagen scaffolds used for nerve cell repair [106], spinal cord repair [107], and embryonic nerve cell culture [108] has shown excellent results. Scaffold fabricated with collagen and glycosaminoglycan encouraged proliferation, migration, and diversity in neural precursor cells after surgically implanting into brain trauma [109]. Typically before going to any surgical procedures, sterilization is required and Graziana et al. [110] examined the influence of three sterilization approaches viz., dry heat (DHS), ethylene oxide (EtO) and electron beam radiation (β) on the properties of collagen scaffolds explicitly designed for peripheral nerve regeneration using rat Schwann cell line RSC96. No major changes in morphology and compressive stiffness were witnessed among scaffolds steril- ized by the dissimilar methods; however, a slight increase of chemical crosslinking upon sterilization (EtO < DHS < β) was detected. Fukai et al. [111] introduced neural stem/progenitor cells (NS/PCs) for restoring facial nerve (FN) injuries as a substitute approach for nerve gap reconstruction by using rat- tail collagen anchored with bFGF to increase the therapeutic effects of cell transplantation. The repair outcomes including vibrissae movements, electrophysiological tests, immune- histochemistry, and remyelination study proved natural nerve conduits were useful for FN reconstruction. Similar results were achieved by fabricating a scaffold containing PCL microfibers supplemented with collagen and human umbilical cord serum (hUCS); found suggestively greater bioactivities in vitro and in vivo, equaled to pure PCL and PCL/collagen fibrous conduits. Since PCL/collagen/hUCS fibrous conduit affords extra favorable micro-environmental situations for FN regeneration, has additional therapeutic perspective than the autograft technique [112]. Compared to nerve cell culture and neuron regeneration, spinal cord regeneration is always challenging because of plentiful inhibitory molecules, weak neurotrophic stimulation and deficient intrinsic regenerative responses involved in the existing methods. To overcome these problems, Xing et al. [113] developed a porous collagen scaffold precisely functionalized using neutralizing proteins (CBD-EphA4LBD, CBD-PlexinB1LBD and NEP1-40) and collagen-binding neurotrophic factors (CBD-BDNF and CBD-NT3) to concurrently neutralize myelin inhibitory molecules (ephrinB3, Sema4D and Nogo) and exert neurotrophic stimulation. The results confirmed the newborn neurons generated in the lesion area formed the neuronal relay and improved the locomotion recovery after severe spinal cord injury. On the other hand, neuronal regeneration of neural stem cells (NSCs) residing in the spinal cord could be an ideal strategy for replenishing the lost neurons and restore the function of the spinal cord. These results indicated that collagen scaffold could be an ideal matrix for spinal cord regeneration after acute SCI.

### 4.2.1.2   ENZYME IMMOBILIZATION

Enzymes are the biological catalyst that catalysis many chemical/biochemical reactions [19]. Due to their ease of production, capacity to catalyze responses in mild conditions with a great degree of substrate specificity and green chemistry these biocatalyst are extensively used in innumerable industries such as food [114], textile [115], paper, and pulp making [116], detergents [117], waste management [118], health care [119, 120], and pharmaceuticals [121]. However, their lack of enduring operational stability, shelf life and their reusability and recovery are often hindering their widespread industrial applications [122]. These problems can be overcome by a special strategy called enzyme immobilization.

Immobilization of enzyme refers to the procedure of incarcerating the enzymes in or on an inert support/matrix for their stability and functional reuse [123]. Immobilized enzymes retain their structural conformation necessary for catalysis; thereby suitable to be more efficient and economical for their industrial use [124]. Although the basic methods of enzyme immobilization can be categorized into adsorption, covalent binding, cross-linking, and entrapment; hundreds of variations, based on combinations of these original methods have been developed [125]. Correspondingly, a variety of carriers (matrix) as bio-immobilizations and bio-separations were designed with the difference in physical and chemical properties [19]. Ideal properties for matrix comprise physical resistance to compression, enzyme inertness, hydrophilicity, biocompatibility, antimicrobial activity, and cost-effective [126]. Several natural polymer materials like chitosan, chitin, cellulose, collagen, starch, pectin, carrageenan, alginate, sepharose, and other natural polymer materials are generally used as support materials [127].

1.  **Chitosan Matrix:** Chitosan due to its exclusive physicochemical and biological properties with its ability to bind to specific constituents comprising enzymes, proteins, fats, cholesterols, metal ions and even tumor cells [128]. Chitosan is a gifted immobilization matrix due to its membrane-forming ability, good adhesion, economic, low immunogenicity, non-toxic, hydrophilicity, great mechanical strength, and stability [129]. Results of numerous studies understood, chitosan was expansively used in immobilization of countless enzymes groups for its several characteristics like enhanced resistance to chemical degradation, circumventing disturbance of metal ions to the enzyme and antibacterial property [130]. Qingqing et al. [131] has immobilized hydroperoxide lyase to 1,6-hexamethylenediamine attached chitosan-κ-carrageenan hydrogel and found as a suitable carrier due to its extreme activity of 7.49 ± 0.19 U/g and a yield of 94% in optimal conditions. The $K_m$ value of hydroperoxide lyase decreased from 108.61 to 79.98 μM for 13-hydroperoxy-linoleic-acid and practically unmoved for 13-hydroperoxy-linolenic-acid, confirms enzyme and substrate affinity and was not reduced after immobilization. Similarly, horseradish peroxidase was immobilized on chitosan crosslinked with cyanuric chloride for reusing and increasing resistance towards harmful compounds. Immobilization of HRP moderately protected them from metallic ions while shifting pH from 5.5 to 5.0, optimum temperature from 30°C to 35°C and thermally stable till 45°C, respectively [132]. Everton et al. [133] immobilized laccase (*Aspergillus* sp.) on chitosan by cross-linking via physical adsorption and investigated its application in batch reactor-based bioconversion of phenolic compounds. In immobilization of various enzymes like-glycosyltransferase, chitosan was used [134], β-glucanase [135], acetyl xylan esterase [136], pectinase [137], urease [138] Keratinase [139], lipase [140], amylase [141], acetylcholinesterase (AChE) [142], papaya laccase [143], glucose-6-phosphatedehydrogenase[144],β-ᴅ-galactosidase[145], pullulanase [146], laccase [147], invertase [148], and inulinase [149]. With the advancement of technology and the introduction

of nanotechnology principles, immobilization of enzymes on the chitosan matrix also taken a new direction and involvement of microspheres and nanoparticles were found in several recent studies.

Uttam et al. [150] have immobilized pectinase onto chitosan magnetic nanoparticles (CMNPs) by dextran polyaldehyde as a macromolecular cross-linking agent. Thermal stability for immobilized pectinase exhibited two folds improvement and $V_{max}$ and $K_m$ values were found to be nearly equal to native with residual activity of 86% after seven successive cycles of reuse, while it retained up to 89% residual activity on storage up to fifteen days. Muhammad et al. [151] successfully trapped laccase produced by *Trametes versicolor* onto chitosan microspheres using GA as a cross-linking agent. Microspheres developed from 2.5% chitosan (w/v) activated by 1.5% (v/v) GA exhibited greatest laccase immobilization effectiveness and showed maximum activity (at pH 6 and 60°C), also retained 80.21% of its activity after ten continuous decolorization cycles reflecting its potential use in industries. Recently magnetic nanocomposites have attracted researches to trap enzymes, for which carboxymethylcellulose and chitosan-coated $Fe_3O_4$ nanocomposites were used to immobilize peroxidase enzyme and achieved a purity of 82.55% [152].

2. **Collagen Matrix:** Collagen, with its distinctive structure with desirable properties like high hydrophilicity and ability to swell and de-swell forms an outstanding matrix for enzyme immobilization. These qualities prevent collagen from denaturation of bound enzymes and favor the accessibility of substrates. Numerous enzymes were immobilized on collagen matrices via protein-protein interactions like multiple salt linkage, hydrogen bonds, and van der Waals interactions. Countless methods were reported regarding the coupling of enzymes on collagen both in the native state and with graft copolymers. Mascini et al. [153] prepared polyvinyl alcohol-collagen membranes for immobilization of glucose oxidase attached to amperometric electrodes for measuring the oxygen concentration in various glucose samples. Results were obtained within 2–3 min of time with a response rate of 80% for 0.1 *M* glucose solution. Panduranga [154] have immobilized urease and trypsin to collagen graft copolymers. A

novel adsorbent was developed for immobilization of lysozyme on Fe(III)-collagen fiber matrix. The adsorption capacity was established to be 398 mg/g at 303 K with a preliminary concentration of 2.5 mg/ml of lysozyme. Moreover, Fe(III)-immobilized collagen fiber has admirable column adsorption kinetic properties, great binding capacity and remained unchanged in adsorption-desorption cycles [155]. Collagen was used for immobilization of catalase employing $Fe^{3+}$ support by retaining significant activity even after 26 reuses [156]. Na et al. [157] reported immobilization of catalase on Zr(IV)-modified collagen by adsorption, the addition of Zr(IV) increased the denaturation temperature from 37 to 75.6°C. The quantity of catalase immobilized on Zr-CF was 45.3 mg/g and the $Km$ and $V_{max}$ values were 23.2 mM and $3.5 \times 10^4$ U/mg for free catalase and 30.2 mM and $1.3 \times 10^4$ U/mg for immobilized catalase, respectively. Above all Zr-collagen-catalase could be reclaimed over 72 times before total deactivation and preserve 86.5% of its original activities being at RT for 12 days. Lipase extracted from *Candida rugosa* was immobilized onto collagen fibers through GA cross-linking method. At ideal immobilization conditions, the activity of the enzyme reached 342 U/g with 28.3% recovery [158].

### 4.2.1.3   DRUG DELIVERY MECHANISMS

Drug delivery refers to strategies, formulations, technologies, and systems for transporting a pharmaceutical compound in the body without losing its desired therapeutic effect [159]. Several pharmaceutical companies are now focusing on controlled/sustained delivery technologies to advance present therapeutic agents than developing new drugs [160]. These technologies control the bloodstream-entering rate, consequently plummeting overdosage [161]. Biopolymers are easily engineered for the growth of controlled delivery devices for a choice of uses related to drugs, food-related bioactive ingredients, and genes. The bioactive agents' release from a biopolymer matrix may be through the diffusion- or degradation-controlled or environmental trigger. Even though biopolymers are biocompatible, non-toxic, and biodegradable;

a major shortcoming of biopolymers is their susceptibility to microbial contamination [162].

1. **Chitosan Matrixes for Drug Release:** Chitosan and its derivatives were produced in the various forms-hydrogels, microparticles, and nanoparticles/ capsules/ spheres/ beads for the controlled release of active biomolecules. Hydrophilic nature of the matrix, cross-linking density, particle size, nature of the drug, and its composition play a significant part in knowing the drug diffusion rate. Peng et al. [163] reported the thermosensitive chitosan/GP hydrogels for the sustained delivery of venlafaxine HCl (VH) and the optimization of this formulation. Both in vitro drug release and in vivo pharmacokinetic studies were investigated and demonstrated for a better-sustained delivery of drug over 24 h. A mucoadhesive hydrogel to improve the efficacy of rectal sulphasalazine (SSZ) administration was engineered using catechol modified-chitosan (Cat-CS) crosslinked by genipin. The efficacy of gels was evaluated on a mouse model of UC and found equivalent histological scores, and induced a lesser plasma concentration of the potential toxicity of sulphapyridine (by-product). Results suggest SSZ/Cat-CS rectal hydrogels are further effective and safer formulations for UC treatment than oral SSZ [164]. Chitosan microspheres fashioned in the water-in-oil emulsion and stabilized by cross-linking agents were used for the release of several therapeutic agents like diclofenac sodium, nifedipine, mitoxantrone, prednisolone sodium phosphate, progesterone, and so on [165]. Hydrogel beads were developed using chitosan derivatives (CSD)/rGO blending with alginate for small-molecule drug delivery. The ideal CSD/reduced GO/ alginate beads displayed a great drug-loading efficacy of 81.6% on small-molecule fluorescein Na (FL-Na), the outstanding sustainable release of 70.8% for 150 h at a physiological pH and quick-release of 81.2% drug content at 20 h in acidic medium [166]. Chitosan nanoparticles ionically crosslinked with tripolyphosphate salts in combination with 5-fluorouracil (5-FU) were efficiently encapsulated and its efficacy was tested against normal cells, fibroblasts (FHB) and human glioblastoma A-172 showed that they were successfully up taken into cell lines. The

use of this in A-172 cells resulted in cell viability of 67–75% and re-growth populations in 4 h. This outcome establishes the latent of CSNPs for the enhancement of MH treatments [178]. In similar lines, chitosan was used with various crosslinkers/combinations/drugs and extended its applications into various fields.

2. **Collagen for Drug Release:** Collagen is a chief constituent with an extensive range of drug delivery systems and biomaterial applications due to their unique physical and structural properties, together with its biocompatibility, stumpy immunogenicity, usual turnover, and effectiveness. Furthermore, to its material properties, collagen also acts together with enzymes tangled in biosynthesis and degradation, as well as matrix metalloproteinases. Moreover, collagen can be a smart site for drug targeting since it is over-expressed in common disease processes such as lung and liver fibrosis, scleroderma, and psoriasis [167].

Collagen has been efficaciously formulated into various materials that include microparticles, hydrogels, coatings, films, pellets, and sponges for transporting minor chemical molecules to DNA, proteins, and even cells [168]. Collagen-HAP composites act as delivery systems for the release of tetracycline, ciprofloxacin [169], norfloxacin, gentamicin, and vancomycin antibiotics for treatment of various diseases. Collagen-HAP scaffolds loaded with tetracycline, ciprofloxacin, norfloxacin, and gentamicin through absorption process had released 79.8%, 27.5%, 95.4% and 48.1%, respectively of the drug within a period of 72–180 hr. The quantity of drug released was larger than the minimal inhibitory concentration required (for inhibiting bacterial growth).

For metastasis-associated drug delivery, a polymer prodrug-embedded collagen gel attached with doxorubicin (DOX) via a pH-degradable linkage was developed [170]. Compared with free Dox, the diffusion of the dendrimer prodrug from the collagen gel was repressed and greatly invasive MDA-MB-231 cells showed extra sensitivity with drug-embedded collagen gel attached with Dox. The collagen hybrid gel acted as a perfect drug carrier, suppressed the tumor growth, and attenuated metastatic activity in vivo. Synthesis and characterization of biomaterials comprehending collagen cross-linked with GA for carrying chloramphenicol for dentistry were reported by Graţiela et al. [171]. The sponges displayed resistance to collagenase degradation adequate water uptake and robust activity countering bacteria. These properties of the designed formulations validate that collagen as drug delivery and adequate for the treatment of infected lesions at the dental level.

A shield based on NP cross-linked collagen towards sustained delivery of pilocarpine HCl was established for glaucoma. Since surviving therapy comprises regular application of eye drops, often resulting in meager patient adherence and therapeutic outcomes. So Yosra et al. [172] demonstrated the release of pilocarpine HCl using metal oxide nanoparticles for two weeks, proposing a promising sustained release treatment option for glaucoma. Phototherapies include photodynamic therapy (PDT) and photothermal therapy (PTT) has shown great potential in non-invasive tumor treatments, but most of the drugs used in PTT are light sensitive and leading to the failure of treatment. To overcome this problem, Jiajia et al. [173] reported an approach to attain synergistic PDT and PTT based on collagen-gold hybrid hydrogels, by incorporating gold nanoparticles as photothermal agents for PTT and photosensitive drugs are entrapped as photodynamic agents for PDT.

## 4.3  CONCLUSION AND FUTURE SCOPE

Natural polymers were proven to be a potential biomaterial due to their biodegradability, biocompatibility, simple processing methods, minimal toxic nature, and reasonably low cost. Although a lot of literature is available on extraction, standard characterization, and applications of these two biomaterials separately, there are no reports on comparative information on chitosan and collagen. Natural biopolymers hold decent biocompatibility and display outstanding bioactivity due to the components of the ECM, and present in abundance, effortlessly available from a variety of sources, say, forest products, grasses, tunicates, crustacean, and stalks.

Chitosan is predominantly used mainly in a widest possible range of biopharmaceutical and biomedical applications including food science and technology. Collagen is a fibrillar protein, an abundant in countless of the living organisms due to its connective role in biological structures follows the conjunctive and connective tissues, principally skin, joints, and bones. In view of its exceptional biocompatibility, biodegradability, non-toxicity, and adsorption assets; indicate as a potentially suitable functional material. In this chapter, some of the natural biopolymers, such as chitosan and were put together towards biomedical applications.

Bio-based polymers are in line and in prime to the conventional polymers than before. Future demand for biopolymers is overwhelming. The biopolymer applications could remarkably increase as the more dependable form for the expansion and manufacture costs remains affordable. Applications by the use of innovative materials utilize the properties of these polymers and the products developed. In this chapter, various biomedical applications such as scaffolds for tissue engineering, enzyme immobilization, and drug delivery mechanisms of chitosan and collagen-based materials have been covered. We guess that this chapter shall deliver insights into the usage of these biomaterials for researchers and scientists working in the field of biomedical sciences and engineering.

## AUTHOR CONTRIBUTIONS

Aparna Tirumalasetti and Murthy Chavali wrote the chapter; Kesana Surendra Babu and Mannam Krishnamurthy initiated and contributed to the scope of the manuscript; Murthy Chavali collected and designed the data analysis; performed the analysis; Enamala Manoj Kumar planned the review of the literature and reorganized the chapter; Murthy Chavali critically reviewed the manuscript. All the authors contributed to this book chapter.

## CONFLICTS OF INTEREST

The authors declare no conflict of interest.

## KEYWORDS

- **biomaterials**
- **biomedical applications**
- **chitosan**
- **collagen**
- **molecular weight**
- **polyurethane**

## REFERENCES

1. Butcher, A. L., Giovanni, S. O., & Michelle, L. O., (2014). Nanofibrous hydrogel composites as mechanically robust tissue engineering scaffolds. *Trends Biotechnol., 32*, 564–570.
2. Yangchao, L., & Qiaobin, H., (2017). 7 - Food-derived biopolymers for nutrient delivery. In: Alexandru, M. G., (ed.), *Nanotechnology in the Agri-Food Industry* (pp. 251–291). Academic Press.
3. Paula, J. P. E., Wen-Xian, D., Avena-Bustillos, R. D. J., Nilda, D. F. F. S., & Tara, H. M., (2014). Edible films from pectin: Physical-mechanical and antimicrobial properties: A review. *Food Hydrocolloids, 35*, 287–296.
4. Manson, J. A., (2012). *Polymer Blends and Composites*. Springer Science and Business Media.
5. Niaounakis, M., (2013). *Biopolymers: Reuse, Recycling, and Disposal*. William Andrew..
6. Sionkowska, A., (2011). Current research on the blends of natural and synthetic polymers as new biomaterials: Review. *Progress in Polymer Science, 36*(9), 1254–1276.
7. Luckachan, G. E., & Pillai, C. K. S., (2011). Biodegradable polymers: A review on recent trends and emerging perspectives. *Journal of Polymers and the Environment, 19*(3), 637–676.
8. Lasprilla, A. J., Martinez, G. A., Lunelli, B. H., Jardini, A. L., & Maciel, F. R., (2012). Poly-lactic acid synthesis for application in biomedical devices: A review. *Biotechnology Advances, 30*(1), 321–328.
9. Gentile, P., Chiono, V., Tonda-Turo, C., Ferreira, A. M., & Ciardelli, G., (2011). Polymeric membranes for guided bone regeneration. *Biotechnology Journal, 6*(10), 1187–1197.
10. Duncan, R., & Vicent, M. J., (2013). Polymer therapeutics-prospects for the 21st century: The end of the beginning. *Advanced Drug Delivery Reviews, 65*(1), 60–70.
11. Guo, B., & Ma, P. X., (2014). Synthetic biodegradable functional polymers for tissue engineering: A brief review. *Science China Chemistry, 57*(4), 490–500.

12. Prasanna, K., Subburaj, T., Jo, Y. N., Lee, W. J., & Lee, C. W., (2015). Environment-friendly cathodes using biopolymer chitosan with enhanced electrochemical behavior for use in lithium-ion batteries. *ACS Applied Materials and Interfaces, 7*(15), 7884–7890.

13. Mülhaupt, R., (2013). Green polymer chemistry and bio-based plastics: Dreams and reality. *Macromolecular Chemistry and Physics, 214*(2), 159–174.

14. Valerio, O., (2014). *Synthesis and Use of Glycerol Based Hyperbranched Biopolyesters as Impact Modifiers for Poly (Butylene Succinate) Matrix (Doctoral dissertation).*

15. Senel, S., & McClure, S. J., (2004). Potential applications of chitosan in veterinary medicine. *Adv. Drug Deliv. Rev., 56*, 1467–1480.

16. Berger, J., Reist, M., Mayer, J. M., Felt, O., Peppas, N. A., & Gurny, R., (2004). Structure and interactions in covalently and ionically crosslinked chitosan hydrogels for biomedical applications. *Eur. J. Pharm. Biopharm., 57*, 19–34.

17. Kong, M., Chen, X. G., Xing, K., & Park, H. J., (2010). Antimicrobial properties of chitosan and mode of action: A state of the art review. *International Journal of Food Microbiology, 144*(1), 51–63.

18. Liu, Z., Ge, X., Lu, Y., Dong, S., Zhao, Y., & Zeng, M., (2012). Effects of chitosan molecular weight and degree of deacetylation on the properties of gelatine-based films. *Food Hydrocolloids, 26*(1), pp.311–317.

19. Ahmad, R., & Sardar, M., (2015). Enzyme immobilization: An overview on nanoparticles as immobilization matrix. *Biochem. Anal. Biochem., 4*(2), 178–186.

20. Mudasir, A., Shakeel, A., Babu, L. S., & Saiqa, I., (2015). Adsorption of heavy metal ions: The role of chitosan and cellulose for water treatment. *Int. J. Pharmacogn., 2*, 280–289.

21. Keong, L. C., & Halim, A. S., (2009). In vitro models in biocompatibility assessment for biomedical-grade chitosan derivatives in wound management. *Int. J. Mol. Sci., 10*, 1300–1313.

22. Kaya, M., Dudakli, F., Asan-Ozusaglam, M., Cakmak, Y. S., Baran, T., Mentes, A., & Erdogan, S., (2016). Porous and nanofiber α-chitosan obtained from blue crab (*Callinectes sapidus*) tested for antimicrobial and antioxidant activities. *LWT-Food Science and Technology, 65*, 1109–1117.

23. Crespo, M. P., Martínez, M. V., Hernández, J. L., & Yusty, M. L., (2006). High-performance liquid chromatographic determination of chitin in the snow crab, *Chionoecetes opilio. Journal of Chromatography A, 1116*(1), 189–192.

24. Benhabiles, M. S., Salah, R., Lounici, H., Drouiche, N., Goosen, M. F. A., & Mameri, N., (2012). Antibacterial activity of chitin, chitosan and its oligomers prepared from shrimp shell waste. *Food Hydrocolloids, 29*(1), 48–56.

25. Mukku, S. R., & Willem, F. S., (2005). Chitin production by *Lactobacillus* fermentation of shrimp biowaste in a drum reactor and its chemical conversion to chitosan. *J. Chem. Technol. Biotechnol., 80*, 1080–1087.

26. Monreal, J., & Reese, E. T., (1969). The chitinase of Serratia marcescens. *Canadian Journal of Microbiology, 15*(7), 689–696.

27. Wassila, A., Leila, A., Lydia, A., & Abdeltif, A., (2013). Chitin recovery using biological methods. *Food Technol. Biotechnol., 51*(1) 12–25.

28. Islam, Y., Sawssen, H., Véronique, F., Marguerite, R., Kemel, J., & Moncef, N., (2014). Chitin extraction from shrimp shell using enzymatic treatment. Antitumor,

antioxidant and antimicrobial activities of chitosan. *International Journal of Biological Macromolecules, 69,* 489–498.

29. Malinin, T. I., (2013). Vivex biomedical Inc. *Self-assembly of Collagen Fibers from Dermis, Fascia and Tendon for Tissue Augmentation and Coverage of Wounds and Burns.* U.S. Patent Application 13/955,226.

30. Liu, D., Liang, L., Regenstein, J. M., & Zhou, P., (2012). Extraction and characterization of pepsin-solubilized collagen from fins, scales, skins, bones and swim bladders of bighead carp (*Hypophthalmichthys nobilis*). *Food Chemistry, 133*(4), 1441–1448.

31. Matmaroh, K., Benjakul, S., Prodpran, T., Encarnacion, A. B., & Kishimura, H., (2011). Characteristics of acid-soluble collagen and pepsin soluble collagen from the scale of spotted golden goatfish (*Parupeneus heptacanthus*). *Food Chemistry, 129*(3), 1179–1186.

32. Almora-Barrios, N., & De Leeuw, N. H., (2010). Modelling the interaction of a hyp-pro-gly peptide with hydroxyapatite surfaces in the aqueous environment. *Cryst. Eng. Comm., 12*(3), 960–967.

33. Muralidharan, N., Shakila, R. J., Sukumar, D., & Jeyasekaran, G., (2013). Skin, bone and muscle collagen extraction from the trash fish, leather jacket (*Odonus niger*) and their characterization. *Journal of Food Science and Technology, 50*(6), 1106–1113.

34. Shigemura, Y., Akaba, S., Kawashima, E., Park, E. Y., Nakamura, Y., & Sato, K., (2011). Identification of a novel food-derived collagen peptide, hydroxypropyl-glycine, in human peripheral blood by pre-column derivatization with phenyl isothiocyanate. *Food Chemistry, 129*(3), 1019–1024.

35. Damodaran, S., Parkin, K., & Fennema, O. R., (2010). *Química de alimentos de fennema* (4th edn., pp. 726–730). São Paulo: Artmed.

36. Srivastava, A., Srivastava, A., Srivastava, A., & Chandra, P., (2015). Marine biomaterials in therapeutics and diagnostics. *Handbook of Marine Biotechnology* (pp. 1247–1263). Springer Berlin Heidelberg.

37. Schrieber, R., & Gareis, H., (2007). *Gelatine Handbook: Theory and Industry Practice,* 347. Wiley Publications, ISBN: 978-3-527-61097-6.

38. Gómez-Guillén, M. C., Giménez, B., López-Caballero, M. A., & Montero, M. P., (2011). Functional and bioactive properties of collagen and gelatin from alternative sources: A review. *Food Hydrocolloids, 25*(8), 1813–1827.

39. Schmidt, M. M., Dornelles, R. C. P., Mello, R. O., Kubota, E. H., Mazutti, M. A., Kempka, A. P., & Demiate, I. M., (2016). Collagen extraction process. *International Food Research Journal, 23*(3), 913–922.

40. Liu, D., Wei, G., Li, T., Hu, J., Lu, N., Regenstein, J. M., & Zhou, P., (2015). Effects of alkaline pretreatments and acid extraction conditions on the acid-soluble collagen from grass carp (*Ctenopharyngodon idella*) skin. *Food Chemistry, 172,* 836–843.

41. Yang, H., & Shu, Z., (2014). The extraction of collagen protein from pigskin. *Journal of Chemical and Pharmaceutical Research, 6*(2), 683–687.

42. Wang, L., Yang, B., Du, X., Yang, Y., & Liu, J., (2008). Optimization of conditions for extraction of acid-soluble collagen from grass carp (*Ctenopharyngodon idella*) by response surface methodology. *Innovative Food Science and Emerging Technologies, 9*(4), 604607.

43. Wang, L., Liang, Q., Chen, T., Wang, Z., Xu, J., & Ma, H., (2014). Characterization of collagen from the skin of Amur sturgeon (*Acipenser schrenckii*). *Food Hydrocolloids, 38*, 104–109.
44. Nagai, T., (2015). Characterization of collagen from emu (*Dromaius novaehollandiae*) skins. *Journal of Food Science and Technology, 52*(4), 2344–2351.
45. Metreveli, G., Wågberg, L., Emmoth, E., Belák, S., Strømme, M., & Mihranyan, A., (2014). A size-exclusion nanocellulose filter paper for virus removal. *Adv. Healthcare Mater., 3*(10), 1546–1550.
46. Pina, S., Oliveira, J. M., & Reis, R. L., (2015). Natural-based nanocomposites for bone tissue engineering and regenerative medicine: A review. *Adv. Mat., 27*(7), 1143–1169.
47. Kim, H. L., Jung, G. Y., Yoon, J. H., Han, J. S., Park, Y. J., Kim, D. G., Zhang, M., & Kim, D. J., (2015). Preparation and characterization of nano-sized hydroxyapatite/alginate/chitosan composite scaffolds for bone tissue engineering. *Mat. Sci. and Engg. C, 54*, 20–25.
48. Saad, B. Q., Shahriar, H., Ying, H., Maksym, P., Volodymyr, D., Mykola, L., Andrew, R., & Ihtesham, U. R., (2017). *In-vitro* and *in-vivo* degradation studies of freeze gelated porous chitosan composite scaffolds for tissue engineering applications. *Polymer Degradation and Stability, 136*, 31–38.
49. Ming-Lei, Z., Ji, C., Ye-Chen, X., Ruo-Feng, Y., & Xu, F., (2017). Raloxifene microsphere-embedded collagen/chitosan/β-tricalcium phosphate scaffold for effective bone tissue engineering. *International Journal of Pharmaceutics, 518*(1/2), 80–85.
50. Aminabhavi, T. M., Dharupaneedi, S. P., & More, U. A., (2017). 1-The role of nanotechnology and chitosan-based biomaterials for tissue engineering and therapeutic delivery. In: Amber, J. J., & Joel, D. B., (eds.), *Chitosan-Based Biomaterials 2* (pp. 1–29). Woodhead Publishing.
51. Tan, M. L., Shao, P., Friedhuber, A. M., Van, M. M., Elahy, M., Indumathy, S., Dunstan, D. E., et al., (2014). The potential role of free chitosan in bone trauma and bone cancer management. *Biomaterials, 35*, 7828–7838.
52. Shayan, G., Fathollah, M., Nooshin, H., Leila, G., Fatemeh, B., Mohammad, A. S., & Zahra, A., (2017). Preparation and characterization of novel functionalized multiwalled carbon nanotubes/chitosan/β-Glycerophosphate scaffolds for bone tissue engineering. *International Journal of Biological Macromolecules, 97*, 365–372.
53. Shamsa, A., Ali, Z., & Masoud, M., (2017). Super-paramagnetic responsive silk fibroin/chitosan/magnetite scaffolds with tunable pore structures for bone tissue engineering applications. *Materials Science and Engineering: C, 70*(1), 736–744.
54. Zhou, C., Ye, X., Fan, Y., Ma, L., Tan, Y., Qing, F., & Zhang, X., (2014). Biomimetic fabrication of a three-level hierarchical calcium phosphate/collagen/hydroxyapatite scaffold for bone tissue engineering. *Biofabrication, 6*(3), 035013.
55. Ning, L., Malmström, H., & Ren, Y. F., (2015). Porous collagen-hydroxyapatite scaffolds with mesenchymal stem cells for bone regeneration. *J. Oral Implantol., 41*(1), 45–49.
56. Rahmatullah, C., Santosh, K. P., Francesca, G., Gayatri, U., Graziana, M., Alessandro, S., & Antonio, L., (2016). Scaffolds for bone regeneration made of hydroxyapatite

microspheres in a collagen matrix. *Materials Science and Engineering: C, 63,* 499–505.

57. Supaporn, S., Suttatip, K., Wen-Lin, C., & Jirut, M., (2016). A biofunctional-modified silk fibroin scaffold with mimic reconstructed extracellular matrix of decellularized pulp/collagen/fibronectin for bone tissue engineering in alveolar bone resorption. *Materials Letters, 166,* 30–34.

58. Chetana, D., Seow, T. O., Neeraj, D., Silvia, M. D., Jayarama, R. V., Balachandar, N., Mobashar, H. U. T. F., et al., (2016). Bio-inspired in situ crosslinking and mineralization of electrospun collagen scaffolds for bone tissue engineering. *Biomaterials, 104,* 323–338.

59. Thalita, M. V., Elisandra, G. C., Maíssa, H. S. C., Martins-Júnior, P. A., Lívia, M. O. S., Patrícia, P. S., Luiz, O. L., & Gregory, T. K., (2016). A novel 3D bone-mimetic scaffold composed of collagen/MTA/MWCNT modulates cell migration and osteogenesis. *Life Sciences, 162,* 115–124.

60. Gayathri, S., Callan, B., & Yildirim-Ayan, E., (2015). Nanofibrous yet injectable polycaprolactone-collagen bone tissue scaffold with osteoprogenitor cells and controlled release of bone morphogenetic protein-2. *Materials Science and Engineering: C, 51,* 16–27.

61. Valderrabano, V., & Steiger, C., (2011). Treatment and prevention of osteoarthritis through exercise and sports. *J. Aging Res.,* 374653.

62. Bhosale, A. M., & Richardson, J. B., (2008). Articular cartilage: Structure, injuries and review of management. *Br. Med. Bull., 87,* 77–95.

63. Luria, A., & Chu, C. R., (2014). Articular cartilage changes in maturing athletes: New targets for joint rejuvenation. *Sports Health, 6*(1), 18–30.

64. Freyria, A. M., Mallein-Gerin, F., (2012). Chondrocytes or adult stem cells for cartilage repair: The indisputable role of growth factors. *Injury, 43*(3), 259–265.

65. Kedong, S., Liying, L., Wenfang, L., Yanxia, Z., Zeren, J., Mayasari, L., Meiyun, F., et al., (2015). Three-dimensional dynamic fabrication of engineered cartilage based on chitosan/gelatin hybrid hydrogel scaffold in a spinner flask with a special designed steel frame. *Materials Science and Engineering: C, 55,* 384–392.

66. Jong, E. L., Ko, E. K., Ick, C. K., Hyun, J. A., Sang-Hoon, L., Hyunchul, C., Hee, J. K., et al., (2004). Effects of the controlled-released TGF-β1 from chitosan microspheres on chondrocytes cultured in a collagen/chitosan/ glycosaminoglycan scaffold. *Biomaterials, 25*(18), 4163–4173.

67. Kinner, B., Capito, R. M., & Spector, M., (2005). Regeneration of articular cartilage. *Adv. Biochem. Engg. Biotechnol., 94,* 91–123.

68. Sophia, F. A. J., Bedi, A., & Rodeo, S. A., (2009). The basic science of articular cartilage: Structure, composition, and function. *Sports Health, 1*(6), 461–468.

69. Amos, M., Tanya, J. L., O'Brien, F. J., & John, P. G., (2012). Addition of hyaluronic acid improves cellular infiltration and promotes early-stage chondrogenesis in a collagen-based scaffold for cartilage tissue engineering. *Journal of the Mechanical Behavior of Biomedical Materials, 11,* 41–52.

70. Birgit, H., Anne, B., Anja, L., Sascha, H., Judith, S., Matthias, K., Holger, N., & Michael, G., (2014). Jellyfish collagen scaffolds for cartilage tissue engineering. *Acta Biomaterialia, 10*(2), 883–892.

71. Jingyu, Y., Xuening, C., Tun, Y., Xiao, Y., Yujiang, F., & Xingdong, Z., (2017). Regulation of the secretion of immunoregulatory factors of mesenchymal stem cells (MSCs) by collagen-based scaffolds during chondrogenesis. *Materials Science and Engineering: C, 70*(Part 2), 983–991.

72. Wenda, D., Naoki, K., Xiaoting, L., Jian, D., & Guoping, C., (2010). The influence of the structural design of PLGA/collagen hybrid scaffolds in cartilage tissue engineering. *Biomaterials, 31*(8), 2141–2152.

73. Hu, M. S., Maan, Z. N., Wu, J. C., Rennert, R. C., Hong, W. X., Lai, T. S., Cheung, A. T., et al., (2014). Tissue engineering and regenerative repair in wound healing. *Ann. Biomed. Eng., 42*, 1494–1507.

74. MacNeil, S., (2008). Biomaterials for tissue engineering of skin. *Mater. Today, 11*, 26–35.

75. Naves, L. B., Almeida, L., & Rajamani, L., (2017). 11-Nanofiber composites in skin tissue engineering, In: *Nanofiber Composites for Biomedical Applications* (pp. 275–300). Woodhead Publishing.

76. Mihail, C., Tripp, L., Joseph, M., & Dennis, O., (2016). Chapter 8: Natural biomaterials for skin tissue engineering. In: Mohammad, Z. A., & James, H. H. IV., (eds.), *Skin Tissue Engineering and Regenerative Medicine* (pp. 145–161). Academic Press, Boston.

77. Morimoto, M., Saimoto, H., Usui, H., Okamoto, Y., Minami, S., & Shigemasa, Y., (2001). Biological activities of carbohydrate-branched chitosan derivatives. *Biomacromolecules, 2*, 1133–1136.

78. Raafat, D., Von, B. K., Haas, A., & Sahl, H. G., (2008). Insights into the mode of action of chitosan as an antibacterial compound. *Applied and Environ. Microbiology, 74*, 3764–3773.

79. Deng, C., Zhang, P., Vulesevic, B., Kuraitis, D., Li, F., Yang, A. F., Griffith, M., et al., (2010). A collagen-chitosan hydrogel for endothelial differentiation and angiogenesis. *Tissue Engineering Part A, 16*, 3099–3109.

80. Shalumon, K. T., Anulekha, K. H., Chennazhi, K. P., Tamura, H., Nair, S. V., & Jayakumar, R., (2011). Fabrication of chitosan/poly(caprolactone) nanofibrous scaffold for bone and skin tissue engineering. *International Journal of Biological Macromolecules, 48*(4), 571–576.

81. Beatriz, V., Daniela, S. C., Paulo, F. D., Marcelo, M., Ribeiro-Do-Valle, R. M., & Lopes-Da-Silva, J. A., (2012). Nanofibrous poly(3-hydroxybutyrate-co-3-hydroxyvalerate)/chitosan scaffolds for skin regeneration. *International Journal of Biological Macromolecules, 51*(4), 343–350.

82. Yunyun, L., Lie, M., & Changyou, G., (2012). Facile fabrication of the glutaraldehyde crosslinked collagen/chitosan porous scaffold for skin tissue engineering. *Materials Science and Engineering: C, 32*(8), 2361–2366.

83. Rafael, B. T., Cecília, B. W., José, A. F. D. S., & Ângela, M. M., (2017). Electro spun multilayer chitosan scaffolds as potential wound dressings for skin lesions. *European Polymer Journal, 88*, 161–170.

84. Yannas, I. V., (2013). Emerging rules for inducing organ regeneration. *Biomaterials, 34*, 321–330.

85. Morshed, M., (2014). *The Currently Available Biomaterials Being Used for Skin Tissue Engineering, 3*, 17–22.

86. Yannas, I. V., Tzeranis, D. S., Harley, B. A., & So, P. T. C., (2010). Biologically active collagen-based scaffolds advances in processing and characterization. *Philos. Trans. A Math. Phys. Eng. Sci., 368*, 2123–2139.

87. Xingang, W., Qiyin, L., Xinlei, H., Lie, M., Chuangang, Y., Yurong, Z., Huafeng, S., et al., (2012). Fabrication and characterization of poly(l-lactide-co-glycolide) knitted mesh-reinforced collagen-chitosan hybrid scaffolds for dermal tissue engineering. *J. of the Mechanical Behavior of Biomedical Materials, 8*, 204–215.

88. Farah, H. Z., Fathima, S. J. H., Mohammad, S. B. A. R., & Mashitah, M. Y., (2014). *In vitro* degradation study of novel HEC/PVA/collagen nanofibrous scaffold for skin tissue engineering applications. *Polymer Degradation and Stability, 110*, 473–481.

89. Sneh, G., Chia-Fu, C., Amit, K. D., Pravin, D. P., & Narayan, C. M., (2014). Surface modification of nanofibrous polycaprolactone/gelatin composite scaffold by collagen type I grafting for skin tissue engineering. *Materials Science and Engineering: C, 34*, 402–409.

90. Sadeghi, A. R., Nokhasteh, S., Molavi, A. M., Khorsand-Ghayeni, M., Naderi-Meshkin, H., & Mahdizadeh, A., (2016). Surface modification of electro spun PLGA scaffold with collagen for bioengineered skin substitutes. *Materials Science and Engineering: C, 66*, 130–137.

91. Huan, C., Ming-Mao, C., Yan, L., Yuan-Yuan, L., Yu-Qing, H., Jian-Hua, W., Jing-Di, C., & Qi-Qing, Z., (2015). Fish collagen-based scaffold containing PLGA microspheres for controlled growth factor delivery in skin tissue engineering. *Colloids and Surfaces B: Biointerfaces, 136*, 1098–1106.

92. Pathum, C., Seok-Chun, K., Gun-Woo, O., Van-Tinh, N., You-Jin, J., Bonggi, L., Chul, H. J., et al., (2015). Fish collagen/alginate/chitooligosaccharides integrated scaffold for skin tissue regeneration application. *Int. J. of Biolog. Macromolecules, 81*, 504–513.

93. Giriprasath, R., Sivakumar, S., Thangavelu, M., Sitalakshmi, T., Paramasivan, T. P., & Uma, T. S., (2017). Design and characterization of 3D hybrid collagen matrixes as a dermal substitute in skin tissue engineering. *Materials Science and Engineering: C, 72*, 359–370.

94. Amado, S., Simoes, M. J., Armada, D. S. P. A. S., Luýs, A. L., Shirosaki, Y., Lopes, M. A., Santos, J. D., et al., (2008). Use of hybrid chitosan membranes and N1E-115 cells for promoting nerve regeneration in an axonotmesis rat model. *Biomaterials., 29*, 4409–4419.

95. Sundback, C. A., Shyu, J. Y., Wang, Y., Faquin, W. C., Langer, R. S., Vacanti, J. P., & Hadlock, T. A., (2005). Biocompatibility analysis of poly(glycerol sebacate) as a nerve guide material. *Biomaterials, 26*, 5454–5464.

96. Cristiana, R. C., López-Cebral, R., Silva-Correia, J., Joana, M. S., João, F. M., Tiago, H. S., Thomas, F., et al., (2017). Investigation of cell adhesion in chitosan membranes for peripheral nerve regeneration. *Materials Science and Engineering: C, 71*(1), pp. 1122–1134.

97. Chuang-Yu, L., Li-Tzu, L., & Wen-Ta, S., (2014). Three-dimensional chitosan scaffolds influence the extracellular matrix expression in Schwann cells. *Materials Science and Engineering: C, 42*, 474–478.

98. Fatemeh, M., Mehdi, F., Vahid, M., Mohammad, Z., Adeleh, D., & Mohammad, A. S., (2011). Enhancement of neural cell lines proliferation using nano-structured chitosan/

poly(vinyl alcohol) scaffolds conjugated with nerve growth factor. *Carbohydrate Polymers, 86*(2), 526–535.

99. Hossein, B., Ahmad, R. S. A., & Shohreh, M., (2015). Fabrication and characterization of conductive chitosan/gelatin-based scaffolds for nerve tissue engineering. *International Journal of Biological Macromolecules, 74*, 360–366.

100. Guicai, L., Luzhong, Z., Caiping, W., Xueying, Z., Changlai, Z., Yanhong, Z., Yaling, W., et al., (2014). Effect of silanization on chitosan porous scaffolds for peripheral nerve regeneration. *Carbohydrate Polymers, 101*, 718–726.

101. Yun, G., Jianbin, Z., Chengbin, X., Zhenmeiyu, L., Fei, D., Yumin, Y., & Xiaosong, G., (2014). Chitosan/silk fibroin-based, Schwann cell-derived extracellular matrix-modified scaffolds for bridging rat sciatic nerve gaps. *Biomaterials, 35*(7), 2253–2263.

102. Guicai, L., Luzhong, Z., & Yumin, Y., (2015). Tailoring of chitosan scaffolds with heparin and γ-aminopropyltriethoxysilane for promoting peripheral nerve regeneration. *Colloids and Surfaces B: Biointerfaces, 134*, 413–422.

103. Guo, J. S., Qian, C. H., Ling, E. A., & Zeng, Y. S., (2014). Nanofiber scaffolds for the treatment of spinal cord injury. *Curr. Med. Chem., 1*, 4282–4289.

104. Suzuki, A., Iwama, A., Miyashita, H., Nakauchi, H., & Taniguchi, H., (2003). Role of growth factors and extracellular matrix components in controlling differentiation of prospectively isolated hepatic stem cells. *Development, 130*, 2513–2524.

105. Gu, W. L., Fu, S. L., Wang, Y. X., Li, Y., Lü, H. Z., Xu, X. M., & Lu, P. H., (2009). Chondroitin sulfate proteoglycans regulate the growth, differentiation and migration of multipotent neural precursor cells through the integrin signaling pathway. *BMC Neurosci., 10*, 128–148.

106. Mollers, S., Heschel, I., Olde, D. L. H. H., Schugner, F., Deumens, R., Muller, B., Bozkurt, A., et al., (2009). Cytocompatibility of novel longitudinally microstructured collagen scaffold intended for nerves tissue repair. *Tissue Eng., 15*, 461–472.

107. Haktan, A., Sven, M., Tobias, F., Ronald, D., Ahmet, B., Ingo, H., Leon, H. H. O. D., et al., (2014). Functional improvement following implantation of a micro-structured, type I collagen scaffold into experimental injuries of the adult rat spinal cord. *Brain Res., 1585*, 37–50.

108. Pietrucha, K., Szymanski, J., & Drobnik, J., (2015). The behavior of embryonic neural cells within the 3D micro-structured collagen-based scaffolds. *IFMBE Proc., 45*, 549–552.

109. Huang, K. F., Hsu, W. C. H., Chiu, W. T., & Wang, J. Y., (2012). Functional improvement and neurogenesis after collagen-GAG matrix implantation into surgical brain trauma. *Biomat., 33*, 2067–2075.

110. Graziana, M., Rahmatullah, C., Luca, S., Marta, M., & Alessandro, S., (2017). Sterilization of collagen scaffolds designed for peripheral nerve regeneration: Effect on microstructure, degradation and cellular colonization. *Materials Science and Engineering: C, 71*, 335–344.

111. Fukai, M., Tongming, Z., Feng, X., Zhifu, W., Yongtao, Z., Qisheng, T., Luping, C., et al., (2016). Neural stem/progenitor cells on collagen with anchored basic fibroblast growth factor as potential natural nerve conduits for facial nerve regeneration. *Acta Biomaterialia.* doi: 10.1016/j.actbio.11.064.

112. Chul, H. J., Hyeongjin, L., Min, S. K., & Geun-Hyung, K., (2016). Effect of polycaprolactone/collagen/hUCS microfiber nerve conduit on facial nerve regeneration. *International Journal of Biological Macromolecules, 93, Part B,* 1575–1582.

113. Xing, L., Jin, H., Yannan, Z., Wenyong, D., Jianshu, W., Jiayin, L., Sufang, H., et al., (2016). Functionalized collagen scaffold implantation and cAMP administration collectively facilitate spinal cord regeneration. *Acta Biomaterialia, 30,* 233–245.

114. Sirma, Y., (2017). Single-step purification and characterization of an extremely halophilic, ethanol tolerant and acidophilic xylanase from *Aureobasidium pullulans* NRRL Y-2311-1 with application potential in the food industry. *Food Chemistry, 221,* 67–75.

115. Amit, M., & Chakraborty, J. N., (2017). Developments in the application of enzymes for textile processing. *Journal of Cleaner Production, 145,* 114–133.

116. Liping, F., Minghui, Z., Guorui, L., Yuyang, Z., Wenbin, L., Linyan, H., & Li, G., (2017). Unexpected promotion of PCDD/F formation by enzyme-aided $Cl_2$ bleaching in non-wood pulp and paper mill. *Chemosphere, 168,* 523–528.

117. Altaf, A. S., Abdul, S. Q., Imrana, K., Chaudhry, H. A., Safia, L., Muhammad, A. B., Ghulam, S. M., & Changrui, L., (2017). Production and partial characterization of α-amylase enzyme from *Bacillus sp.* BCC 01-50 and potential applications. *BioMed Research International,* 1–9. Article ID: 9173040.

118. Arun, C., & Sivashanmugam, P., (2017). Study on optimization of process parameters for enhancing the multi-hydrolytic enzyme activity in garbage enzyme produced from pre-consumer organic waste. *Bioresource Technology, 226,* 200–210.

119. Matthew, D. M., & Lee-Ann, J., (2017). Development of a recombinase polymerase amplification assay for detection of epidemic human noroviruses. *Scientific Reports, 7,* 40244. doi: 10.1038/srep40244.

120. Eswara, R. T., Imchen, M., & Kumavath, R., (2017). Marine enzymes: Production and applications for human health. *Advances in Food and Nutrition Research,* Academic Press. ISSN: 1043-4526, http://dx.doi.org/10.1016/bs.afnr.2016.11.006 (accessed on 4 November 2020).

121. Roger, A. S., (2017). The E factor 25 years on the rise of green chemistry and sustainability. *Green Chem., 19,* 18–43.

122. Prakash, O., & Jaiswal, N., (2011). Immobilization of a thermostable α-amylase on agarose and agar matrices and its application in starch stain removal. *World Applied Sciences Journal, 13*(3), 572–577.

123. Singh, V., Sardar, M., & Gupta, M. N., (2013). Immobilization of enzymes by bioaffinity layering. In: *Immobilization of enzymes and cells: Methods Mol. Biol.,* (Vol. 1051, pp. 129–137). doi: 10.1007/978-1-62703-550-7_9.

124. Hartmann, M., & Kostrov, X., (2013). Immobilization of enzymes on porous silicas-benefits and challenges. *Chem. Soc. Rev., 42,* 6277–6289.

125. Min, K., & Yoo, Y. J., (2014). Recent progress in nanobiocatalysis for enzyme immobilization and its application. *Biotechnology and Bioprocess Engineering, 19,* 553–567.

126. Brena, B. M., & Batista-Viera, F., (2006). Immobilization of enzymes. In: *Immobilization of Enzymes and Cells* (pp. 15–30). Springer.

127. Datta, S., Christena, L. R., & Rajaram, Y. R. S., (2013). Enzyme immobilization: An overview of techniques and support materials. *3 Biotech., 3*, 1–9.

128. Grenha, A., Seijo, B., & Remunan-Lopez, C., (2005). Microencapsulated chitosan nanoparticles for lung protein delivery. *Eur. J. Pharmaceutical Sci., 25*, 427–437.

129. Colonna, C., Conti, B., Perugini, P., Pavanetto, F., & Modena, T., et al., (2008). *Ex vivo* evaluation of prolidase loaded chitosan nanoparticles for the enzyme replacement therapy. *Eur. J. Pharmaceutics Biopharmaceutics, 70*, 58–65.

130. Tang, Z. X., Qian, J. Q., & Shi, L. E., (2006). Characterizations of immobilized neutral proteinase on chitosan nanoparticles. *Process Biochem., 41*, 1193–1197.

131. Qingqing, L., Yufei, H., Xiangzhen, K., Caimeng, Z., & Yeming, C., (2013). Covalent immobilization of hydroperoxide lyase on chitosan hybrid hydrogels and production of C6 aldehydes by the immobilized enzyme. *Journal of Molecular Catalysis B: Enzymatic, 95*, 89–98.

132. Saleh, A. M., Al-Malki, A. L., Taha, A. K., & El-Shishtawy, R. M., (2013). Horseradish peroxidase and chitosan: Activation, immobilization and comparative results. *International Journal of Biological Macromolecules, 60*, 295–300.

133. Everton, S., Mylena, F., Maria, D. L. B. M., Gustavo, F. D. S., & Jair, J. J., (2014). Substrate specificity and enzyme recycling using chitosan immobilized laccase. [Carlos Henrique Lemos Soares and Agenor Fúrigo júnior]. *Molecules, 19*, 16794–16809.

134. Schöffer, J. D. N., Klein, M. P., Rodrigues, R. C., & Hertz, P. F., (2013). Continuous production of beta-cyclodextrin from starch by highly stable cyclodextrin glycosyltransferase immobilized on chitosan. *Carbohydrate Polymers, 98*, 1311–1316.

135. Beibei, W., Xueping, J., Haiyan, Z., Na, W., Xianrui, L., Ruixing, N., & Yuheng, L., (2014). An amperometric β-glucan biosensor based on the immobilization of bi-enzyme on Prussian blue-chitosan and gold nanoparticles-chitosan nanocomposite films. *Biosensors and Bioelectronics, 55*, 113–119.

136. Thiyagarajan, S., Thayumanavan, P., Dae-Hyuk, K., & Seung-Moon, P., (2014). Optimized immobilization of peracetic acid-producing recombinant acetyl xylan esterase on chitosan-coated-$Fe_3O_4$ magnetic nanoparticles. *Process Biochemistry, 49*(11), 1920–1928.

137. Haneef, U. R., Mohammad, A. N., Afsheen, A., Abdul, H. B., & Shah, A. U. Q., (2014). Immobilization of pectinase from *Bacillus licheniformis* KIBGE-IB21 on chitosan beads for continuous degradation of pectin polymers. *Biocatalysis and Agricultural Biotechnology, 3*(4), 282–287.

138. Yasemin, I. D., İlyas, D., Mustafa, T., & Bedrettin, M., (2014). $TiO_2$ beads and $TiO_2$-chitosan beads for urease immobilization. *Materials Science and Engineering: C, 42*, 429–435.

139. Ivana, A. C., Contreras-Esquivel, J. C., & Sebastián, F. C., (2014). Immobilization of a keratinolytic protease from *Purpureocillium lilacinum* on genipin activated-chitosan beads. *Process Biochemistry, 49*(8), 1332–1336.

140. Xiang-Yu, W., Xiao-Ping, J., Yue, L., Sha, Z., & Ye-Wang, Z., (2015). Preparation $Fe_3O_4$@chitosan magnetic particles for covalent immobilization of lipase from *Thermomyces lanuginosus*. *International Journal of Biological Macromolecules, 75*, 44–50.

141. Garima, S., Sonam, R., & Arvind, M. K., (2015). Immobilization of fenugreek β-amylase on chitosan/PVP blend and chitosan-coated PVC beads: A comparative study. *Food Chemistry, 172*, 844–851.

142. Naghme, D., Nasrin, N. S., Mehdi, J., Hamid, G., & Seyed-Omid, R. S., (2015). Surface modification of chitosan/PEO nanofibers by air dielectric barrier discharge plasma for acetylcholinesterase immobilization. *App. Sur. Sci., 349*, 940–947.

143. Nivedita, J., Veda, P. P., & Upendra, N. D., (2016). Immobilization of papaya laccase in chitosan led to improved multipronged stability and dye discoloration. *International Journal of Biological Macromolecules, 86*, 288–295.

144. Selmihan, S., & Ismail, O., (2016). Determination of optimum conditions for glucose-6-phosphate dehydrogenase immobilization on chitosan-coated magnetic nanoparticles and its characterization. *Journal of Molecular Catalysis B: Enzymatic, Supplement, 133*(S-1), S25–S33. doi: 10.1016/j.molcatb.2016.11.004.

145. Manuela, P. K., Camila, R. H., André, S. G. L., Rafael, C. R., Tania, M. H. C., Jorge, L. N., & Plinho, F. H., (2016). Chitosan crosslinked with genipin as a support matrix for application in food process: Support characterization and β-d-galactosidase immobilization. *Carbohydrate Polymers, 137*(10), 184–190.

146. Jie, L., Enbo, X., Xingfei, L., Zhengzong, W., Fang, W., Xueming, X., Zhengyu, J., et al., (2016). Effect of chitosan molecular weight on the formation of chitosan-pullulanase soluble complexes and their application in the immobilization of pullulanase onto $Fe_3O_4$-κ-carrageenan nanoparticles. *Food Chemistry, 202*, 49–58.

147. Fei, Z., Bao-Kai, C., Xue-Jun, W., Ge, M., Hong-Xia, L., & Jing, S., (2016). Immobilization of laccase onto chitosan beads to enhance its capability to degrade synthetic dyes. *International Biodeterioration and Biodegradation, 110*, 69–78.

148. Waifalkar, P. P., Parit, S. B., Chougale, A. D., Subasa, C. S., Patil, P. S., & Patil, P. B., (2016). Immobilization of invertase on chitosan-coated γ-$Fe_2O_3$ magnetic nanoparticles to facilitate magnetic separation. *Journal of Colloid and Interface Science, 482*, 159–164.

149. Singh, R. S., Singh, R. P., & Kennedy, J. F., (2017). Immobilization of yeast inulinase on chitosan beads for the hydrolysis of inulin in a batch system. *International Journal of Biological Macromolecules, 95*, 87–93.

150. Uttam, V. S., Shamraja, S. N., & Virendra, K. R., (2017). Immobilization of pectinase onto chitosan magnetic nanoparticles by macromolecular cross-linker. *Carbohydrate Polymers, 157*, 677–685.

151. Muhammad, A., Sadia, N., & Muhammad, B., (2017). Enhancing the catalytic functionality of *Trametes* versicolor IBL-04 laccase by immobilization on chitosan microspheres. *Chemical Engineering Research and Design, 119*, 1–11.

152. Belma, Z. K., Fatih, U., & Zehra, D., (2017). Chitosan and carboxymethyl cellulose-based magnetic nanocomposites for application of peroxidase purification. *International Journal of Biological Macromolecules, 96*, 149–160.

153. Mascini, M., Mateescu, M. A., & Pilloton, R., (1986). Polyvinylalcohol-collagen membranes for enzyme immobilization. *Bioelectrochemistry and Bioenergetics, 16*(1), 149–157.

154. Panduranga, R. K., (1996). Recent developments of collagen-based materials for medical applications and drug delivery systems, *Journal of Biomaterials Science, Polymer Edition, 7*(7), 623–645.

155. Ai, X. L., Xue, P. L., Rong, Q. Z., & Bi, S., (2007). Preparation of Fe(III)-immobilized collagen fiber for lysozyme adsorption. *Colloids and Surfaces A: Physicochemical and Engineering Aspects, 301*(1–3), 85–93.

156. Sheng, W., Gong, C., & Xue, B., (2011). *Immobilization of Catalase on Fe (III) Modified Collagen Fiber, 27*(7), 1076–1081.

157. Na, S., Shuang, C., Xin, H., Xuepin, L., & Bi, S., (2011). Immobilization of catalase by using Zr(IV)-modified collagen fiber as the supporting matrix. *Process Biochemistry, 46*(11), 2187–2193.

158. Dewei, S., Min, C., & Haiming, C., (2016). Collagen-immobilized lipases show good activity and reusability for butyl butyrate synthesis. *Appl. Biochem. Biotechnol., 180*, 826.

159. Pal, K., Paulson, A. T., & Rousseau, D., (2012). 14 biopolymers in controlled-release delivery systems. *Handbook of Biopolymers and Biodegradable Plastics: Properties, Processing and Applications*, 329.

160. Namdev, B. S., Roshan, J., Cato, T. L., & Sangamesh, G. K., (2014). Polysaccharide biomaterials for drug delivery and regenerative engineering. *Polym. Adv. Technol., 25*, 448–460.

161. Brannon-Peppas, L., (1997). Polymers in controlled drug delivery. *Medical Plastics and Biomaterials Magazine*, 34.

162. Matalanis, A., Jones, O. G., & McClements, D. J., (2011). Structured biopolymer-based delivery systems for encapsulation, protection, and release of lipophilic compounds. *Food Hydrocolloids, 25*(8), 1865–1880.

163. Peng, Y., Li, J., Li, J., Fei, Y., Dong, J., & Pan, W., (2013). Optimization of thermosensitive chitosan hydrogels for the sustained delivery of venlafaxine hydrochloride. *International Journal of Pharmaceutics, 441*(1), 482–490.

164. Jinke, X., Mifong, T., Sepideh, S., Sophie, L., Jake, B., Mary, M. S., & Marta, C., (2017). Mucoadhesive chitosan hydrogels as rectal drug delivery vessels to treat ulcerative colitis. *Acta Biomaterialia, 48*, 247–257.

165. Jameela, S. R., Kumary, T. V., Lal, A. V., & Jayakrishnan, A., (1998). Progesterone-loaded chitosan microspheres: A long-acting biodegradable controlled delivery system. *Journal of Controlled Release, 52*(1), 17–24.

166. Kaihang, C., Yunzhi, L., Cong, C., Xiaoyun, L., Xiao, C., & Xiaoying, W., (2016). Chitosan derivatives/reduced graphene oxide/alginate beads for small-molecule drug delivery. *Materials Science and Engineering: C, 69*, 1222–1228.

167. Fang, M., Yuan, J., Peng, C., & Li, Y., (2014). Collagen as a double-edged sword in tumor progression. *Tumor Biol., 35*, 2871–2882.

168. Wallace, D. G., & Rosenblatt, J., (2003). Collagen gel systems for sustained delivery and tissue engineering. *Adv. Drug Deliv. Rev., 55*, 1631–1649.

169. Martins, V. C., Goissis, G., Ribeiro, A. C., Marcantônio, Jr. E., & Bet, M. R., (1998). The controlled release of antibiotic by hydroxyapatite: Anionic collagen composites. *Artificial Organs, 22*(3), 215–221.

170. Chie, K., Tomoyuki, S., Kenji, W., Mikako, O., Ayano, F., Eiko, N., Atsushi, H., et al., (2013). Doxorubicin-conjugated dendrimer/collagen hybrid gels for metastasis-associated drug delivery systems. *Acta Biomaterialia, 9*(3), 5673–5680.

171. Graţiela, T. T., Camelia, U., Răzvan, C. B., Roxana, G. Z., Ileana, R., Aurelia, M., Mădălina, G. A., & Mihaela, V. G., (2015). Chloramphenicol collagen sponges for local drug delivery in dentistry. *Comptes. Rendus. Chimie., 18*(9), 986–992.

172. Yosra, A., Jiaxin, L., Sujay, P., Ali, S., & Ilva, D. R., (2016). Nanoparticle cross-linked collagen shields for sustained delivery of pilocarpine hydrochloride. *International Journal of Pharmaceutics, 501*(1, 2), 96–101.

173. Jiajia, S., Ying, G., Ruirui, X., Tifeng, J., Qianli, Z., & Xuehai, Y., (2017). Synergistic *in vivo* photodynamic and photothermal antitumor therapy based on collagen-gold hybrid hydrogels with the inclusion of photosensitive drugs. *Colloids and Surfaces A: Physicochemical and Engineering Aspects, 514*, 155–160.

174. Yu, Y., Zhang, H., Sun, H., et al. (2013). Nano-hydroxyapatite formation via co-precipitation with chitosan-g-poly(N-isopropylacrylamide) in coil and globule states for tissue engineering application. *Front. Chem. Sci. Eng. 7*, 388–400. https://doi.org/10.1007/s11705-013-1355-0.

175. McDaniel, J.S., Pilia, M., Raut, V. et al. (2016). Alternatives to autograft evaluated in a rabbit segmental bone defect. *International Orthopaedics (SICOT), 40*, 197–203. https://doi.org/10.1007/s00264-015-2824-5.

176. Oh, S. H., Park, I. K., Kim, J. M., &Lee, J. H. (2007). In vitro and in vivo characteristics of PCL scaffolds with pore size gradient fabricated by a centrifugation method. *Biomaterials.* Mar; *28*(9), 1664–1671. doi: 10.1016/j.biomaterials.2006.11.024. Epub 2006 Dec 28. PMID: 17196648.

177. Shuping Wang, Changkai Sun, Shui Guan, Wenfang Li, Jianqiang Xu, Dan Ge, Meiling Zhuang, Tianqing Liua, & Xuehu Ma, (2017). Chitosan/gelatin porous scaffolds assembled with conductive poly(3,4-ethylenedioxythiophene) nanoparticles for neural tissue engineering. *J. Mater. Chem. B., 5*, 4774–4788.

178. Zamora-Mora, V., Fernández-Gutiérrez, M., González-Gómez, Á., Sanz, B., Román, J. S., Goya, G. F., Hernández, R., & Mijangos, C. (2017). Chitosan nanoparticles for combined drug delivery and magnetic hyperthermia: From preparation to in vitro studies. *Carbohydr Polym.* Feb 10; *157*, 361–370. doi: 10.1016/j.carbpol.2016.09.084. Epub 2016 Sep 28. PMID: 27987939.

**CHAPTER 5**

# Biosensor and Drug Delivery Application by the Utilization of Green Nanotechnology

MEEGLE S. MATHEW,[1] APPUKUTTAN SARITHA,[2] and KURUVILLA JOSEPH[1]

[1]Department of Chemistry, Indian Institute of Space Science and Technology, Valiyamala, Thiruvananthapuram, Kerala, India, E-mails: meeglesmathew@gmail.com (M. S. Mathew), sarithatvla@gmail.com (A. Saritha)

[2]Department of Chemistry, School of Arts and Sciences, Amrita Vishwa Vidyapeetham, Amritapuri, Clappana, Kollam, Kerala, India, E-mail: kjoseph.iist@gmail.com

## ABSTRACT

Green nanotechnology enables the synthesis and development of nano-materials through safer fabrication routes with low toxicity so that the utilization of these materials in biomedical applications is constantly gaining momentum. The advent of green initiatives in nanotechnology has revolutionized the biosensor and drug delivery arena, and biosensors are now considered powerful analytical tools for selective and sensitive detection and examination of many analytes and diseases. Apart from nanomaterials, nanoclusters, hybrid nanomaterials, biological molecules, microbes, and nanocomposites are also involved in the active fabrication of biosensors and drug delivery agents. This chapter focuses on the various green strategies used for the fabrication of potential nanoclusters that could be employed in the fields of bio-detection and drug delivery. Though there are many review articles that point out the utility of nanomaterials in biosensing and drug delivery, yet a few reports concentrate exclusively on nanoclusters. Hence our earnest approach is to bridge the gap in the literature. The chapter also concentrates on the various mechanisms through which these biosensors and drug delivery agents operate.

## 5.1　INTRODUCTION

Green synthesis is an emerging tool for the synthesis of nanomaterials [1]. The nanomaterials exhibiting fluorescent behavior has grabbed attention in nanobiotechnology, owing to their exceptional and attractive optoelectronic and functional properties. Noble metal quantum clusters (NMQC) have lately gained the attention of contemporary material scientists. These are clusters consisting of several tens of metal atoms in the sub-nanometer core sized dimension (1–2 nm) [2]. Unlike the nanoparticles that exhibit surface plasmon resonance, the exhibit molecule like optical features [2b, 3]. Various advantages like low toxicity, chemical stability, photostability, tunable fluorescent emissions, and the ultra-small sizes enabling easy drain out after in vivo treatment make them promising candidates in biosensing and drug delivery [3a, 4, 5]. The structure of clusters comprises of a core-shell type of structure with the functioning as core and ligands serving as a shell (Figure 5.1) [2b, 6]. Several ligands, as well as bulky molecules [2b], are currently employed as protecting agents in the fabrication of these materials. The green synthesized protein protected clusters have aqueous solubility, outstanding biocompatibility, functionalization susceptibility, and characteristic structures for specific bio-recognition [7]. The protein stabilized AuQCs synthesized through the biomineralization process was first reported in 2009 [8].

## 5.2　BIOSENSOR

Biosensors are devices or materials used for the recognition of specific components of interest. With the advent of nanomaterials, the field of biosensors has outgrown into an independent research arena with application in almost every walk of life. The major applications of biosensors are in the field of metal detection, food safety, wastewater treatment, medical diagnostics, and many other fields.

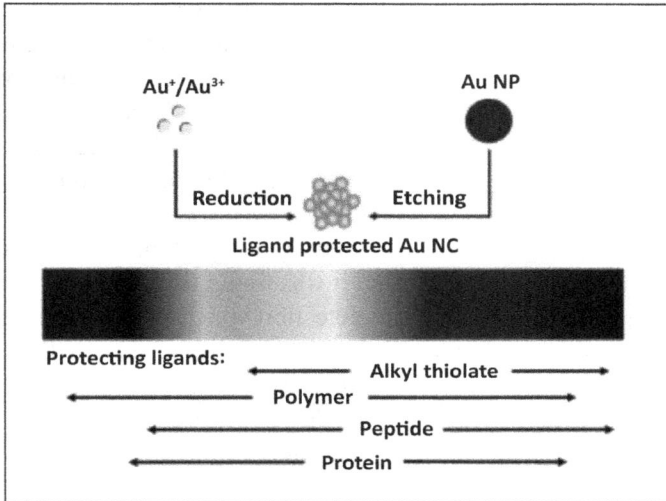

**FIGURE 5.1**    The illustration of the quantum cluster formation using various ligands [3c]. *Source:* Reprinted with permission from Ref. [3]. Copyright ©2015, American Chemical Society.

The mechanism of biosensing in a nanocluster is based on fluorescent sensing, and the strategies involved are fluorescence quenching/turn-off sensing, inner filter effect (IFE), fluorescent enhancement/turn-on sensing, and ratiometric sensing [9].

## 5.2.1   METAL ION SENSING

The sensing of metal ions using green synthesized materials is highly mandatory to lessen the toxicity in biological samples. Xie et al. carried out the recognition of $Hg^{2+}$ using $Au_{25}$@BSA employing a quenching strategy [10]. The excellent selectivity exhibited can be attributed to the specific interaction of $Hg^{2+}$ with $Au^+$. Protein protected metal QCs have been used by many groups for the detection of mercury [11, 12]. Bimetallic QC offers promising properties like a higher quantum yields and a greater sensitivity for sensing [13]. Sensitive detection of Hg (II) was done by many researchers [14]. AuQC-Graphene quantum dot nanocomposite was developed for Hg (II) detection by incorporating the fillers into electrospun PVA. The colorimetric sensing platform thus developed is depicted in Figure 5.2 [15]. Durgadas et al. have described the process of copper ion detection using BSA-protected gold clusters using the quenching of fluorescence [16]. HSA stabilized fluorescent nanocrystals containing gold and silver atoms were used for copper ion detection using redox-based fluorescent quenching [17]. In another interesting work, CdTe, silica, and AuQCs were clubbed in the form of hybrid spheres for copper ion detection [18].

Li et al. designed gold clusters containing 16 atoms with BSA protection for the detection of (Ag (I), and it was found that the system exhibited a detection limit of 0.10 mM. The detection was carried out via a turn-on fluorescence sensing strategy (Figure 5.3). The blue shift in fluorescence occurs because of the reaction between the Ag(I) and the cluster system, which causes a change in the surface electron energy of $Au_{16}QCs$. In 2013 they found that the actual sensing was due to the formation of a bimetallic cluster Au@AgQCs [19b]. This observation is further supported by the increase in the binding energy of Au (I) in XPS.

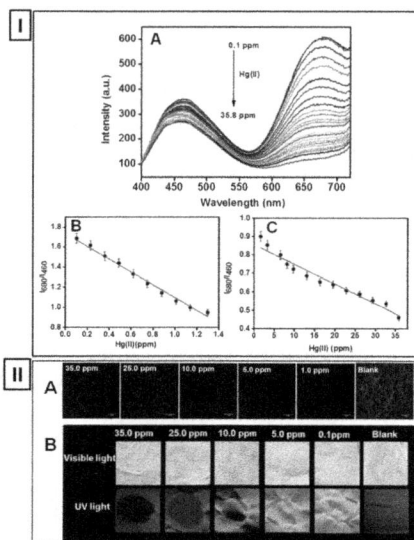

**FIGURE 5.2**   I(A) Fluorescence behavior of the bimetallic quantum cluster with different concentrations of Hg. I (B) and (C) shows the fluorescence intensity ratio (I680/I460) of AuQC@GQD versus Hg (II) concentrations in a range of (0.1–1.3 ppm) and (1.6–35.8 ppm), respectively.
*Source:* Reprinted with permission from Ref. [15]. Copyright ©2018 Wiley-VCH Verlag GmbH and Co. KGaA, Weinheim.

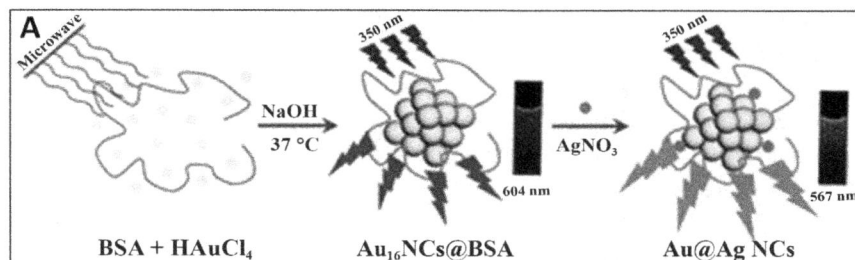

**FIGURE 5.3** (A) Synthesis of BSA protected AuQC and its conversion into Au@ Ag bimetallic Quantum cluster. II (A) shows the CLSM image of AuQC@GQD-PVA nanofiber mat with different concentration of Hg (II). II(B) Shows the photograph of AuQC@GQD-PVA mat with different concentration of Hg (II) (35.0 ppm – 0.1 ppm) taken under visible light and UV light.
*Source:* Reprinted with permission from Ref. [19b]. Copyright ©2016, American Chemical Society.

Chromium(VI) sensor with a recognition boundary of 0.6 nM was developed using AuQC@BSA [20]. A sensor for Zn (II) with a detection limit of 29.28 nM was developed by Lui et al. AuQC@BSA contains amino groups capable of interacting with the salicylic acid and subsequently led to quenching of fluorescence. A recovery of fluorescence was noticed upon the addition of zinc ions into the system [21]. Bothra et al. employed a similar mechanism for sensing Zn(II) with the help of gold QC protected by lysozyme. The AuQCs@Lyso system exhibited a red to yellow emission, which in turn showed turn-on recognition of $Zn^{2+}$ ions [22]. AuQC@ BSA was used by Lee et al. for the detection of $Pb^{2+}$. They proposed a quenching mechanism with a detection limit of 4.8 nM [23]. A bimetallic QC based on gold and silver, which functioned on quenching strategy using aggregation, was designed for sensing of Pb (II). The bimetallic system was stabilized using BSA and had a detection limit of 2 nM [24].

## 5.2.2 ANION SENSING

Sensing of various anions like $CN^-$ chloride, Iodate, etc., are carried out using the versatile platform of protein-protected clusters (QCs) [25]. BSA stabilized AuQCs was developed for cyanide detection in which the etching of Au by $CN^-$ causes fluorescent quenching [26]. Nitrite sensor using the same system was developed by many research groups [27–29].

The quenching of fluorescence occurs via the conversion of zero-valent gold to Au(I) by $NO^+$. Similar strategies were employed for the detection of $I^-$ ions [30]. A sulfide ion sensor was developed by the utilization of Au-S chemistry. The formation of $Au_2S$ during the process of sensing causes the quenching of fluorescence and enables the sensing of sulfide ions. The detection limit was found to be 0.029 $\mu M$ [31]. In another work, three different types of silver quantum clusters protected with lysozyme were employed for the detection of $S_2^-$ through different strategies [32].

### 5.2.3   SMALL BIOMOLECULE SENSING

Numerous biomolecules have a vital role in the biochemical functioning of various body parts, and hence an abnormal amount might prove fatal in many cases. Quantum clusters protected by proteins are excellent platforms for sensing biomolecules. Xia et al. employed gold QC for glucose detection. They used glucose oxidase for protecting the clusters. The $H_2O_2$ liberated during the conversion of glucose oxidase in the presence of glucose causes aggregation of the clusters leading to quenching of fluorescence [33]. Similar strategies were employed by several groups later for glucose sensing [34, 35]. AuAg@BSA was employed for the recognition of uric acid utilizing the phenomenon known as IFE. The phenomenon occurring between 2,3-diaminophenazine and the cluster helped in the recognition process [36], and the reaction is taking place in the presence of horse radish peroxidase. Catalase conjugated gold cluster functioned as an effective system for sensing many other useful materials [37]. Red emitting gold clusters were used for the sensing of hydrogen peroxide in another interesting work [38]. The mimetic activity exhibited by these clusters was utilized effectively for sensing clinically important biomolecules [36]. Several biomolecules like xanthine [39], cholesterol, dopamine [40–42, 44]. The absorber/fluorophore pair was constituted by the BSA protected gold nanoclusters, and the PVP protected nanogold particles for the detection of cholesterol. In the presence of cholesterol oxidase, $H_2O_2$ was generated, and the interaction of $H_2O_2$ with AuNP causes an expansion of AuNP size. The surface Plasmon band of the nanoparticles undergoes a shift with an increase in the concentration of $H_2O_2$ and, led to the quenching of the fluorescence of the nanocluster due to the overlap excitation of the gold nanocluster and the surface Plasmon absorption of the nanoparticle [44] (Figure 5.4).

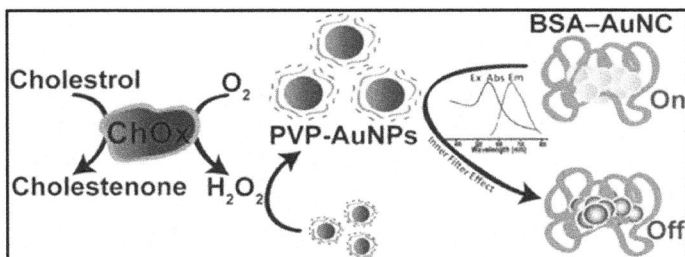

**FIGURE 5.4** Cholesterol detection due to the quenching of fluorescence of the nanoclusters.
*Source:* Reprinted with permission from Ref. [44]. Copyright ©2015, American Chemical Society.

Acetylcholine (ACh), an important neurotransmitter, was detected using $Au_{QC}$@BSA in conjugation with acetylcholinesterase (AChE) by quenching of fluorescence. The sensor had the power of detecting acetylcholine to a low concentration of 10 nM. (Figure 5.5) [45].

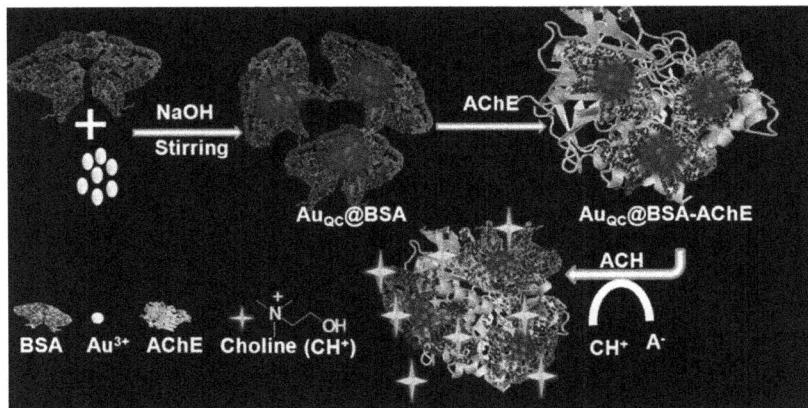

**FIGURE 5.5** Sensing of acetylcholine using BSA protected gold quantum clusters.
*Source:* Reprinted with permission from Ref. [45], Copyright ©2016, Elsevier.

The detection of glutathione (GSH) was enabled using blue-emitting $Au_8QC$ stabilized using lysozyme [46]. Many studies were done on the detection of enzyme activity [47, 48] and enzymes like trypsin [49], Cystatin C [50], Ovalbumin [51], and molecules like Creatinine [52].

### 5.2.4 BACTERIA DETECTION

Detection of bacteria using metal nanocluster was well studied [53]. Wu et al. fabricated an arrangement of sensors for the screening of protein and bacteria. They have used a metal ion-protein nanocluster adduct for the screening of nine different proteins and five different bacteria. The nanocluster gives a unique fluorescence response with each analyte. AuQC stabilized by lysozyme has the ability to sense *E. coli*, while the gold nanoclusters, which were protected by BSA, could not detect the presence of *E. coli* [54]. Interestingly, the gold nanoclusters stabilized by HAS could be employed successfully for the recognition of *Staphylococcus aureus* and methicillin-resistant *S. aureus* [54b]. The development of an assortment of sensors for the detection of bacteria was developed using protein stabilized Au quantum clusters. They have synthesized four different protein stabilized nanocluster. Based on the specific interaction between the protein and bacteria, each nanocluster gives a different response with bacteria [54c]. An *E. coli* detection was carried out using BSA stabilized nanocluster by an on-off-on sensing strategy. The interaction of Cu(II) ion quenches the fluorescence of AuNCs by direct interaction of Cu and amino acid present in the BSA. Thereafter, in the presence of *E. coli* bacteria, the bacteria replace the Cu (II) and again recovered the fluorescence (Figure 5.6) [54d].

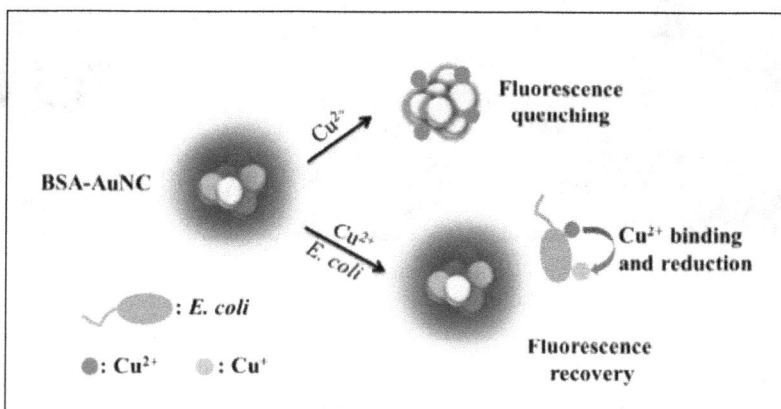

**FIGURE 5.6**   The schematic representation for the development of an on-off-on sensing strategy for *E. coli* detection.
*Source:* Reproduced from Ref. 54(d). Copyright ©2018, American Chemical Society.

## 5.3 DRUG DELIVERY

Nanomaterials are considered excellent materials for drug delivery applications, but the presence of organic molecules, which are employed as reducing agents as well as capping agents in the preparative steps, reduce the eco-friendly nature of the systems. Hence there is an urge to replace these chemicals with biomolecules. One of the emerging areas that have grabbed the interest of researchers in recent years is the utilization of green synthesized quantum clusters in drug delivery applications. Novel biocompatible clusters with unique cell internalization characteristics as well as excellent fluorescent emissions are slowly replacing traditional nanomaterial-based sensor platforms. Shichao Wu et al. devised an environmentally benign method to fabricate flower-shaped gold nanoclusters using epigallocatechin gallate, an ingredient in tea leaves [55]. They used these nanoclusters to deliver the drugs methotrexate (MTX) and doxorubicin (DOX) by conjugating them to the cluster via a cysteine bridge (Figure 5.7).

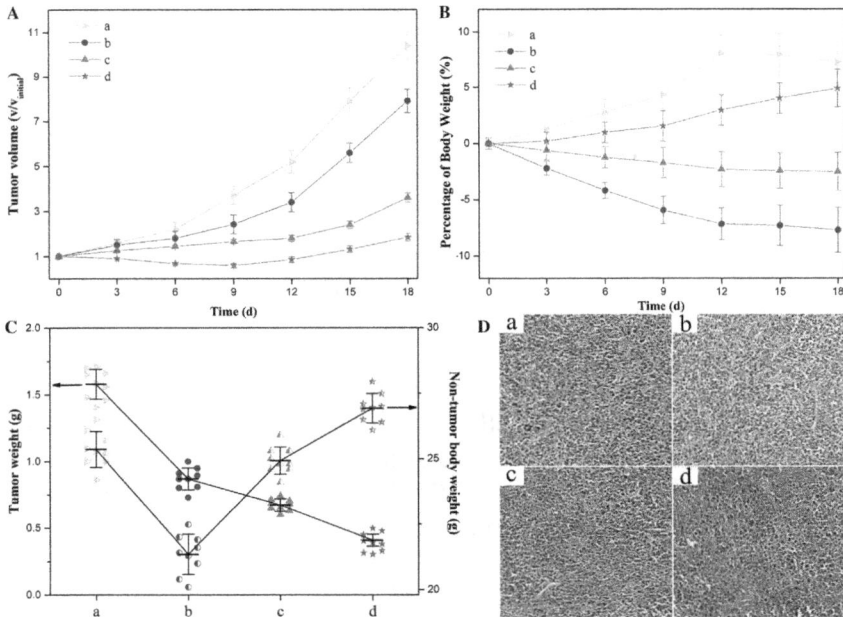

**FIGURE 5.7** Anticancer effects of different formulations [55].
*Source:* Open access.

Hang Ding et al. synthesized protein-gold hybrid nanocubes containing both fluorescent and vehicle function, which could serve the dual purpose of delivery of drugs and imaging [56]. The blue system with approximately 100 nm was fabricated using bovine serum albumin (BSA), gold clusters, and tryptophan as precursors. These hybrid nanomaterials have exhibited high internalization by cells, less cytotoxicity, and were found to act as an excellent vehicle for the delivery of drugs. Figure 5.8 represents the synthesis of the biosensor and its subsequent application in bioimaging and delivery of drugs.

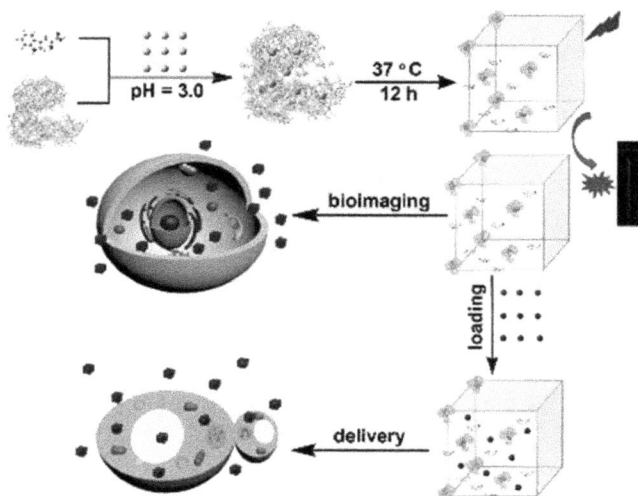

**FIGURE 5.8**  Synthesis of gold nanocubes for bioimaging and drug delivery applications. *Source:* Reprinted with permission from Ref. [56]. Copyright ©2015, American Chemical Society.

An array of characterization techniques were employed to stud the gold nanoclusters with and without drug loading. The cluster formation was confirmed by the additional factor like the absence of SPR peak.

Yong Yu et al. [57] detected the binding of drugs like ibuprofen, warfarin, phenytoin, and sulfanilamide to protein-protected Au NCs and monitored the kinetics of the binding process. The proteins employed for the protection of clusters were HSA and BSA. Figure 5.9 shows the photoemission features of the quantum cluster, both inclusive as well as devoid of the drugs.

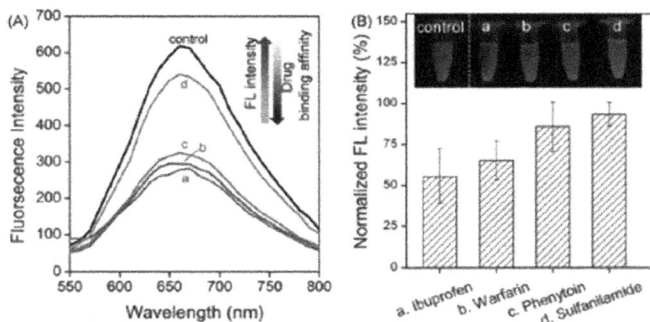

**FIGURE 5.9**   Photoemission from HAS capped Au NCs containing different drug samples. *Source:* Reprinted with permission from Ref. [57], Copyright ©2014, Royal Society of Chemistry.

Usually, drug release from nanosystems involves thiol/disulfide exchange, and GSH is a very promising candidate in the area of drug delivery. Zhang and co-workers studied the drug delivery of histidine protected AuNCs by GSH exchange [58]. Choi and Wong studied the crucial role-played by GSH in the targeted drug delivery to cancer cells [59]. Chattoraj et al. monitored the release of DOX into breast cancer cells (Figure 5.10) by means of lysozyme protected AuNCs and explained the mechanism using FRET [60].

Intracellular GSH will be substituted by GSH, leading to the formation of GSH-capped AuNCs, and thus, cancer cells show an elevated uptake of silver nanoparticles. A higher content of GSH in breast cancer cells will facilitate the ligand exchange leading to the delivery of the loaded drug.

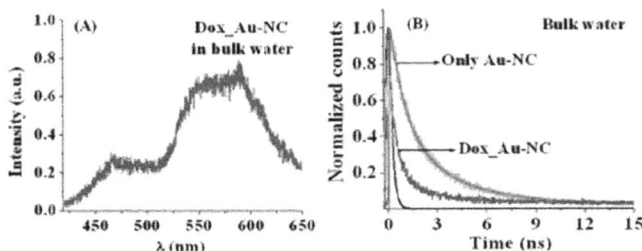

**FIGURE 5.10**   (A) Doxorubicin-loaded AuNCs coated with lysozyme showing fluorescent emission. (B) Comparison of fluorescence decay of lysozyme-coated AuNCs in bulk water in the absence (green) and the presence (blue) of doxorubicin. *Source:* Reprinted with permission from Ref. [60], Copyright ©2016, Wiley-VCH Verlag GmbH, and Co. KGaA, Weinheim.

Fangyuan Zhou and his group [61] have used a theranostic system like gold nanoclusters associated with cisplatin and folic acid for the delivery of drugs into breast cancer cells (Figure 5.11). The cisplatin could be delivered into the cancer cells by the reduction using GSH.

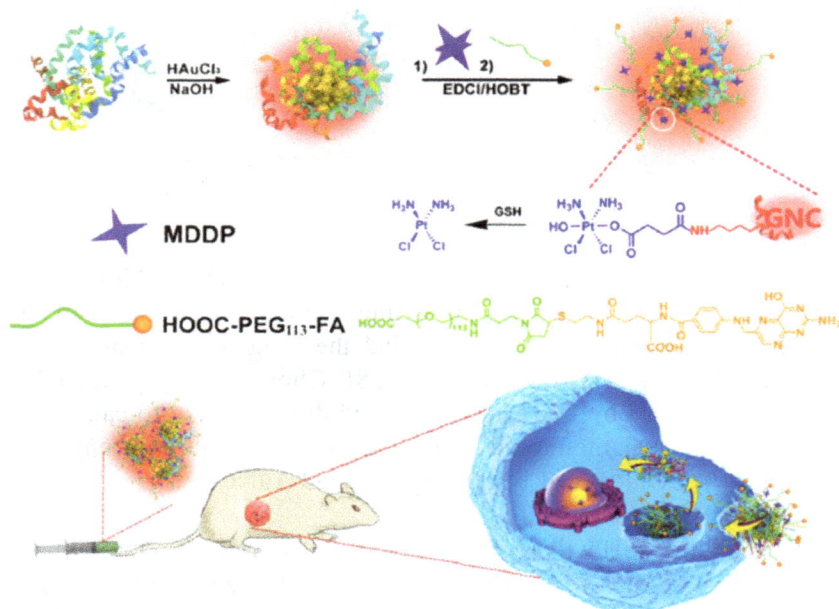

**FIGURE 5.11**    Graphic representation of gold nanocluster based theranostic nanoplatform [61].
*Source:* Open access.

## 5.4    CONCLUSIONS AND OUTLOOK

Nanomaterials have emerged as the most capable candidates in the field of nanomedicine, biosensing, and theranostics as they possess superior properties over the existing materials. Green synthesis of nanoclusters and their subsequent utilization in biosensing and drug delivery are discussed in detail throughout the chapter. The real mechanism of action, as well as toxicity involved in these processes, is yet to be studied in detail and hence would open up new avenues for research in the area. The biosensor technology will revolutionize the food, agricultural, and packaging industry in the coming years. Cost-effective biosensors that can simultaneously detect two toxins are more challenging and is yet to become a reality. Another deficit in this field of research that is yet to be addressed is the fabrication of field portable sensors. Hitherto we have succeeded in the detection of various biomolecules using protein-protected bimetallic quantum clusters, and the challenge lies in the scaling up and integration of the lab-scale process into cost-effective sensor fabrication, which is under progress. This research on green synthesized nanosystems would definitely lead to the creation of novel systems with efficient biosensing as well as enhanced theranostic capabilities.

## KEYWORDS

- **acetylcholine**
- **biosensor**
- **drug delivery**
- **green nanotechnology**
- **inner filter effect**
- **noble metal quantum clusters**

## REFERENCES

1. (a) Cheng, L., Wang, C., Feng, L., Yang, K., & Liu, Z., (2014). Functional nanomaterials for phototherapies of cancer. *Chemical Reviews, 114*(21), 10869–10939; (b) Dwivedi, N., Kumar, S., Carey, J. D., & Dhand, C., (2015). Functional nanomaterials for electronics, optoelectronics, and bioelectronics. *Journal of Nanomaterials*, 2; (c) Liu, J. M., Hu, Y., Yang, Y. K., Liu, H., Fang, G. Z., Lu, X., & Wang, S., (2018). Emerging functional nanomaterials for the detection of food contaminants. *Trends in Food Science and Technology, 71*, 94–106.
2. (a) Lu, Y., & Chen, W., (2012). Sub-nanometer sized metal clusters: From synthetic challenges to the unique property discoveries. *Chemical Society Reviews, 41*(9), 3594–3623; (b) Mathew, A., & Pradeep, T., (2014). Noble metal clusters: Applications in energy, environment, and biology. *Part. Part. Syst. Charact.*
3. (a) Shahsavari, S., Hadian-Ghazvini, S., Hooriabad, S. F., Menbari, O. I., Hasany, M., Simchi, A., & Rogach, A. L., (2019). Ligand functionalized copper nanoclusters for versatile applications in catalysis, sensing, bioimaging, and optoelectronics. *Materials Chemistry Frontiers, 3*(11), 2326–2356; (b) Hu, Y., Guo, W., & Wei, H., (2015). Protein- and peptide-directed approaches to fluorescent metal nanoclusters.

*Israel Journal of Chemistry, 55*(6/7), 682–697; (c) Li-Yi, C., Chia-Wei, W., & Zhiqin, Y., (2015). Fluorescent gold nanoclusters: Recent advances in sensing and imaging. *Anal. Chem., 87*(1), 216–229.

4. (a) Li, H., Li, H., & Wan, A., (2020). Luminescent gold nanoclusters for *in vivo* tumor imaging. *Analyst, 145*(2), 348–363; (b) Jiang, X., Du, B., Huang, Y., & Zheng, J., (2018). Ultrasmall noble metal nanoparticles: Breakthroughs and biomedical implications. *Nano Today, 21*, 106–125.

5. (a) Tao, Y., Li, M., Ren, J., & Qu, X., (2015). Metal nanoclusters: Novel probes for diagnostic and therapeutic applications. *Chemical Society Reviews, 44*(23), 8636–8663; (b) Bhattacharyya, K., & Mukherjee, S., (2018). Fluorescent metal nanoclusters as next generation fluorescent probes for cell imaging and drug delivery. *Bulletin of the Chemical Society of Japan, 91*(3), 447–454.

6. Yu, P., Wen, X., Toh, Y. R., Ma, X., & Tang, J., (2015). Fluorescent metallic nanoclusters: Electron dynamics, structure, and applications. *Particle and Particle Systems Characterization, 32*(2), 142–163.

7. (a) Chevrier, D. M., Chatt, A., & Zhang, P., (2012). Properties and applications of protein-stabilized fluorescent gold nanoclusters: Short review. *J. Nanophoton., 6*(1), 064504-1-064504-16; (b) Xavier, P. L., Chaudhari, K., Baksi, A., & Pradeep, T., (2012). Protein-protected luminescent noble metal quantum clusters: An emerging trend in atomic cluster nanoscience. *Nano Reviews, 3*(1), 14767.

8. Xie, J., Zheng, Y., & Ying, J. Y., (2009). Protein-directed synthesis of highly fluorescent gold nanoclusters. *J. Am. Chem. Soc., 131*(3), 888–889.

9. Nawrot, W., Drzozga, K., Baluta, S., Cabaj, J., & Malecha, K., (2018). A fluorescent biosensors for detection vital body fluids' agents. *Sensors, 18*(8), 2357.

10. Xie, J., Zheng, Y., & Ying, J. Y., (2010). Highly selective and ultrasensitive detection of $Hg^{2+}$ based on fluorescence quenching of Au nanoclusters by $Hg^{2+}$–$Au^+$ interactions. *Chemical Communications, 46*(6), 961–963.

11. (a) Yang, G., Zhang, H., Wang, Y., Liu, X., Luo, Z., & Yao, J., (2017). Enhanced stability and fluorescence of mixed-proteins-protected gold/silver clusters used for mercury ions detection. *Sensors and Actuators B: Chemical, 251*, 773–780; (b) Shi, H., Ou, M. Y., Cao, J. P., & Chen, G. F., (2015). Synthesis of ovalbumin-stabilized highly fluorescent gold nanoclusters and their application as an $Hg^{2+}$ sensor. *RSC Advances, 5*(105), 86740–86745; (c) Guo, C., & Irudayaraj, J., (2011). Fluorescent Ag clusters via a protein-directed approach as a Hg(II) ion sensor. *Anal. Chem., 83*(8), 2883–2889; (d) Pyng, Y., Xiaoming, W., Yon-Rui, T., Jane, H., & Jau, T., (2013). Metallophilic bond-induced quenching of delayed fluorescence in Au25@ BSA nanoclusters. *Particle and Particle Systems Characterization, 30*(5), 467–472.

12. Hu, D., Sheng, Z., Gong, P., Zhang, P., & Cai, L., (2010). Highly selective fluorescent sensors for $Hg^{2+}$ based on bovine serum albumin-capped gold nanoclusters. *Analyst, 135*(6), 1411–1416.

13. Zheng, B., Zheng, J., Yu, T., Sang, A., Du, J., Guo, Y., Xiao, D., & Choi, M. M. F., (2015). Fast microwave-assisted synthesis of AuAg bimetallic nanoclusters with strong yellow emission and their response to mercury(II) ions. *Sensors and Actuators B: Chemical, 221*, 386–392.

14. Zhao, J., Huang, M., Zhang, L., Zou, M., Chen, D., Huang, Y., & Zhao, S., (2017). Unique approach to develop carbon dot-based nanohybrid near-infrared ratiometric

fluorescent sensor for the detection of mercury ions. *Analytical Chemistry*, *89*(15), 8044–8049.

15. Mathew, M. S., Sukumaran, K., & Joseph, K., (2018). Graphene carbon dot assisted sustainable synthesis of gold quantum cluster for bio-friendly white light emitting material and ratiometric sensing of mercury ($Hg^{2+}$). *Chemistry Select*, *3*(33), 9545–9554.

16. Durgadas, C. V., Sharma, C. P., & Sreenivasan, K., (2011). Fluorescent gold clusters as nanosensors for copper ions in live cells. *Analyst*, *136*(5), 933–940.

17. Gui, R., & Jin, H., (2013). Aqueous synthesis of human serum albumin-stabilized fluorescent Au/Ag core/shell nanocrystals for highly sensitive and selective sensing of copper(ii). *Analyst*, *138*(23), 7197–7205.

18. Wang, Y. Q., Zhao, T., He, X. W., Li, W. Y., & Zhang, Y. K., (2014). A novel core-satellite CdTe/Silica/Au NCs hybrid sphere as dual-emission ratio metric fluorescent probe for $Cu^{2+}$. *Biosensors and Bioelectronics*, *51*, 40–46.

19. (a) Yue, Y., Liu, T. Y., Li, H. W., Liu, Z., & Wu, Y., (2012). Microwave-assisted synthesis of BSA-protected small gold nanoclusters and their fluorescence-enhanced sensing of silver(i) ions. *Nanoscale*, *4*(7), 2251–2254; (b) Li, H. W., Yue, Y., Liu, T. Y., Li, D., & Wu, Y., (2013). Fluorescence-enhanced sensing mechanism of BSA-protected small gold-nanoclusters to silver(I) ions in aqueous solutions. *J. Phys. Chem. C*, *117*, 16159–16165.

20. (a) Jian-Feng, G., Chang-Jun, H., Mei, Y., Dan-Qun, H., & Huan-Bao, F., (2016). Ultra-sensitive fluorescence determination of chromium (VI) in aqueous solution based on selectively etching of protein-stabled gold nanoclusters. *RSC Advances*, *6*(106), 104693–104698; (b) Zhang, J. R., Zeng, A. L., Luo, H. Q., & Li, N. B., (2016). Fluorescent silver nanoclusters for ultrasensitive determination of chromium (VI) in aqueous solution. *Journal of Hazardous Materials*, *304*, 66–72.

21. Liu, X., Fu, C., Ren, X., Liu, H., Li, L., & Meng, X., (2015). Fluorescence switching method for cascade detection of salicylaldehyde and zinc(II) ion using protein protected gold nanoclusters. *Biosensors and Bioelectronics*, *74*, 322–328.

22. Bothra, S., Babu, L. T., Paira, P., Ashok, K. S., Kumar, R., & Sahoo, S. K., (2018). A biomimetic approach to conjugate vitamin B6 cofactor with the lysozyme cocooned fluorescent AuNCs and its application in turn-on sensing of zinc(II) in environmental and biological samples. *Analytical and Bioanalytical Chemistry*, *410*(1), 201–210.

23. Lee, C. Y., Hsu, N. Y., Wu, M. Y., & Lin, Y. W., (2016). Microwave-assisted synthesis of BSA-stabilized gold nanoclusters for the sensitive and selective detection of lead(ii) and melamine in aqueous solution. *RSC Advances*, *6*(82), 79020–79027.

24. Wang, C., Cheng, H., Sun, Y., Xu, Z., Lin, H., Lin, Q., & Zhang, C., (2015). Nanoclusters prepared from a silver/gold alloy as a fluorescent probe for selective and sensitive determination of lead(II). *Microchimica Acta*, *182*(3), 695–701.

25. (a) Xiong, X., Tang, Y., Zhang, L., & Zhao, S., (2015). A label-free fluorescent assay for free chlorine in drinking water based on protein-stabilized gold nanoclusters. *Talanta*, *132*, 790–795; (b) Li, R., Xu, P., Fan, J., Di, J., Tu, Y., & Yan, J., (2014). Sensitive iodate sensor based on fluorescence quenching of gold nanocluster. *Analytica Chimica Acta*, *827*, 80–85.

26. Liu, Y., Ai, K., Cheng, X., Huo, L., & Lu, L., (2010). Gold-nanocluster-based fluorescent sensors for highly sensitive and selective detection of cyanide in water. *Adv. Funct. Mater.*, *20*(6), 951–956.

27. Liu, H., Yang, G., Abdel-Halim, E., & Zhu, J. J., (2013). Highly selective and ultrasensitive detection of nitrite based on fluorescent gold nanoclusters. *Talanta, 104*, 135–139.

28. Yue, Q., Sun, L., Shen, T., Gu, X., Zhang, S., & Liu, J., (2013). Synthesis of fluorescent gold nanoclusters directed by bovine serum albumin and application for nitrite detection. *J. Fluoresc.,* 1–6.

29. Unnikrishnan, B., Wei, S. C., Chiu, W. J., Cang, J., Hsu, P. H., & Huang, C. C., (2014). Nitrite ion-induced fluorescence quenching of luminescent BSA-Au25 nanoclusters: Mechanism and application. *Analyst, 139*(9), 2221–2228.

30. (a) Sun, J., & Jin, Y., (2014). Fluorescent Au nanoclusters: Recent progress and sensing applications. *Journal of Materials Chemistry C, 2*(38), 8000–8011; (b) Zhang, J., Chen, C., Xu, X., Wang, X., & Yang, X., (2013). Use of fluorescent gold nanoclusters for the construction of a NAND logic gate for nitrite. *Chem. Commun., 49*(26), 2691–2693; (c) Cao, X. L., Luo, Y. N., Lian, L. L., Wu, Y. Q., & Lou, D. W., (2015). Selective detection of iodine/iodide using BSA-stabilized gold nanoclusters-based fluorescence probe. *Chemistry Letters, 44*(10), 1392–1394.

31. Liu, J. M., Cui, M. L., Wang, X. X., Lin, L. P., Jiao, L., Zheng, Z. Y., Zhang, L. H., & Jiang, S. L., (2013). A promising gold nanoclusters fluorescence sensor for highly sensitive and selective detection of $S^{2-}$. *Sens. Actuators, B: Chemical.*

32. Gao, Z., Liu, F., Hu, R., Zhao, M., & Shao, N., (2016). Lysozyme-stabilized Ag nanoclusters: Synthesis of different compositions and fluorescent responses to sulfide ions with distinct modes. *RSC Advances, 6*(70), 66233–66241.

33. Xia, X., Long, Y., & Wang, J., (2013). Glucose oxidase-functionalized fluorescent gold nanoclusters as probes for glucose. *Anal. Chim. Acta, 772*(0), 81–86.

34. Wang, C., Shu, S., Yao, Y., & Song, Q., (2015). A fluorescent biosensor of lysozyme-stabilized copper nanoclusters for the selective detection of glucose. *RSC Advances, 5*(123), 101599–101606.

35. (a) Li, M., Yang, D. P., Wang, X., Lu, J., & Cui, D., (2013). Mixed protein-templated luminescent metal clusters (Au and Pt) for $H_2O_2$ sensing. *Nanoscale Res. Lett., 8*(1), 182; (b) Liu, F., Bing, T., Shangguan, D., Zhao, M., & Shao, N., (2016). Ratio metric fluorescent biosensing of hydrogen peroxide and hydroxyl radical in living cells with lysozyme-silver nanoclusters: Lysozyme as stabilizing ligand and fluorescence signal unit. *Analytical Chemistry, 88*(21), 10631–10638.

36. Wang, X. Y., Zhu, G. B., Cao, W. D., Liu, Z. J., Pan, C. G., Hu, W. J., Zhao, W. Y., & Sun, J. F., (2019). A novel ratiometric fluorescent probe for the detection of uric acid in human blood based on $H_2O_2$-mediated fluorescence quenching of gold/silver nanoclusters. *Talanta, 191*, 46–53.

37. Meng, F., Yin, H., Li, Y., Zheng, S., Gan, F., & Ye, G., (2018). One-step synthesis of enzyme-stabilized gold nanoclusters for fluorescent ratio metric detection of hydrogen peroxide, glucose, and uric acid. *Microchemical Journal, 141*, 431–437.

38. Wen, F., Dong, Y., Feng, L., Wang, S., Zhang, S., & Zhang, X., (2011). Horseradish peroxidase functionalized fluorescent gold nanoclusters for hydrogen peroxide sensing. *Anal. Chem., 83*(4), 1193–1196.

39. Wang, X. X., Wu, Q., Shan, Z., & Huang, Q. M., (2011). BSA-stabilized Au clusters as peroxidase mimetics for use in xanthine detection. *Biosensors and Bioelectronics, 26*(8), 3614–3619.

40. Tao, Y., Lin, Y., Ren, J., & Qu, X., (2013). A dual fluorometric and colorimetric sensor for dopamine based on BSA-stabilized Au nanoclusters. *Biosens. Bioelectron.*, *42*(0), 41–46.

41. Govindaraju, S., Ankireddy, S. R., Viswanath, B., Kim, J., & Yun, K., (2017). Fluorescent gold nanoclusters for selective detection of dopamine in cerebrospinal fluid. *Scientific Reports, 7*, 40298.

42. Miao, Z., Hou, W., Liu, M., Zhang, Y., & Yao, S., (2018). BSA capped bi-functional fluorescent Cu nanoclusters as pH sensor and selective detection of dopamine. *New Journal of Chemistry, 42*(2), 1446–1456.

43. Hu, L., Yuan, Y., Zhang, L., Zhao, J., Majeed, S., & Xu, G., (2013). Copper nanoclusters as peroxidase mimetics and their applications to $H_2O_2$ and glucose detection. *Anal. Chim. Acta, 762*(0), 83–86.

44. Chang, H. C., & Ho, J. A. A., (2015). Gold nanocluster-assisted fluorescent detection for hydrogen peroxide and cholesterol based on the inner filter effect of gold nanoparticles. *Analytical Chemistry, 87*(20), 10362–10367.

45. Mathew, M. S., Baksi, A., Pradeep, T., & Joseph, K., (2016). Choline-induced selective fluorescence quenching of acetylcholinesterase conjugated Au@ BSA clusters. *Biosensors and Bioelectronics, 81*, 68–74.

46. (a) Chen, T. H., & Tseng, W. L., (2012). (Lysozyme type VI)-Stabilized Au8 clusters: Synthesis mechanism and application for sensing of glutathione in a single drop of blood. *Small, 8*(12), 1912–1919; (b) Zhai, Q., Xing, H., Fan, D., Zhang, X., Li, J., & Wang, E., (2018). Gold-silver bimetallic nanoclusters with enhanced fluorescence for highly selective and sensitive detection of glutathione. *Sensors and Actuators B: Chemical, 273*, 1827–1832.

47. (a) Xu, S., Feng, X., Gao, T., Wang, R., Mao, Y., Lin, J., Yu, X., & Luo, X., (2017). A novel dual-functional biosensor for fluorometric detection of inorganic pyrophosphate and pyrophosphatase activity based on globulin stabilized gold nanoclusters. *Analytica Chimica Acta, 958*, 22–29; (b) Rong, L., Zhaoyang, W., Yuanlian, Y., Shuzhen, L., & Ruqin, Y., (2018). Application of gold-silver nanocluster based fluorescent sensors for determination of acetylcholinesterase activity and its inhibitor. *Materials Research Express, 5*(6), 065027; (c) Selvaprakash, K., & Chen, Y. C., (2014). Using protein-encapsulated gold nanoclusters as photoluminescent sensing probes for biomolecules. *Biosensors and Bioelectronics, 61*, 88–94; (d) Halawa, M. I., Gao, W., Saqib, M., Kitte, S. A., Wu, F., & Xu, G., (2017). Sensitive detection of alkaline phosphatase by switching on gold nanoclusters fluorescence quenched by pyridoxal phosphate. *Biosensors and Bioelectronics, 95*, 8–14.

48. Zhou, Q., Lin, Y., Xu, M., Gao, Z., Yang, H., & Tang, D., (2016). Facile synthesis of enhanced fluorescent gold-silver bimetallic nanocluster and its application for highly sensitive detection of inorganic pyrophosphatase activity. *Analytical Chemistry, 88*(17), 8886–8892.

49. Wang, G. L., Jin, L. Y., Dong, Y. M., Wu, X. M., & Li, Z. J., (2015). Intrinsic enzyme mimicking activity of gold nanoclusters upon visible light triggering and its application for colorimetric trypsin detection. *Biosensors and Bioelectronics, 64*, 523–529.

50. Lin, H., Li, L., Lei, C., Xu, X., Nie, Z., Guo, M., Huang, Y., & Yao, S., (2013). Immune-independent and label-free fluorescent assay for cystatin C detection based on protein-stabilized Au nanoclusters. *Biosensors and Bioelectronics, 41*, 256–261.

51. Li, Y., Chen, Y., Huang, L., Ma, L., Lin, Q., & Chen, G., (2015). A fluorescent sensor based on ovalbumin-modified Au nanoclusters for sensitive detection of ascorbic acid. *Analytical Methods, 7*(10), 4123–4129.

52. Rajamanikandan, R., & Ilanchelian, M., (2018). Protein-protected red emissive copper nanoclusters as a fluorometric probe for highly sensitive biosensing of creatinine. *Analytical Methods, 10*(29), 3666–3674.

53. Li, D., Kumari, B., Makabenta, J. M., Gupta, A., & Rotello, V., (2019). Effective detection of bacteria using metal nanoclusters. *Nanoscale, 11*(46), 22172–22181.

54. Wu, Y., Wang, B., Wang, K., & Yan, P., (2018). Identification of proteins and bacteria based on a metal ion-gold nanocluster sensor array. *Analytical Methods, 10*(32), 3939–3944; (a) Liu, J., Lu, L., Xu, S., & Wang, L., (2015). One-pot synthesis of gold nanoclusters with bright red fluorescence and good biorecognition Abilities for visualization fluorescence enhancement detection of *E. coli. Talanta, 134*, 54–59; (b) Chan, P. H., & Chen, Y. C., (2012). Human serum albumin stabilized gold nanoclusters as selective luminescent probes for staphylococcus aureus and methicillin-resistant staphylococcus aureus. *Analytical Chemistry, 84*(21), 8952–8956; (c) Ji, H., Wu, L., Pu, H., Ren, J., & Qu, X., (2018). Point-of-care identification of bacteria using protein-encapsulated gold nanoclusters. *Adv. Healthcare Mater., 7*, 1701370; (d) Yan, R., Shou, Z., Chen, J., Wu, H., Zhao, Y., Qiu, L., Jiang, P., et al., (2018). *ACS Sustainable Chem. Eng., 6*, 4504–4509.

55. Wu, S., Yang, X., Luo, F., Wu, T., Xu, P., Zou, M., & Yan, J., (2018). Biosynthesis of flower-shaped Au nanoclusters with EGCG and their application for drug delivery. *Journal of Nanobiotechnology, 16* (1), 90.

56. Ding, H., Yang, D., Zhao, C., Song, Z., Liu, P., Wang, Y., Chen, Z., & Shen, J., (2015). Protein-gold hybrid nanocubes for cell imaging and drug delivery. *ACS Applied Materials and Interfaces, 7*(8), 4713–4719.

57. Yu, Y., New, S. Y., Xie, J., Su, X., & Tan, Y. N., (2014). Protein-based fluorescent metal nanoclusters for small molecular drug screening. *Chemical Communications, 50*(89), 13805–13808.

58. Zhang, X., Wu, F. G., Liu, P., Gu, N., & Chen, Z., (2014). Enhanced fluorescence of gold nanoclusters composed of HAuCl$_4$ and histidine by glutathione: Glutathione detection and selective cancer cell imaging. *Small, 10*(24), 5170–5177.

59. Wong, P. T., & Choi, S. K., (2015). Mechanisms of drug release in nanotherapeutic delivery systems. *Chemical Reviews, 115*(9), 3388–3432.

60. Chattoraj, S., Amin, A., Jana, B., Mohapatra, S., Ghosh, S., & Bhattacharyya, K., (2016). Selective killing of breast cancer cells by doxorubicin-loaded fluorescent gold nanoclusters: CONFOCAL microscopy and FRET. *Chem. Phys. Chem., 17*(2), 253–259.

61. Zhou, F., Feng, B., Yu, H., Wang, D., Wang, T., Liu, J., Meng, Q., et al., (2016). Cisplatin prodrug-conjugated gold nanocluster for fluorescence imaging and targeted therapy of the breast cancer. *Theranostics, 6*(5), 679–687.

# CHAPTER 6

# New, Simple, and Cost-Effective Synthesis of Green Nanotechnology in Anti-Microbial Applications

TEAN ZAHEER

*Department of Parasitology, University of Agriculture, Faisalabad, Pakistan, E-mail: teanzaheer942@gmail.com*

## ABSTRACT

Green nanotechnology is the science of nanoparticle (<100 nm) synthesis, using biological resources including plants, bacteria, fungi, viruses, algae, yeasts, cell lines, etc. The process of green nanoparticles (GNPs) synthesis is more facile, biodegradable, sustainable, renewable, environment friendly, and less toxigenic, among other methods. There are several biomedical applications of GNPs. Most widely used GNPs are of plant origin, mediated by using various parts viz. leaf, stem, bark, fruit, latex, seed, root, etc. Pathogens and vectors of human and animal diseases have significantly increased the disease and death tolls worldwide. Non-judicious use of conventional antimicrobials has led to the development of antimicrobial-resistant populations of pathogens and vectors. The chapter deals with the potential of GNPs in tackling pathogens, including bacteria, viruses, fungi, and parasites and vectors of these diseases. In addition, the areas of prospective research in the field have been highlighted.

## 6.1 INTRODUCTION

The science of synthesizing nanoparticles (<100 nm size) using biological machinery of various organisms (plants/algae/yeast, etc.) is known as "green nanotechnology" or "nanobiotechnology." The biological method of nanoparticle synthesis follows a bottom-up approach, involving redox reactions. The green synthesis of nanoparticles is a single step, biocompatible, time saving, more economical, having lower environmental hazards, and renewable procedure, among other approaches [1]. Additionally, the approach to green nanoparticles (GNPs) is more simplistic yet adequately bio-functional, involving a limited number of reagents required. The ability of biological machinery to bring forward redox reactions and serve as capping agents eliminates the use of toxic chemicals.

GNPs have wide-ranging biomedical applications, including use in nutraceuticals, diagnostics, treatment (drug loading and delivery), surgery, prophylaxis (vaccination), gene delivery, nanorobotics, etc., [2]. The rise in the superbug population of microbes and parasites exhibiting antimicrobial, multidrug, and anti-parasitical resistance has focused research towards alternative control options. The presence of antibiotic/ antiparasitic residues in milk and meat of farmed animals may lead to serious health consequences in human consumers. GNPs have provided a great promise in these areas by virtue of their efficient particle properties, cost-effectiveness, and ease of administration. This chapter deals with cost-effective and efficient ways of production and applications of GNPs against various microbes, e.g., bacteria, parasites, viruses, and fungi. GNPs are analyzed using UV-*vis* spectrophotometer (UV-*vis*), Fourier transforms infrared spectroscopy (FTIR), Electron microscopy (transmission and scanning), atomic force microscopy (AFM), x-ray diffraction analysis (XRD), dynamic light scattering (DLS), scanning tunneling microscopy (STM), scanning tunneling spectroscopy (STS), chromatography, filtration techniques, inductively coupled plasma-mass spectrometry (ICPMS), graphite furnace atomic absorption spectroscopy (GFAAS), selected area diffraction, Z-potential, inductively coupled plasma-optical emission spectrometry (ICPES), laser-induced breakdown detection technique (LIBS), and capillary exclusion [3, 4]. Major sources of green nanoparticle synthesis have been illustrated in Figure 6.1.

Most widely, the GNPs have been synthesized using various types of plants, including lavender, neem, fern, alfalfa, aloe vera, false daisy, tea, lemon, coffee, gooseberry, oat, metel, bamboo, coconut, fig, garlic, sorghum, oak, potato, orange, banana, pineapple, papaya, rambutan, mango, sapodilla, moringa, peanut, cashew, sugar apple, lilies, euphorbia, soursop, blue dawn flower, indigo, orchid tree, mokryeon, chrysanthemum, jasmine, mustard, lotus, claudius, red clover, tansy, cannabis, mangrove, white cedar, cinnamon, pistachio, eucalyptus, soapnut, thyme, hibiscus, etc. [5]. Different plant active materials can function as both reducing and stabilizing agents during the green synthesis of nanoparticles making the process simpler and cost-effective. Major plant actives that mediate antimicrobial and antioxidative pathways have been shown in Figure 6.2.

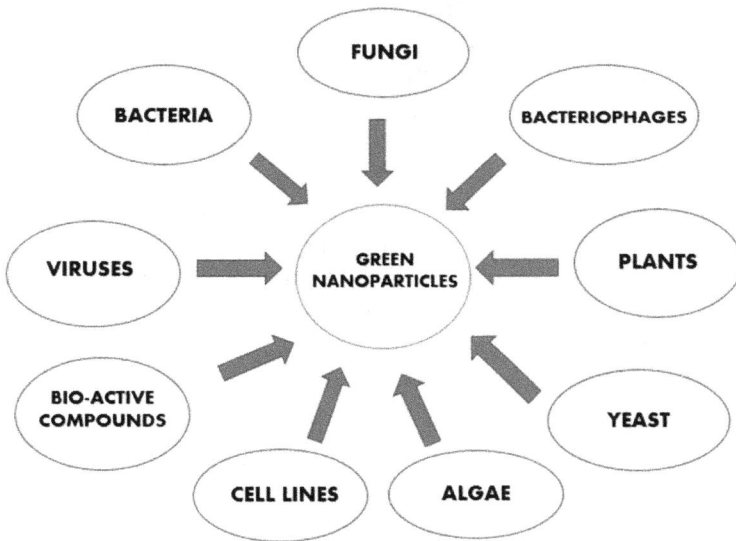

**FIGURE 6.1**   Various sources of green nanoparticles.

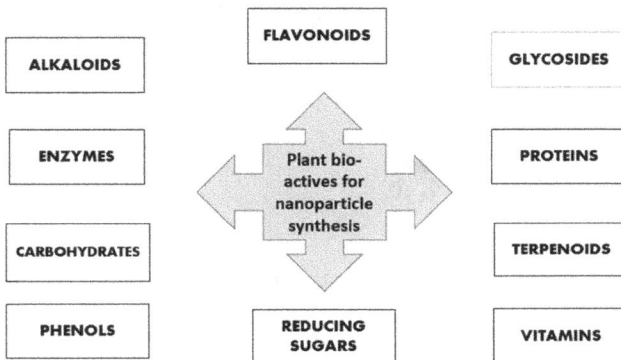

**FIGURE 6.2**   Some antimicrobial/antioxidative plant bioactives mediating nanoparticle synthesis.

Some bacteria (*Actinobacter* sp., *Aeromonas* sp., *Bacillus* sp., *Corynebacterium* sp., *Pseudomonas* sp. etc.), viruses (plant: cowpea mosaic, papaya mosaic, tobacco mosaic; animal viruses, e.g., adenoviruses, and bacteriophages, e.g., M13), some strains of yeast (*Candida* sp., *Rhodosporidium* sp.), fungi (*Aspergillus* sp., *Fusarium* sp., *Trichoderma*, etc.), algae (*Chlorella* sp., *Lyngbya* sp., *Naviculla* sp., *Sargassum* sp., etc.), human cell lines (e.g., epithelial cell lines), and other bioactive compounds of biological origin (mannose, chitosan, soluble starch, glucose) have also been utilized to synthesize GNPs [6].

Various GNPs having metallic ions like aluminum (Al), Argentum (Ag), aurum (Au), bismuth (Bi), carbon (C), copper (Cu), cobalt (Co), iron (Fe), indium (In), lead (Pb), magnesium (Mg), nickel (Ni), nitrogen (N), palladium (Pd), platinum (Pt), antimony (Sb), selenium (Se), sulfur (S), silicon (Si), tellurium (Te), titanium (Ti), and zinc (Zn) have been synthesized using biological machinery [7]. Most frequently used GNPs in biomedical applications are of plant origin. A brief overview of selected plant-mediated nanoparticle synthesis utilizing different parts of plants have been illustrated (Figure 6.3).

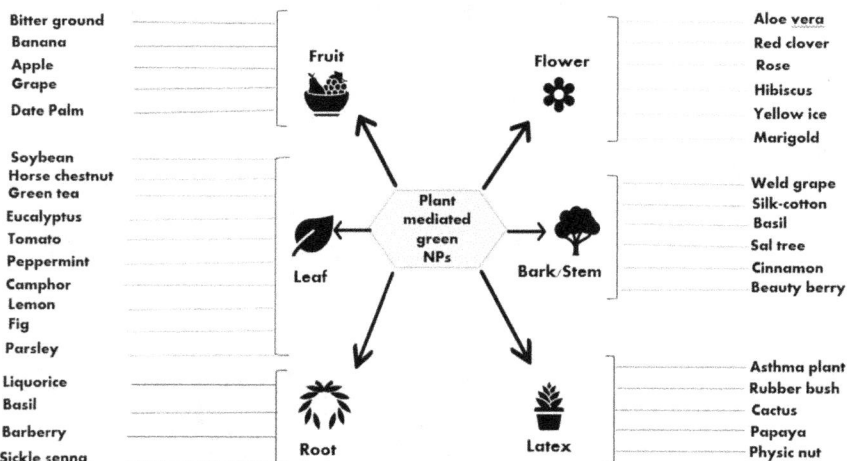

**FIGURE 6.3**   Selected review of some plant-mediated nanoparticle synthesis through extracts from various plant parts.

The nanobioparticles are extracted from different parts of the plant like leaves, stems, seeds, bran, roots, shoots, flowers, fruits, hulls, and barks. Table 6.1 presents a brief overview of some GNPs having various biomedical applications.

**TABLE 6.1** Some Recent Green Nanoparticles Showing Antimicrobial and Anti-Parasitical Properties

| Green Nanoparticle | Source | Properties (Active) | Application | References |
|---|---|---|---|---|
| Argentum (Ag) | Cyanobacteria (*Leptolyngbya JSC-1*) | Hydroxyl, carboxyl, and amide groups | Anti-cancer Antibacterial | [8] |
| Aurum (Au) | Algae (*Galaxaura elongate*) | Andrographolide, Alloaromadendrene oxide and others | Antibacterial | [9] |
| Copper (Cu) | Algae (*Botryococcus braunii*) | Bioactive compounds | Antibacterial | [10] |
| Nickel (Ni) | Plant (*Cocos nucifera*) | 3-methoxycinnamic acid | Anti-larval Anti-pest | [11] |
| Palladium (Pd) | Plant (*Filicium decipiens*) | Glycosides and saponins | Antibacterial | [5] |
| Selenium (Se) | Fungus (*Trichoderma atroviride*) | Hydroxyl and amides | Anti-mycotic | [12] |
| Titanium (Ti) | Plant (*Euphorbia prostrata*) | 2,3-Dihydrobenzofuran | Antiparasitic | [13] |
| Zinc (Zn) | Plant (Aloe vera) | Phenolic compounds, terpenoids, proteins | Antibacterial and anti-biofilm | [3] |

## 6.2   MECHANISM OF ACTION OF GREEN NANOPARTICLES (GNPS) AGAINST MICROBES AND PARASITES

Different metals act through various pathways leading to the prevention or treatment of target pathogens. However, some generalized pathways attributable as the mode of action of nanoparticles could be described in the following paragraphs.

### 6.2.1   PATHOGEN TOXICITY

Green nanoparticle conjugated antimicrobials or anti-parasitical aid the target dose-dependent drug response against the pathogen. The exact mechanism of toxicity in target species is not completely understood. However, some explanations of GNPs in pathogen toxicity and death have been presented. Primarily, the nanoparticles show an electrostatic interaction with cellular membranes, leading to membrane disruption. The antimicrobial potential of GNPs highly depends on the size, i.e., having <10 nm is more electrically reactive to the membrane molecules on target. This interaction also leads to the production of reactive oxygen species (ROS), e.g., $\alpha$-oxygen, peroxides, hydroxyl radical, superoxide, and others. These free radicals may further cause membrane damage, hampered protein function, disruption of DNA material, inhibition of the respiratory chain, and release of more free radicals. Nanoparticles of polycationic character may induce signal transduction leading to programmed cell death. Some GNPs have an affinity for specific sites in target species; for instance, selenium, copper, zinc, and silver nanoparticles particularly bind the sulfur-containing proteins. This may lead to dysregulation of protein functions and hinder Adenosine triphosphate (energy) synthesis, eventually leading to decreased cellular activity and cell death [8]. In addition, some nanomaterials may be photo-catalytic, and some may produce RNS for cell destruction. The pathogen toxicity is further enhanced by the antioxidant nature of GNPs that also acts as an immune booster (improved immunological response) to the host.

### 6.3   GREEN NANOPARTICLES (GNPS) AGAINST BACTERIA

In synergy with non-judicious use of drugs, diverse genetic properties, and several other factors, various bacteria have become resistant to many antimicrobials at previously effective therapeutic doses. From a broader perspective, this has led to many issues affecting all levels of food chains and entire eco-healthy. The application of GNPs against both gram-positive and gram-negative bacteria have provided a useful alternative to anti-microbials. Inhibition of growth and multiplication in bacteria, including those listed in Figure 6.4.

```
                                        ┌─ Corynebacterium
                                        │   Staphylococcus
                                        │   Mycobacterium
                                        │   Streptococcus
          ┌─ Gram positive Bacteria    │   Lactobacillus
          │                             │   Helicobacter
          │                             │   Listeria
          │                             └─ Bacillus
Bacteria ─┤
          │                             ┌─ Pseudomonas
          │                             │   Salmonella
          │                             │   Escherichia
          │                             │   Citrobacter
          │                             │   Klebsiella
          └─ Gram negative Bacteria     │   Serratia
                                        │   Proteus
                                        └─ Vibrio
```

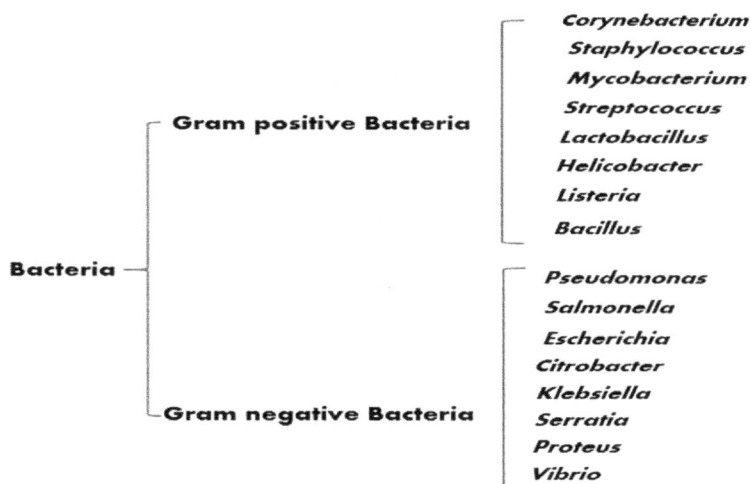

**FIGURE 6.4**    Documented use of green nanoparticles against bacteria.

GNPs have also shown large promise in successful inhibition of growth and multiplication of drug-resistant bacteria, including *Escherichia coli*, *Bacillus cereus*, MRSA (Methicillin Resistant *Staphylococcus aureus*), *Mycobacterium* sp. causing multidrug resistant tuberculosis (MDR-TB), Extended spectrum beta lactmase (ESBL) producing gram-negative bacteria, Methicillin-Resistant *Staphylococcus epidermidis* (MRSE) [14].

Fungi mediated GNPs of silver (having higher catechins, apigenins, prochatechuic acid, etc.), can inhibit growth of clinically significant bacteria like *Staphylococcus aureus* and *Escherichia coli*. This composition further acts as potential antibacterial and antioxidative (reducing disease severity inside the host) [15]. The bio-inspired green nanoscience approach towards a broad spectrum of bacterial microbes infecting animals, humans, and plants have added valuable insights for tackling emerging antibiotic resistance, biogenetical implementation. The presence of biogenic silver nanoparticles has shown increased susceptibility of single or multidrug-resistant bacterial strains (*Streptococcus mutans*, *Acinetobacter baumannii*, respectively) towards antibiotic and GNP combination [16].

Coating of antimicrobial peptides (AMPs) with nano-liposomes, dextrans, chitosan improves in-vivo antibacterial efficacy of AMPs. A similar approach has been applied against foodborne bacteria of prime concern, including *Salmonella, Escherichia, Listeria,* and *Enterococcus* species. Using nanocoated AMPs has increased anti-microbial (against *Listeria* sp.) drug delivery up to 2000 folds [17]. The sustained and targeted release of antimicrobials by nano-drug delivery system possess highly desirable qualities like adaptability, biodegradation, sustained release, non-toxic residues, and others. The multidrug-resistant bacteria present a great clinical challenge that is difficult to counter in both human and animal cases. In this scenario, enhanced antimicrobial activity may be achieved by deploying GNPs in synergy with anti-biotics. In addition, the antimicrobial adjuvants may be designed using GNPs for therapy and vaccine against single or multidrug-resistant bacterial pathogens.

## 6.4   GREEN NANOPARTICLES (GNPS) AGAINST VIRUSES

The viruses, particularly RNA viruses, can mutate their genome fragments to show up as a new field of a challenge during/between subsequent disease outbreaks. This mutagenic ability of viruses makes them difficult to control via antiviral therapies and vaccines. The GNPs offer a highly customized, multi-dimensional, and safer inhibition of many human and animal viruses. Specific binding to envelop proteins of the virus, interference with genomic material (DNA/RNA) synthesis by pathway inhibition has shown the control of CoxB4 (Coxsackievirus), HAV-10 (Hepatitis A Virus), HSV-1 (Herpes Simplex Virus), H1N1 (Influenza Virus), Hepatitis B virus and others at lab scale [4]. Bacteria borne siRNA have been utilized to inhibit the respiratory syncytial virus genes in lab trials. The antiviral property of GNPs is exhibited at different stages of the viral life cycle. The inhibition of viral entry, internalization, and propagation may be disrupted by green mediated metal nanomaterials.

The organic lipid molecules offering genomic treatment against the hepatitis B virus have been marketed with the name ARB-001467 TKM-HBV® [18]. Some polyethylene glycolated interferons have been marketed for use against hepatitis B virus and hepatitis C virus. Organic nanocoated short interfering RNA (SiRNA) provides therapeutic gene silencing for Human Influenza Virus (H1N1, H5N1, H7N3) and Human Papilloma virus (HPV) [19]. All these therapeutic preparations provide better immunogenic coverage due to stabilized proteins/antigens. Similarly, the nano-lipid coated antiviral drugs are being trialed and validated against human viruses of prime concern, including, i.e., Zika virus, Ebola virus, herpes simplex virus, human parainfluenza virus, respiratory syncytial virus, human norovirus, and human immunodeficiency virus. The *in ovo* injection provided reasonable antiviral activity against one of the most important viruses of poultry (New Castle's Disease Virus) [20].

Bacteria (*E. coli*) expressed self-assembling virus like particles have been shown to offer protective immunity against swine influenza and swine circo viruses simultaneously. The economical industrial-scale production of nano-vaccines has been a concern. Recently, a non-invasive, intra-nasal, and broader spectrum of immunogenicity offering vaccines has been trialed against the influenza virus. The matrix protein from influenza virus was utilized to produce nanoparticle vaccine offering immune protection against both homosubtypic and heterosubtypic influenza virus [21]. Among other GNPs, silver nanoparticles have been most widely applied as antivirals in various lab trials. The molecular-scale study of protein docking by nanoparticles inside host could help validate them as safe. The associated concerns regarding toxicity and the level of protein-specific binding ability of GNPs need further probing. These would lead to commercialization of green nanoparticle approach against human, animal, and zoonotic viruses.

## 6.5   GREEN NANOPARTICLES (GNPS) AGAINST FUNGI

Fungi have been tested as both source and target for green nanoparticle synthesis. Fungi are unique eukaryotes that possess enzymes and proteins, capable of action as an efficient reducing and capping agents in nanoparticle synthesis. Plant-mediated green nano-synthesis has exhibited a broad zone of inhibition against *Aspergillus flaws, Aspergillus terreus, Candida albicans, Fusarium oxysperium, Penicillium camemeri, Trichophyton,* and *Rhizopus sp.* Fungal infections in human and animals present a great challenge in terms of local and systemic disease symptoms, reduced weight gains, secondary infectious diseases, resistance towards routine sanitation, and disinfection. Mycotoxicosis is a huge economic burden and difficult to tackle condition in livestock/poultry farming. Produced by one or more fungal strains, some of the important mycotoxins (toxic substances produced by fungi) are aflatoxins, fumonisins, ochratoxins, ergotamine, patulin, citrinin, trichothecenes, and zearalenone. Fungus (*Aspergillus niger*) mediated GNPs have exhibited their potential to inhibit pathogenic strains of fungi including: *Aspergillus flavus, Aspergillus fumigatus, Candida albicans, Candida tropicalis, Candida parapsilosis,* and *Candida krusei*. Similarly, the *Aspergillus niger* mediated nanoparticles having minimum inhibitory concentration (MIC) as low as 0.5–10 µL can arrest growth of *Fusarium oxysporum, Aspergillus flavus,* and *Penicillin digitatum*. The probable mechanism of toxicity induced in fungi is due to membrane damage, oxidative stress that eventually leads to cell death in the target species [22–24].

## 6.6   GREEN NANOPARTICLES (GNPS) AGAINST PARASITES

Parasites are the type of organisms that thrive at the expense of another organism by living inside or at the organism (host). Several species of parasites are known to cause heavy losses in terms of treatment costs, decreased production and performance, deaths, and associated preventive measures. Collectively, each year the parasites are affecting several billion people across the globe. The parasites are broadly classified into two major groups, namely ectoparasites (mosquitoes, ticks, lice, fleas, flies, mites, etc.), and endo-parasites (*Leishmania, Enterobius, Filaria, Setaria, Onchocerca, Ancylostoma,* etc.), based on their preferred location for utilizing food, shelter or other resources of the host. Apart from high disease and death toll, some parasites have become tolerant and/ or resistant to routinely used antiparasitic drugs. Consequently, this has shown aftermath in the form of hazardous residues in milk and meat of inadequately treated animals. The ultimate solution to this problem was to develop new groups of antiparasitic drugs, which could be time taking. However, among others, one of the most workable solutions is the use of green nanotechnology. It has shown widespread potential in diagnosing, treating, and preventing parasitic diseases.

Parasitic vectors like mosquitoes, ticks, fleas, lice, flies not only damage the skin/ hide of the host but also transmit widely spread infectious diseases of global concern (Malaria, Dengue virus, Zika virus, Crimean Congo hemorrhagic fever, River blindness, Leishmaniasis, Filariasis, etc.). The use of GNPs has shown success in the control of various life cycle stages of blood-feeding parasites and vectors of several pathogenic diseases, including ticks, mosquitoes, fleas, flies, lice, fresh-water snails, etc. The entomopathogenic fungus (*Isaria fumosorosea*) mediated green synthesis has shown $LC_{90}$ (lethal concentration at which 90% of population is killed) as low as 0.065 against larval stages of mosquitoes *Aedes aegypti* and *Culex quinquefasciatus*. The GNPs have shown to be 90–99% effective in controlling some species of ticks known to be a vector (living organism transmitting infectious disease/s) for human, livestock, and zoonotic diseases [25]. Some green nanoemulsions have also been shown to posses prolonged mosquito repellent properties, stable droplet size, and higher safety profile.

Several endo-parasites have been treated with GNPs *in vitro* and the studies have revealed a large promise in many gastrointestinal parasites (*Giardia, Echinococcus, Cryptosporidium, Entamoeba, Fasciola, Raillietina, Toxoplasma*, etc.), blood parasites (*Leishmania, Plasmodium*) as shown in Figure 6.5. One of the most significant application of this approach is anti-malarial and anti-leishmanial nano-delivered drugs for human use. Both parasitic diseases are of prime significance and endemic in many regions of the world. Silver GNPs have been shown to regulate pro-inflammatory cytokines, upregulate the anti-oxidation genes, proven as novel anti-toxoplasma therapeutic agent [1]. The use of biogenic nanoparticles can augment the in vitro efficacy of certain antiparasitic drugs, e.g., the effect of miltefosine was enhanced many times at lower doses using plant origin silver nanoparticles [26].

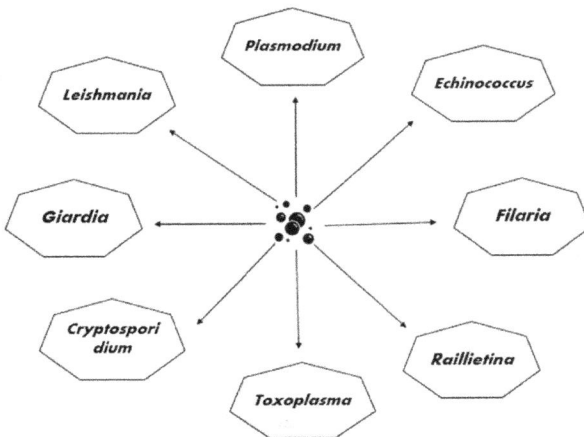

**FIGURE 6.5**   Green nanotechnology against endo-parasitic species.

Treatment of both ecto- and endo-parasites has been successfully carried out using green nanotechnology. The sole treatment of parasitic diseases of public health and veterinary significance has paved the way for the development of nanoparticles-conjugated drugs. Another avenue in the treatment of parasitic diseases is the use of nano-delivered drugs. Toxoplasmosis in humans could be prevented by the use of protein-based nano-vaccines. This vaccine basically enhances the ability of the host's immunity to present the parasite antigens in a repetitive manner, leading to self-assembling protein nanoparticle (SAPN) mediated immune response. Similarly, the green nanoparticle vaccine adjuvants have been shown to act as potential immune protectants in commercially significant diseases of livestock, e.g., chicken coccidiosis. Another potential use of nanoparticles in parasitology is the use in diagnostic testing. The green nanotechnology is yet to be trialed for use in diagnostic testing against vector-borne diseases of humans.

## 6.7　MISCELLANEOUS APPLICATIONS OF GREEN NANOMATERIALS

GNPs have exhibited efficacy in treating and preventing carcinoma (cancer) of immune, nervous, reproductive, and musculoskeletal system. Xiang et al. [27] have reported the use of polystyrene nanoparticle (PSNP) vaccine conjugated to human proteins (E7, SV, and WT1) to generate and potentiate host immunity towards human gynecological cancers, as demonstrated in animal models. Also, the immune-stimulating complexes (ISCOMS) of <40 nm size have shown enhanced host immunity against many types of cancers. Recently, the use of soya bean oil-based nanoemul-sion has shown protective immune efficacy against a food allergy [28]. The work on cancer nano-vaccines are progressively heading to clinical trials in humans. However, there is limited success in terms of preven-tion. More research is being directed to tackle the clinical challenges thus associated. The GNPs are being probed for their potential use as anti-microbial adjuvants, offering sustainable, easily biodegradable, and less hazardous solutions against pathogens. The use of green nanotechnology in composite treatment may also be channelized in the same manner as directed pathogen killing has been achieved using nanoparticles of metallic origin. The use in gene therapies, tissue engendering, diagnostics, and imaging is also underway, as indicated in Figure 6.6.

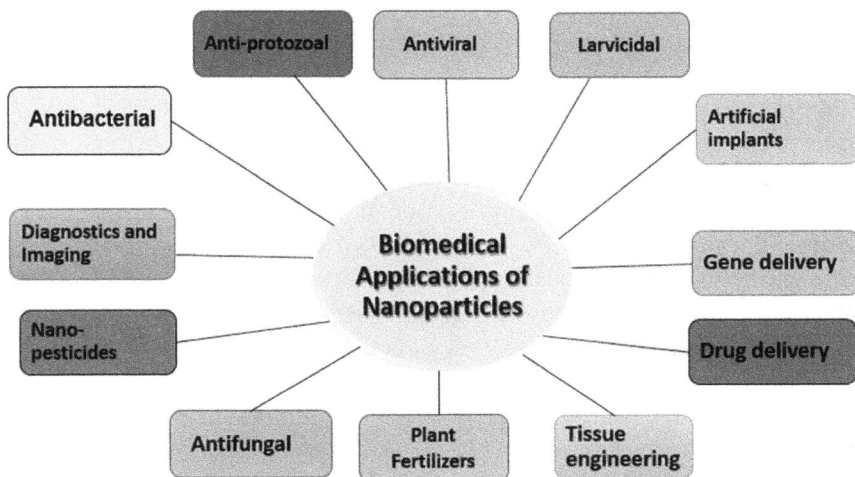

**FIGURE 6.6** Biomedical applications of nanoparticles.

## 6.8 CONCERNS ASSOCIATED WITH GREEN NANOTECHNOLOGY

As for metallic nanoparticle synthesis, the toxic potential of reactants is questionable. However, it is presumed and somewhat validated that the biogenetic nanoparticles are more biodegradable, renewable, and least toxigenic compared with metallic NPs. Apart from this, the commercial scalability of green nanotechnology needs to be further strengthened. Extensive use of biological sources (plants/marine life) may lead to disturbance in the eco-biology of the associated niche. Interactions (pharmacokinetics and pharmacodynamics) of nano-therapeutics and nano-vaccines within the host bodies are intricate and not well studied. However, it is presumed that nanoparticles can internalize the cells of the skin, lungs, gastrointestinal tract, and brain. The localization of metals in these organs of the infected host is one of major concern. It is imperative to further investigate the mechanisms of target pathogen toxicity and the development of therapeutic windows. In addition, the development and standardization of model biological organisms for use in diagnostic toxicity assays needs more research focus. Following the one health approach, it is important to not only safely administer, but also adequately dispose-off the nanoparticles and/or their hazardous metabolites.

## 6.9   CONCLUSIONS AND OUTLOOK

There are extensive research efforts globally on green nanotechnology against bacteria, viruses, fungi, and parasites. The combined efforts in this regard have proposed eco-friendly, economical, and safer solutions to the human, animal, and environmental health concerns. Sustainable production in terms of green nanoparticle production is a question to be addressed. In addition, it is imperative to scale-up, commercialize, and materialize the efficient production of GNPs in treating and preventing human, animal, and plant pathogens of concern.

## KEYWORDS

- **atomic force microscopy**
- **dynamic light scattering**
- **Fourier transform infrared spectroscopy**
- **green nanoparticles**
- **parasites**
- **vectors**

## REFERENCES

1. Alajmi, R. A., Al-Megrin, W. A., Metwally, D., Al-Subaie, H., Altamrah, N., Barakat, A. M., Abdel, M. A. E., et al., (2019). Anti-*toxoplasma* activity of silver nanoparticles green synthesized with *Phoenix dactylifera* and *Ziziphus spina-christi* extracts which inhibits inflammation through liver regulation of cytokines in Balb/c mice. *Biosci Rep., 39*(5), BSR20190379.
2. Zdrojewicz, Z., Waracki, M., Bugaj, B., Pypno, D., & Cabała, K., (2015). Medical applications of nanotechnology. *Postepy. Hig. Med. Dosw., 69*, 1196–1204.
3. Ali, K., Dwivedi, S., Azam, A., Saquib, Q., Al-Said, M. S., Alkhedhairy, A. A., & Musarrat, J., (2016). Aloe vera extract functionalized zinc oxide nanoparticles as nanoantibiotics against multidrug resistant clinical bacterial isolates. *J. Colloid. Interf. Sci., 472*, 145–156.

4. Haggag, E. G., Elshamy, E. M., Rabeh, M. A., Gabr, N. M., Salem, M., Youssif, K. A., Samir, A., et al., (2019). Antiviral potential of green synthesized silver nanoparticles of *Lampranthus coccineus* and *Malephora lutea*. *Int. J. Nanomed., 14*, 6217–6229.

5. Sharmila, G., Fathima, M. F., Haries, S., Geetha, S., Kumar, N. M., & Muthukumaran, C., (2017). Green synthesis, characterization, and antibacterial efficacy of palladium nanoparticles synthesized using *Filicium decipiens* leaf extract. *J. Mol. Struct., 1138*(2017), 35–40.

6. Garcia-Moure, M., Martinez-Velez, N., Patino-Garcia, A., & Alonso, M. M., (2017). Oncolytic adenoviruses as a therapeutic approach for osteosarcoma: A new hope. *J. Bone Oncol., 9*, 41–47.

7. Saratale, R. G., Saratale, G. D., Shin, H. S., Jacob, J. M., Pugazhendhi, A., Bhaisare, M., & Kumar, G., (2018). New insights on the green synthesis of metallic nanoparticles using plant and waste biomaterials: Current knowledge, their agricultural and environmental applications. *Environ. Sci. Poll. Res., 25*(11), 10164–10183.

8. Zada, S., Ahmad, A., Khan, S., Yu, X., Chang, K., Iqbal, A., Ahmad, A., et al., (2018). Biogenic synthesis of silver nanoparticles using extracts of *Leptolyngbya* JSC-1 that induce apoptosis in HeLa cell line and exterminate pathogenic bacteria. *Artificial Cells, Nanomedicine, and Biotechnology., 46*, S471–S480.

9. Abdel-Raouf, N., Al-Enazi, N. M., & Ibraheem, I. B. M., (2017). Green biosynthesis of gold nanoparticles using *Galaxaura elongata* and characterization of their antibacterial activity. *Arab. J. Chem., 10*, S3029–S3039.

10. Arya, A., Gupta, K., Chundawat, T. S., & Vaya, D., (2018). Biogenic synthesis of copper and silver nanoparticles using green alga *Botryococcus braunii* and its antimicrobial activity. *Bioorg. Chem., 2018*, 9.

11. Elango, G., Roopan, S. M., Dhamodaran, K. I., Elumalai, K., Al-Dhabi, N. A., & Arasu, M. V., (2016). Spectroscopic investigation of biosynthesized nickel nanoparticles and its larvicidal, pesticidal activities. *J. Photochem. Photobiol. B., 162*(2016), 162–167.

12. Joshi, S. M., Britto, S. D., Jogaiah, S., & Ito, S., (2019). Mycogenic selenium nanoparticles as potential new generation broad-spectrum antifungal molecules. *Biomolecules, 9*, 419.

13. Zahir, A. A., Chauhan, I. S., Bagavan, A., Kamaraj, C., Elango, G., Shankar, J., Arjaria, N., et al., (2015). Green synthesis of silver and titanium dioxide nanoparticles using *Euphorbia prostrata* extract shows shift from apoptosis to G0/G1 arrest followed by necrotic cell death in *Leishmania donovani*. *Antimicrob. Agents Chemother., 59*, 4782–4799.

14. Punjabi, K., Mehta, S., Chavan, R., Chitalia, V., Deogharkar, D., & Deshpande, S., (2018). Efficiency of biosynthesized silver and zinc nanoparticles against multidrug resistant pathogens. *Front. Microbiol., 9*, 2207.

15. Jogaiah, S., Kurjogi, M., Abdelrahman, M., Hanumanthappa, N., & Tran, L. P., (2019). *Ganoderma applanatum*-mediated green synthesis of silver nanoparticles: Structural characterization, and *in vitro* and *in vivo* biomedical and agrochemical properties. *Arab. J. Chem., 12*(7), 1108–1120.

16. Singh, R., Wagh, P., Wadhwani, S., Gaidhani, S., Kumbhar, A., Bellare, J., & Chopade, B. A., (2013). Synthesis, optimization, and characterization of silver nanoparticles from *Acinetobacter calcoaceticus* and their enhanced antibacterial activity when combined with antibiotics. *Int. J. Nanomed., 8*, 4277–4290.

17. Cantor, S., Vargas, L., Rojas, A. O. E., Yarce, C. J., Salamanca, C. H., & Oñate-Garzón, J., (2019). Evaluation of the antimicrobial activity of cationic peptides loaded in surface-modified nanoliposomes against foodborne bacteria. *Int. J. Mol. Sci., 20*(3), 680.

18. Singh, L., Kruger, H. G., Maguire, G. E. M., Govender, T., & Parboosing, R., (2017). The role of nanotechnology in the treatment of viral infections. *Ther. Adv. Infectious Dis., 4*(4), 105–131.

19. Fatima, M., Zaidi, N. U., Amraiz, D., & Afzal, F., (2016). *In vitro* antiviral activity of *Cinnamomum cassia* and its nanoparticles against H7N3 influenza a virus. *J. Microbiol. Biotechnol., 26*(1), 151–159.

20. Yugandhar, P., Vasavi, T., Rao, Y. J., Devi, P. U. M., Narasimha, G., & Savithramma, N., (2018). Cost effective, green synthesis of copper oxide nanoparticles using fruit extract of *Syzygium alternifolium* (Wt.) Walp., characterization and evaluation of antiviral activity. *Clust. Sci., 29*, 743.

21. Qi, M., Sun, X., Zhang, X., Li, W., Zhang, Z., & Cui, Z., (2018). Intranasal nanovaccine confers homo- and hetero-subtypic influenza protection. *Small, 14*, 1703207.

22. Medda, S., Hajra, A., Dey, U., Bose, P., & Mondal, N. K., (2015). Biosynthesis of silver nanoparticles from *Aloe vera* leaf extract and antifungal activity against *Rhizopus* sp. and *Aspergillus* sp. *Appl. Nanosci., 5*, 875–880.

23. Rodríguez-Luis, O. E., Hernandez-Delgadillo, R., Sánchez-Nájera, R. I., Martínez-Castañón, G. A., Niño-Martínez, N., Navarro, M. C. S., Ruiz, F., & Cabral-Romero, C., (2016). Green Synthesis of silver nanoparticles and their bactericidal and antimycotic activities against oral microbes. *J. Nanomater., 2016*, 10.

24. Folorunso, A., Akintelu, S., Oyebamiji, A. K., Ajayi, S., Abiola, B., Abdusalam, I., & Morakinyo, M., (2019). Biosynthesis, characterization, and antimicrobial activity of gold nanoparticles from leaf extracts of *Annona muricate. J. Nanostruct. Chem., 9*, 111.

25. Rajakumar, G., Rahuman, A. A., Roopan, S. M., Chung, I. M., Anbarasan, K., & Karthikeyan, V., (2015). Efficacy of larvicidal activity of green synthesized titanium dioxide nanoparticles using *Mangifera indica* extract against blood-feeding parasites. *Parasitol. Res., 114*, 571–581.

26. Kalangi, S. K., Dayakar, A., Gangappa, D., Sathyavathi, R., Maurya, D. S., & Rao, D. N., (2016). Biocompatible silver nanoparticles reduced from *Anethum graveolens* leaf extract augments the antileishmanial efficacy of miltefosine. *Exp. Parasitol., 170*, 184–192.

27. Xiang, S. D., Wilson, K. L., Goubier, A., Heyerick, A., & Plebanski, M., (2018). Design of Peptide-based nanovaccines targeting leading antigens from gynecological cancers to induce HLA-A2.1 restricted CD8+ T-cell responses. *Front. Immunol., 9*, 2968.

28. O'Konek, J. J., & Baker, J. R., (2020). Treatment of allergic disease with nanoemulsion adjuvant vaccines. *Allergy, 75*, 246–249.

# CHAPTER 7

# Antimicrobial Applications of Green Synthesized Nanoparticles and Nanocomposites of Silver

JAISON JEEVANANDAM,[1] BALA S. C. KORITALA,[2,3]
MALAKONDAIAH SURESH,[4] STEPHEN BOAKYE-ANSAH,[5] and
MICHAEL K. DANQUAH[6]

[1]*Department of Chemical Engineering, Faculty of Engineering and Science, Curtin University, CDT 250, Miri – 98009, Sarawak, Malaysia, E-mail: jaison.jeevanandam@gmail.com*

[2]*Department of Pharmaceutical Sciences, College of Pharmacy and Pharmaceutical Sciences, Washington State University, Spokane, WA – 99202, USA*

[3]*Sleep and Performance Research Center, Washington State University, Spokane, WA – 99210, USA*

[4]*Loyola Institute of Frontier Energy, Post Graduate and Research Department of Advanced Zoology and Biotechnology, Loyola College, Chennai – 600034, Tamil Nadu, India*

[5]*Department of Chemical Engineering, Henry M. Rowan College of Engineering, Rowan University, 201 Mullica Hill Road, Glassboro, NJ – 08028, United States*

[6]*Chemical Engineering Department, University of Tennessee, Chattanooga, TN – 37403, USA*

## ABSTRACT

Nanotechnology has provided numerous exciting materials with a variety of opportunities to be utilized for exclusive applications that are not possible with their bulk counterparts. Metal nanoparticles are the most common nanosized particles that are extensively under research and are currently employed in various commercial applications. Among metal nanoparticles, silver nanoparticles are widely used for biomedical applications, due to their unique optical properties, enhanced stability, bioreactivity, and bioavailability. In addition, the silver nanoparticles are known for their effective microbial cell inhibition ability. The challenges related to the toxicity of chemically and physically synthesized silver nanoparticles can be reduced using green synthesis methods. In addition, the incorporation of different metals with silver to create nanocomposites is reported to increase antimicrobial efficacy. This chapter provides an overview of various green synthesis approaches used for the production of silver nanoparticles and their efficacy in exhibiting antimicrobial activity. Moreover, the potential antimicrobial mechanism of silver nanomaterials and the future of silver nanoparticles are discussed.

## 7.1  INTRODUCTION

There are numerous nanoparticles that are fabricated for biomedical applications due to the advantages in the field of nanotechnology, the need for alternate drugs to replace conventional medicines, and the exclusive biomedical properties of nanosized particles [1]. Metal nanoparticles are the most common and are widely fabricated for various electronic, environmental, and biomedical applications, as they are highly reactive and easy to fabricate [2]. Among metal nanoparticles, silver nanoparticles are extensively fabricated for innumerable applications, especially in biomedical and pharmaceutical fields [3]. Silver nanoparticles are widely fabricated via physical approaches such as laser ablation [4], radiofrequency sputtering [5], and ball milling [6]. Although physical approaches are beneficial in yielding silver nanoparticles (<100 nm in size), the cost involved in yielding large-scale production has led to an economy-based limitation [7]. Chemical methods such as precipitation [8], hydrothermal [9], solvothermal [10], and sol-gel approaches [11] are used to yield nanoparticles (10–100 nm) with less cost, as an alternative to physical methods. However, this approach cannot be utilized to fabricate nanoparticles for biomedical applications, as the chemicals used as reducing and stabilizing agents are toxic to living cells [12]. Thus, researchers are turning toward green synthesis approaches using microbes and plants as a source of non-toxic reducing and stabilizing agents for use in biomedical applications.

Green synthesis approaches are generally sub-classified into microbial and plant-based methods, depending on the organism from which the extracts are obtained [13]. The extracts contain secondary metabolites that, while not essential for the growth of the organism, possess biomolecules which are proven to reduce, initiate nucleation, and stabilize their nanostructure of metal precursors [14]. It is noteworthy that the secondary metabolites of bacteria, fungi, and algae are extensively employed to fabricate silver nanoparticles [15]. Similarly, plant extracts containing phytochemicals, which contain flavonoids, tannins, terpenoids, phenols, and other phytocompounds, are responsible for the formation of silver nanoparticles as well as nanocomposites [16]. Generally, silver is known for its exclusive antimicrobial property, since ancient times [17]. Nanosized silver possesses enhanced antimicrobial efficacy towards a wide variety of microbes, compared to its bulk counterparts [18]. Green, or biosynthesized, silver nanoparticles and nanocomposites are fabricated to exhibit their characteristic antimicrobial properties with minimized toxicity towards other living organisms and the environment [19]. An overview of various green synthesis approaches used for the production of silver nanoparticles and their efficacy in exhibiting antimicrobial activity are discussed in this chapter. And also, the potential antimicrobial mechanism of silver nanomaterial and the future of silver nanoparticles are discussed.

## 7.2 GREEN SYNTHESIS OF NANOSIZED SILVER PARTICLES

Microbes and plants are the major significant source of biological agents that are extensively used for the formation and synthesis of nanosized silver particles. The extracts of these biological organisms, such as enzymes and secondary metabolites, are proven to possess the ability to reduce silver precursors, initiate nucleation to form nanoparticles, and stabilize them to avoid agglomeration, which may lead to increases in size to micro-sized particles. Figure 7.1 shows the Transmission Electron Microscope (TEM) images of various silver nanoparticles that are fabricated via the biological organism-based green approach.

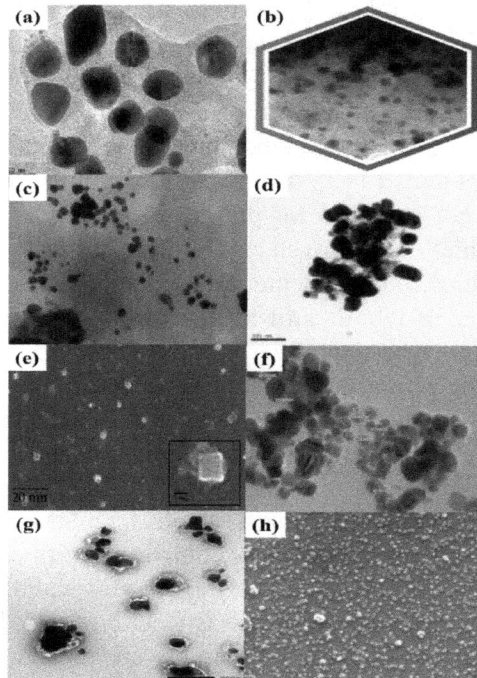

**FIGURE 7.1**   The electron micrograph of biosynthesized silver nanoparticles from the extracts of bacterial strains such as (a) *Nocardiopsis* species [20], (b) *Escherichia coli* [21], algal species of *Sargassum longifolium* [22], (c) *Spirulina platensis* [23], (d) fungal species of *Aspergillus fumigatus* [24], (e) *Fusarium oxysporum* [25] and plant species of (f) *Crinum latifolium* [26] and (g) *Clitoria ternatea* [27].

*Source:* All these images were obtained from the open access articles from Hindawi publications, which are distributed under the Creative Commons Attribution License.

## 7.2.1   *BACTERIA-MEDIATED SYNTHESIS*

There are more than 40 gram-negative and gram-positive bacterial species that have been identified for the fabrication of nanosized silver particles with various sizes and shapes [28, 29]. Although the majority of bacterial species are associated with extracellular synthesis, certain bacterial species such as *Brevibacterium casei, Bacillus cereus*, and the *Idiomarina* species synthesize nanosized silver particles inside the cell [28]. However, few bacterial species are capable of synthesizing nanosized silver via both intra- and extracellular approaches. Interestingly, nanoparticle depositions have been identified in the periplasmic space [30] or cell-free extracts [31] in two distinct *Bacillus* species. The sizes of silver particles that are fabricated via bacterial species are below 200 nm in diameter with morphologies such as spheres, quasi-spheres, triangle, rod, disk, cube, and hexagons. There are various catalytic proteins and cofactors, namely reductases and nicotinamide adenine dinucleotide (NADH), which are involved in bacterial mediated nanosized silver synthesis [32]. Importantly, nitrate reductase is a key enzyme involved in the bioreduction of the ionic silver to produce nanosized silver in several species, including *Enterobacter, Pseudomonas, Escherichia,* and *Bacillus* [33–36]. There are also augmented recovery mechanisms reported with increased pH and bioreduction rate of nanosized silver particles in *Lactobacillus* species [37]. Additionally, visible light is also proven to be an influencing factor in the production of nanosized silver via culture supernatants of *Klebsiella pneumonia* [38]. Based on the known mechanisms, it is noteworthy that the enzymes and cofactors play crucial roles in the bioreduction of silver ions to silver nanoparticles in multiple bacterial species.

Recently, Gurunathan [39] reported that the *Bacillus cereus* culture supernatants can be utilized for the extracellular fabrication of nanosized silver particles. The resultant nanoparticles are 2–16 nm in size with excellent homogeneity and a quasi-spherical shape. Further, the fabricated nanosized silver has exhibited superior wide-spectrum antibacterial efficacy against *Streptococcus mutans* and *Escherichia fergusonii*, similar with conventional antibiotics such as vancomycin and gentamycin [39]. Similarly, Divya et al. [40] isolated extracts from 57 bacterial species from corals and found the isolates of *Alcaligenes* species to be beneficial for silver nanoparticle fabrication. The synthesized nanosized particles are spherical and irregular in shape ranging from 30–50 nm in size. These nanosized particles are further demonstrated to possess efficient antibacterial properties against human urinary tract pathogens such as *Staphylococcus aureus, Escherichia coli, Pseudomonas aeruginosa, Candida albicans, Bacillus* species, and *Klebsiella pneumonia* [40]. Likewise, Almaki, and Khalifa [41] fabricated nanosized silver using extracellular extracts from culture supernatants of the marine *Bacillus* species KFU36 strain. The resultant nanoparticles are 5–15 nm in size with a spherical morphology and are employed to exhibit anticancer ability. The silver nanoparticles synthesized via bacterial extracts showed superior anticancer efficacy by inhibiting 61% of breast cancer cells via dosage-depended toxic reactions

[41]. All these studies demonstrated that the silver nanoparticles fabricated via bacterial extracts, as shown in Figure 7.2, possess enhanced biological properties with biocompatibility and bioavailability.

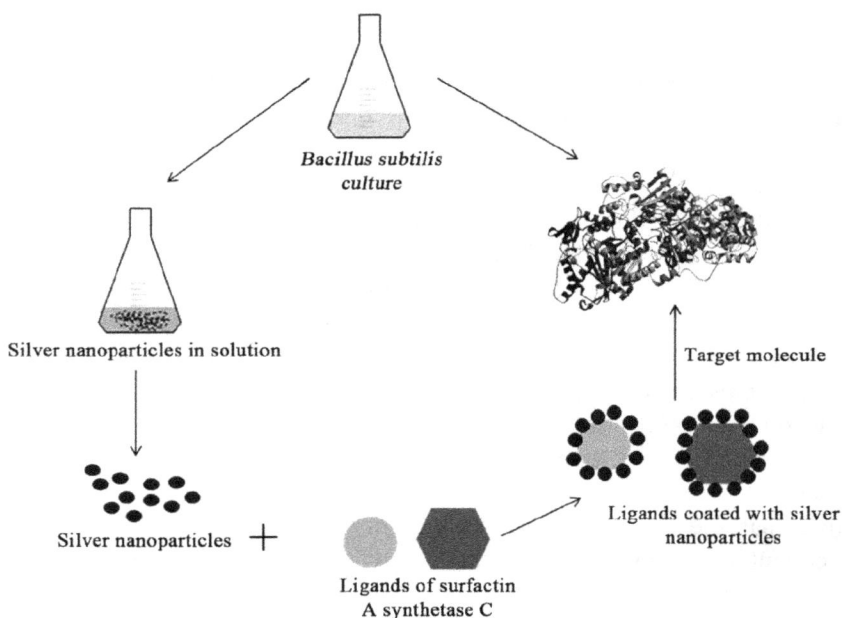

**FIGURE 7.2**    Synthesis of silver nanoparticles using bacterial extracts.
*Source:* Reproduced from [42], IOP Publication.

## 7.2.2   ALGAE-MEDIATED SYNTHESIS

The first algal species used for nanosized silver synthesis was *Plectonema boryanum* [43]. Over the past decade, different classes of micro and macroalgal species (Cyanobacteria, green, red, and brown algae) have been utilized for the fabrication of nanosized silver. Initial findings suggest a metabolism-dependent mechanism in cyanobacteria for the bioreduction of silver nitrate ($AgNO_3$) to generate silver nanoparticles [43]. Further, Xie et al. [44] synthesized nanosized silver particles via unicellular green *Chlorella vulgaris* algal extracts under kinetically controlled processes, where hydroxyl tyrosine groups were involved in the biological reduction of ionic silver, with the shape of the nanosized silver controlled by carboxyl groups of aspartic and glutamic acid [44, 45]. Similarly, Barwal et al. [46] reported that *in vivo* synthesis approaches are comparatively faster than *in vitro* synthesis methods using *Chlamydomonas reinhardtii* biochemical extracts. Their experimental observations suggested that metabolic components alter the size and biosynthesis rate of nanosized silver formation [46]. Furthermore, the amount of both chlorophyll and primary amines are involved in the alteration of nanoparticle size and bioreduction of ionic silver using extracts of *Euglena* species [47]. Incubation temperatures and pH are also reported to be involved in the optimization of size and the production rate of nanosized silver particles [48]. Based on the recent literature, 80 μg/ml of biomass, 1 mM concentration of silver nitrate as precursor, pH of 5.5, temperature of 60C, and 1 h of ultraviolet exposure is considered as favorable conditions for the optimal synthesis of nanosized silver using extracts of *Microchaete* species [49].

Fatima et al. [50] synthesized novel nanosized silver particles via extracts that are obtained from red *Portieria hornemannii*. The results showed that the algal extract led to the formation of spherical nanoparticles with an average size of 60–70 nm. Further, the study revealed that these nanoparticles possess enhanced antibacterial efficacy against pathogens such as *Vibrio harveyii*, *Vibrio anguillarum*, *Vibrio alginolyticus,* and *Vibrio parahaemolyticus* that can infect fishes and cause diseases [50]. Likewise, Bhuyur et al. [51] utilized extracts from marine Padina species macroalgae for the synthesis of silver nanoparticles. The resultant nanoparticles are 25–60 nm in size with irregular shapes and several aggregations. The study also showed that these biosynthesized nanoparticles possess growth inhibition properties against *Pseudomonas aeruginosa* (gram-negative) and *Staphylococcus aureus* (gram-positive) strains of bacteria [51]. Recently, it has been stated by Hamida et al. [52] that the extracellular isolates of *Cyanobacteria desertifilum* species are useful in the fabrication of nanosized silver particles. The study revealed that the utilization of *Cyanobacteria* have led to the formation of 4.5 to 26 nm-sized silver particles with spherical shapes. Further, the findings demonstrated that these nanoparticles are highly efficient as an antibacterial agent that can inhibit five significant bacterial pathogens, including multidrug-resistant strains, with effective anticancer efficacy against liver, breast, and colorectal cancer cells [52]. These studies show the benefits of utilizing algal extracts in the formation of biologically significant silver nanoparticles with properties that are useful for biomedical applications.

### 7.2.3   BIOSYNTHESIS OF SILVER NANOPARTICLES VIA FUNGAL EXTRACTS

Among all other microbes, fungi have enormous potential for the large-scale synthesis of nanosized silver, due to their high tolerance towards metals and their ability to produce huge biomass. Moreover, fungi secrete large amounts of extracellular proteins and enzymes with the potential to reduce ionic silver via fungal filtrates, and help in the sustainable formation of nanosized silver [53]. However, nanosized silver particles that are produced through the utilization of intra or extracellular regions of fungal cultures must be further purified via chemicals, filtration, and centrifugation approaches [54–57]. Although cofactors such as NADH, nicotinamide adenine dinucleotide phosphate (NADPH), and reductase enzymes are reported to be necessary for the bioreduction of ionic silver, while using *Fusarium oxysporum* fungal extracts [58, 59], a recent study suggested that NADPH can drive nanosized particle formation without any need of nitrate reductase enzyme [60]. However, there are more studies required to understand the action of free NADPH in the bioreduction process. Similar to other organisms, the optimal parameters for synthesis of nanoparticles are identified to be biomass, dispersion media, light, pH, temperature, and concentration of precursor [55, 61–64]. Several fungal species used for optimizing the synthesis of nanosized silver include *Aspergillus* [65–68], *Colleotrichum* [69], *Duddingtonia* [70], *Epicoccum* [71], *Fusarium* [62, 72, 73], *Guignardia* [74], *Isaria* [75], *Penicillium* [68, 76, 77], *Rhizoctonia* [56], *Rhizopus* [78], *Sclerotinia* [63], and *Trichoderma* [79–81]. The results from all these studies suggested that distinct culture conditions are responsible for producing silver nanoparticles with specific characteristics, and the exact parameters that influence the individual characteristics of resultant nanoparticles are still unclear. However, the results suggested that optimization methods may vary depending on the fungal species that were utilized for silver nanoparticle fabrication.

Recently, Feroz et al. [82] synthesized 60–80 nm-sized spherical shaped silver particles using metabolites that are extracted from *Penicillium oxalicum* fungal species. These nanoparticles showed enhanced antibacterial activity against pathogenic bacterial strains such as *Staphylococcus aureus*, *Salmonella typhi,* and *Shigella dysenteriae* [82]. Further, Yousef et al. [83] reported that the nanosized silver particles with an average size of 9.8 nm can be fabricated using the supernatant cell filtrate of endophytic

*Alternaria tenuissima* fungi that are isolated from healthy *Ruta graveolans* plant leaves. These spherical nanosized particles are further established to be a potent antimicrobial agent able to inhibit the growth of pathogenic *Candida albicans* and several bacterial strains along with free radical scavenging and antioxidant properties [83]. Likewise, Kobashigawa et al. [84] fabricated nanosized silver particles using the metabolite extract of the white-rot ligninolytic basidiomycete fungi named *Trametes trogii*. The resultant nanoparticles are irregularly shaped with the nanosized spheres as predominant particles being in cluster with an average size of 15 nm. Further, the study showed that the addition of strong basic sodium hydroxide solution to adjust pH has a significant effect in yielding nanosized spherical shaped particles [84]. Moreover, 100 nm-sized silver particles were fabricated via extracts of the endophytic fungi named *Cladosporium cladosporioides* that are isolated from brown *Sargasssum wightii* algae. The findings revealed that the reductase of NADPH is responsible for the nanosized particle formation and facilitates effective antimicrobial and free radical scavenging properties [85]. All these studies emphasized that the fungal extracts support the formation of nanosized silver particles and improve their biological properties.

### 7.2.4   SYNTHESIS OF SILVER NANOPARTICLES VIA PLANT EXTRACTS

Numerous plant materials, including leaves, peels, flowers, seeds, rhizomes, and fruits, are reported to facilitate nanosized silver particle synthesis [86, 87]. The protocol used for the synthesis of nanoparticles via plant material is both economical and eco-friendly. The methods involved in plant-based nanosized silver particle synthesis involve preparation of plant broth, followed by the addition of silver nitrate as precursor to the filtered plant broth to initiate the nucleation process [86]. Biomolecules of plant broth such as amino acids, organic acids, proteins, vitamins, and secondary metabolites are involved in the reduction and stabilization of ionic silver to form nanosized silver. However, the exact mechanisms are not yet known [87] with reports suggesting that components and mechanisms involved in silver nanoparticle fabrication may vary between plant species [88, 89]. Among extracts obtained from distinct plant parts, leaves are considered as the most common substrates to be beneficial for plant-based silver nanoparticle synthesis, due to its economic advantage. In addition to culture conditions such as temperature, higher levels of carbohydrates, flavonoids, steroids, sapogenins, and other phytochemicals play significant roles in the production of stable silver nanoparticles [86].

Recently, there are several studies which have shown plant extracts as potential candidates for nanoparticle fabrication, especially nanosized noble metals including silver. Banasiuk et al. [90] utilized phytochemical extracts from four carnivorous plants, namely *Drosera indica, Drosera spatulata, Drosera binata,* and *Dionaea muscipula* for the synthesis of silver nanoparticles. The resultant nanoparticles are quasi-spherical with 10–60 nm range with the study also confirming that parameters such as the addition of polyvinylpyrrolidone (PVP), heat radiation, and microwave irradiation are responsible for the nanosized particle formation. Further, the study revealed that these nanoparticles possess properties that allow efficient inhibition of human and plant pathogens [90]. Similarly, Nasr et al. [91] demonstrated that the aqueous extract of lemon peel could be a novel and a potent stabilizing and reducing agent for silver nanoparticle fabrication. The presence of exclusive phytochemicals in the peel extracts has led to the formation of spherical, 9.3–20.3 nm-sized silver particles with excellent antibacterial activity against gram-positive *S. aureus* and *B. subtilis* bacterial strains, along with antifungal efficacy against *Candida albicans* and *Aspergillus flavus* [91]. Likewise, Balu et al. [92] recently reported that 30–40 nm-sized silver with heterogenous shapes could be synthesized using aqueous extracts obtained from a medicinal grass variety of *Saccharum spontaneum.* The nanoparticles are stated to be in hexagonal, rod-like, spherical, and triangular shape with effective antibacterial activity against several bacterial pathogens. In addition, the study emphasized that these nanosized silver particles are highly compatible with blood and enhance the proliferation of MG63 osteoblast cells [92]. Further, Aygun et al. [93] also demonstrated that *Ganoderma lucidum* aqueous extract produced with microwave assistance could lead to spherical and 15–22 nm-sized silver particles. These nanoparticles also possess efficient antibacterial properties against both gram-positive and gram-negative strains of bacteria and antifungal efficacy [93]. These studies emphasized that phytochemicals from plants can be extensively utilized for the fabrication of nanosized silver particles in the latest green synthesis modalities as displayed in Figure 7.3.

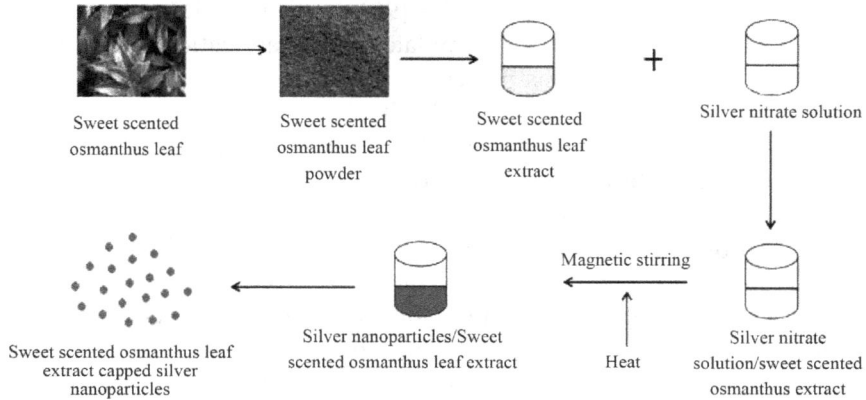

**FIGURE 7.3**   Synthesis of silver nanoparticles via plant extracts.
*Source:* Reproduced from [94], Scientific and Academic Publishing.

## 7.2.5   OTHER NOVEL SYNTHESIS APPROACHES

In recent times, there have been several novel methods that have been introduced for the biosynthesis of nanosized silver particles, which includes utilization of milk proteins, spider web, and extracts from agricultural wastes. Athreya et al. [95] reported that silver nanoparticles could be fabricated by using egg white, pasteurized, and raw milk of cow and lysozyme. This novel synthesis method led to the formation of 20–20 nm-sized silver particles with spherical morphology and showed that the proteins present in these biological substances are responsible for the nanoparticle fabrication by acting as a potential reducing as well as a stabilizing agent. Moreover, the results revealed that these novel nanoparticles possess the ability to inhibit the proliferation of bacterial strains such as *Bacillus subtilis, Escherichia coli, Staphylococcus aureus, Bacillus cereus,* and *Pseudomonas alcaligenes* [95]. Similarly, milk from *Camelus dromedarius* was used as a novel reducing agent for the formation of nanosized silver particles. This camel milk-mediated synthesis approach has led to the formation of 200–300 nm-sized silver particles via casein micelles, kappa casein, insulin, and niacin as major components that might be responsible for their formation by acting as effective reduction and stabilization agents. These nanoparticles also possess enhanced antibacterial efficacy against oral pathogenic *Staphylococcus aureus* and

*Streptococcus mutans* bacterial strains [96]. Further, spider web has been proposed as a novel biomaterial template for the fabrication of nanosized silver particles. The proteins present in the spider web were reported to be the significant factors for the synthesis of spherical and 3–50 nm-sized silver nanoparticles by acting as an efficient capping and reducing agent. Further, the study showed that these novel nanoparticles possess enhanced antibacterial activity against airborne pathogens and are useful for the production of antibacterial emulsion paints [97]. Furthermore, spherical, and 25 nm-sized silver particles have been fabricated using the secondary metabolite extract obtained from dragon fruit peel with effective antibacterial properties [98]. Moreover, extracts that are obtained from market vegetable wastes [99], timber industry wastes [100], and agricultural wastes of *Annona squamosa* peel extract [101] and wastes of grape pomace [102] are under extensive research for use in synthesis of novel silver nanoparticles. Table 7.1 is the summary of various silver nanoparticles that are synthesized via green/biological approaches.

**TABLE 7.1**    Green Synthesized Silver Nanoparticles Using Biological Sources

| Bacteria-Mediated Synthesis of Silver Nanoparticles | | |
|---|---|---|
| **Biological Source** | **Characteristics** | **References** |
| *Bacillus cereus* | Quasi-spherical, 2–16 nm size | [39] |
| *Alcaligenes* species | 30–50 nm in size and spherical as well as irregular morphology | [40] |
| Marine *Bacillus* species KFU36 | 5–15 nm in size with spherical morphology | [41] |
| *Bacillus subtilis* T. | Spherical morphology with antibacterial efficacy | [103] |
| *Bacillus brevis* (NCIM 2533) | 41–68 nm with spherical morphology | [104] |
| *Pseudomonas aeruginosa, Escherichia coli, Acinetobacter baumannii,* and *Staphylococcus aureus* | 11–15 nm-sized with spherical morphology | [105] |
| Bacterial exopolysaccharide | 35 nm-sized with spherical morphology | [106] |
| *Bacillus flexus* and *Bacillus pseudomycoides* | Spherical and pseudo-spherical morphology with 30–70 nm size | [107] |
| *Lactobacillus delbrueckii* subsp. *bulgaricus* | Polyhedral and spherical morphology with 1–9 nm | [108] |
| *Bacillus methylotrophicus* | Spherical morphology with 10–30 nm size | [109] |

**TABLE 7.1**   *(Continued)*

Algae-Mediated Silver Nanoparticle Synthesis

| | | |
|---|---|---|
| Red *Portieria hornemannii* | Spherical shaped 60–70 nm sizes | [50] |
| Marine Padina species macroalgae | Irregular shaped 25–60 nm-sized nanoparticles | [51] |
| Cyanobacteria *Desertifilum* species | Spherical morphology with 4.5 to 26 nm-sized nanoparticles | [52] |
| *Caulerpa serrulata* green algae | 10–12 nm-sized spherical shaped morphology | [110] |
| Marine *Caulerpa racemose* green algae | 25 nm-sized spherical shaped morphology | [111] |
| Algal polysaccharide Ulvan from *Ulva armoricana* green algae | Monodispersed nanoparticles below 100 nm in size | [112] |
| Marine *Spyridia fusiformis* red algae | Crystalline 5–50 nm in size | [113] |
| *Polysiphonia* algae | Spherical 5–25 nm-sized particles | [114] |
| *Botryococcus braunii* | Cubical, truncated triangle and spherical shaped 40–90 nm-sized particles | [115] |
| *Hypnea musciformis* | Morphologies such as triangle, hexagons, pentagons, and spherical shapes with 16–42 nm-sized particles | [116] |

Fungi-Mediated Silver Nanoparticle Synthesis

| | | |
|---|---|---|
| White rot fungi | Spherical to round shaped morphology with 15–25 nm-sized particles | [117] |
| Xylanase from *Aspergillus niger* and *Trichoderma longibrachiatum* | Spherical shaped 15–78 nm-sized nanoparticles | [118] |
| *Beauveria bassiana* | Spherical shaped ~90 nm-sized particles | [119] |
| Encapsulated biomass beads of *Phoma exigua* | Spherical shaped 22 nm-sized particles | [120] |
| *Cladosporium* species | Uniform spherical shaped nanoparticles with 50–100 nm sizes | [121] |
| *Raphanus sativus* | Spherical shaped 4–30 nm-sized particles | [122] |
| *Arthroderma fulvum* | Spherical shaped 15–20 nm-sized particles | [123] |
| *Neurospora crassa* | Quasi-spherical nanoparticles with 2–22 nm size | [124] |

**TABLE 7.1**    *(Continued)*

| | | |
|---|---|---|
| *Aspergillus terreus* | Spherical shaped 16.5 nm-sized particles | [125] |
| *Cladosporium cladosporioides* | Spherical morphology with 30–60 nm-sized particles | [85] |
| **Plant Extract-Mediated Silver Nanoparticle Synthesis** | | |
| *Drosera indica, Drosera spatulata, Drosera binata,* and *Dionaea muscipula* | Quasi-spherical morphology with 10–60 nm size | [90] |
| Aqueous extract of lemon peel | Spherical morphology with 9.3–20.3 nm-sized particles | [91] |
| *Saccharum spontaneum* | Heterogenous morphology such as hexagon, rod, spherical, and triangles with 30–40 nm-sized particles | [92] |
| *Ganoderma lucidum* aqueous extract | Spherical shaped 15–22 nm-sized nanoparticles | [93] |
| *Azadirachta indica* aqueous leaf extract | Spherical and irregular shaped nanoparticles with 34 nm size | [126] |
| *Aloe vera* plant extract | Crystalline nanoparticles with 70–100 nm size | [127] |
| *Crocus sativus* (saffron) wastages | Spherical shaped 15 nm-sized particles | [128] |
| *Origanum vulgare* leaf extract | Polydispersed spherical shaped nanoparticles with 2–25 nm sizes | [129] |
| *Phlomis* species | Spherical nanoparticles with 25 nm size | [130] |
| *Salvia spinosa* | Spherical shaped morphology with 19–125 nm-sized particles | [131] |

## 7.3    GREEN SYNTHESIS OF SILVER NANOCOMPOSITES

Apart from nanoparticles, silver is incorporated with other metals or compounds to fabricate nanosized composites for elevating their exclusive biomedical properties and eliminating their potential limitations [132]. Similar to nanoparticles, green synthesis via biological agents are extensively utilized to improve the exclusive biological properties of silver nanoparticles, especially its antimicrobial property [133].

### 7.3.1  SYNTHESIS OF SILVER NANOCOMPOSITES USING BACTERIA, FUNGI, AND ALGAE

Bacterial cellulose can be mixed with silver nanoparticles to fabricate bio-nanocomposites of silver for potential biomedical and pharmaceutical applications. In a recent study, cellulose extracted from bacteria was incorporated with nanosized silver particles to form nanocomposites of 15–30 nm-sized silver nanoparticles in cellulose fibers. These nanosized composites exhibited 99.9% of antimicrobial efficacy against food-borne pathogens and have been proposed to protect food products from spoilage for 30 days [134]. Similarly, Pinto et al. [135] fabricated 50–100 nm nanosized silver composites in the form of ribbon-like nanofibril 3D structures using cellulose, that are extracted from *Acetobacter xylinum* bacteria with 50–100 nm of width in the form of ribbon-like nanofibril 3D structures. These nanocomposites exhibited enhanced antibacterial activity against *Klebsiella pneumoniae*, *Bacillus subtilis* and *Staphylococcus aureus* at low concentrations [135]. Likewise, Sureshkumar et al. [136] fabricated polydopamine (PDA)-iron oxide-silver nanocomposites via cellulose extracted from *Acetobacter xylinum*. These 30–50 nm-sized spherical shaped nanocomposites embedded in cellulose fibers exhibited magnetic properties along with antimicrobial efficacy against *Escherichia coli* and *Bacillus subtilis* acting as a mild sterilizing agent for fermentation medium [136]. Further, *Gluconacetobacter xylinum* was used to extract cellulose and fabricate silver-silver chloride nanocomposites for potential biological applications. The resultant nanosized composites are spherical, 17.4 nm in size and are randomly embedded in the cellulose fibrous matrix. These nanosized composites exhibited enhanced antibacterial efficacy against *E. coli* and *S. aureus* and are proposed to be beneficial for wound healing applications [137].

There are very few records on the benefits of algal extracts as a reducing agent for the formation of silver nanocomposites. Satheeshkumar et al. [138] fabricated 15–21 nm-sized silver-iron oxide nanocomposites using the algal extracts from micro green *Chlorella vulgaris* algae. These novel silver-based bio-nanocomposites exhibited super paramagnetism property along with effective anticancer efficacy against human IMR-32 neuroblastoma cells [138]. Similar to bacteria, fungi polymers were also used as a matrix for silver nanoparticles or nanocomposites to exhibit biomedical properties. Madhusudhan et al. [139] fabricated 100 nm-sized silver nanocomposites via chitin and chitosan extracted from *Aspergillus niger*. The resultant nanocomposites exhibited antibacterial activity against *Bacillus subtilis* and *Bacillus cereus*, causes of pathogenic infections in *Bombyx mori* (silkworm) and humans, respectively [139]. Further, chitosan-poly vinyl alcohol-silver nanocomposites have been fabricated using a cell-free extract of white-rot fungi as a potential drug carrier. These nanocomposites showed effective antibacterial activity against *Pseudomonas*, *Klebsiella*, *Escherichia*, and *Staphylococcus* bacterial species. In addition, these nanocomposites possess the ability to encapsulate aspirin with the potential to efficiently carry and deliver drugs in a controlled manner [140]. Likewise, asparaginase extracted from fungal strains is utilized as a potential reducing agent for the formation of silver bio-nanocomposites. The resultant nanocomposites are 60–80 nm in size with effective anti-proliferation properties against ovarian (A2780) and lung (A549) cancer cells [141]. Similarly, Sathiyaseelan et al. [142] prepared a novel nanosized biocomposite by synthesizing silver nanoparticles via phytochemical extracts of *Aloe vera* and *Cuscuta reflexa*. These biosynthesized nanoparticles are further loaded with fungal chitosan extracted from *Cunninghamella elegans* by freeze-drying approach for wound dressing applications. These novel nanosized bio-composites exhibited effective antibacterial activity against pathogenic bacteria and are less toxic towards human dermal fibroblast cells [142].

### 7.3.2 SYNTHESIS OF SILVER NANOCOMPOSITES USING PLANT EXTRACTS

Plant extracts are considered the most common and potent biological reducing agent for the formation of nanoparticles, as mentioned in section 2, as well as nanosized composites. Batool et al. [43] fabricated nanosized silver particles using fruit extracts of *Diospyros lotus*. These biosynthesized nanoparticles are embedded with poly vinyl alcohol-starch to form nanosized hydrogel composite membranes for wound dressing applications [143]. Likewise, nanosized silver-montmorillonite composites were prepared via the aqueous leaf extract of *Tarragon*. The resultant nanoparticles were crystalline with an average size of 25.12 nm and exhibited antibacterial efficacy against *E. coli* and *S. aureus* [144]. A similar study was carried out by Ghiassi et al. [145], where nanosized silver particles that are fabricated via phytochemicals extracted from *Satureja hortensis* were embedded with montmorillonite to form 4.88–26.70 nm-sized nanocomposites with antibacterial properties against *Escherichia coli* and *Staphylococcus aureus* [145]. Recently, self-assembled nano-porphyrins with silver nanoparticles as composites are fabricated using *Sesbania sesban* plant extract. These nanocomposites are 15 nm in size and are proposed to be beneficial as a potential heterogenous catalyst [146]. Similarly, reduced graphene oxide (GO)-silver nanocomposites have been fabricated using leaf extract of *Plectranthus amboinicus* via a hydrothermal approach. These nanocomposites are proved to possess an enhanced molecular sensing property and showed efficiency in the detection of hydrogen peroxide as a novel material to be present in nonenzymatic electrochemical sensors [147].

Agricultural plant wastes are also considered a potential source for the fabrication of silver nanocomposites. Song et al. [148] recently utilized metabolic extracts of rice husk as a novel reducing agent for the formation of silver nanoparticles and the extract residues were used to synthesize silica nanoparticles. The study emphasized that the phytochemicals present in rise husk are responsible for the reduction of the silver precursor to form nanosized silver particles with an antioxidant property [148]. Similarly, silver nanoparticles can be synthesized by using the phytochemical extracts from pistachio shell as a significant reducing and capping agent. The nanoparticles are coated with the phytochemicals as a bio-nanocomposite and are 10–15 nm in diameter. These biosynthesized nanocomposites showed effective catalytic reduction of organic dyes without any hazardous reaction towards other living organisms and the environment [149]. Further, Patil et al. [150] fabricated GO-silver nanocomposites using the waste fruit shell extracts of *Moringa oleifera* using sunlight as an energy source. These novel nanocomposites exhibited better selectivity for the detection of lead, chromium, and mercury ions to remove heavy metal contamination in soil and water [150]. All these studies show that microbial and plant extracted secondary metabolites are also beneficial for the formation of silver nanocomposites, similar to silver nanoparticles.

## 7.4    ANTIMICROBIAL PROPERTIES OF SILVER NANOPARTICLES AND NANOCOMPOSITES

Nanosized silver particles are fabricated via green or biosynthesis approaches to make them useful in biomedical applications. The antimicrobial property is one of the prime avenues of use for silver nanoparticles, as silver is known for its efficiency in inhibiting pathogenic microbes. Reduction in the size of silver particles to a nanoscale with the help of biological entities will further enhance their ability to inhibit microbial proliferation. Figure 7.4 is a schematic representation of the probable antimicrobial mechanism exhibited by silver nanoparticles.

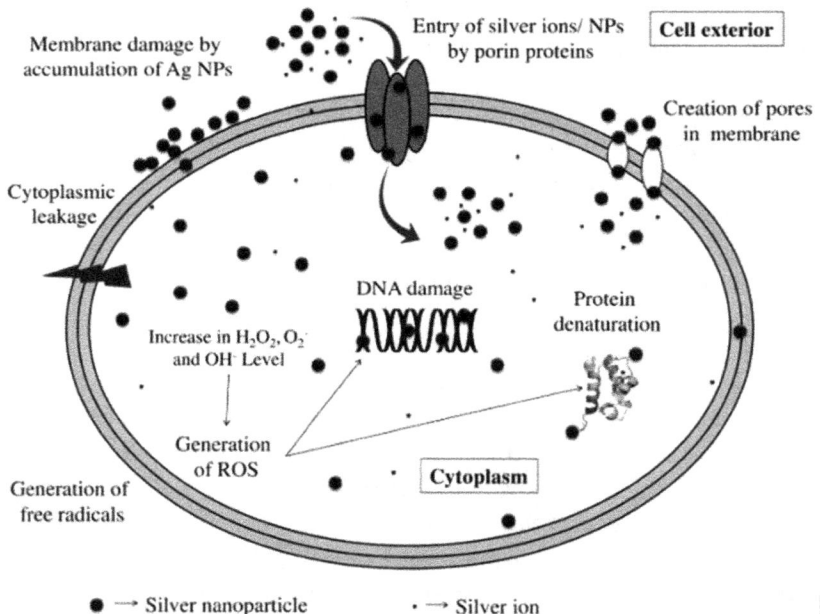

**FIGURE 7.4**    Antimicrobial mechanism of silver nanoparticles.
*Source:* Reproduced from [151], MDPI.

### 7.4.1    ANTIBACTERIAL ACTIVITY

There is a wealth of literatures available in recent times to showcase the antibacterial efficacy of nanosized silver particles. It has been reported by Gomathi et al. [152] that aqueous leaf extracts of *Amorphophallus paeoniifolius* can be used to form spherical-shaped 20–30 nm-sized silver particles at room temperature. These green synthesized silver nanoparticles are revealed to possess enhanced antibacterial efficacy against pathogens such as *Bacillus subtilis* and *Klebsiella pneumoniae* [152]. Similarly, phytochemical extracts of *Jasminum auriculatum* stem are utilized for the fabrication of spherical, 10–20 nm-sized silver particles. The result showed that these biosynthesized nanoparticles possess the ability to inhibit the proliferation of bacterial pathogens such as *P. aeruginosa*, *Enterococcus faecalis*, *Escherichia coli,* and *Staphylococcus aureus* with a 10–12 mm zone of inhibition [153]. Likewise, silver nanoparticles are fabricated using filtered and fresh buttermilk as a novel biological source. These nanoparticles exhibited enhanced antibacterial efficacy against plant pathogenic *Xanthomonas axonopodis* and human or animal pathogenic *Escherichia coli* and *Staphylococcus aureus* [154]. Further, *Neolamarckia cadamba* fruit and leaf extracts are utilized for silver nanoparticle synthesis. The resultant nanoparticles exhibited that the leaf extract synthesized nano-sized particles possess enhanced antibacterial property against both gram strains of four bacterial pathogens that can cause disease in humans [155]. Furthermore, secondary metabolites obtained from the endophytic *Talaromyces purpureogenus* fungus are used for the fabrication of antibacterial nanosized silver particles. The synthesized nanoparticles are 25 nm in size with spherical and triangle morphologies and displayed efficient anti-proliferation activity against both gram-negative and positive bacterial pathogens [156].

Apart from nanosized silver, nanocomposites of silver nanoparticles are also extensively utilized to eliminate pathogenic bacteria via enhanced antibacterial property. Hasan et al. [157] recently reported that dextrin can be used to synthesize nanosized silver particles and grafted with poly (methyl methacrylate) for the fabrication of green nanocomposites. These nanosized composites are revealed to possess enhanced antibacterial activity against multidrug-resistant bacteria such as *S. aureus* resistant to methicillin (MRSA), *Klebsiella pneumoniae* ATCC 700603 and *Pseudomonas aeruginosa* PAO1 producing extended-spectrum b-lactamases [157]. Likewise, a novel spherical and 42 nm-sized silver chloride-silver composite was fabricated using metabolites of an *Arthrobacter* species, that are isolated from a bacteria that grows in Antarctic soil and are non-pathogenic to humans. These nanocomposites also showed enhanced antibacterial efficacy against both gram strains of bacteria, including *Pseudomonas aeruginosa* KPC37 that are resistant to multiple drugs [158]. Similarly, a significant nanocomposite of silver and chitosan has been fabricated using the biodegradable N, N, N-trimethyl chitosan chloride polymer to reduce and stabilize the nucleated nanosized composite. The resultant nanocomposites are 11–17.5 nm-sized and uniformly distributed with spherical morphology. These nanocomposites exhibited enhanced antibacterial activity against *Mycobacterium tuberculosis* with minimum inhibitory concentration (MIC) of 1.95 μg/mL, and maybe a potential drug for the treatment of tuberculosis [159]. Further, phytochemical extracts of two plants, namely *Teucrium polium* and *Ocimum basilicum* from Iran are reported to be beneficial capping and reducing agent for the formation of novel nanosized silver-montmorillonite composites. Initially, the silver particles were 80 and 20 nm, while using *Ocimum basilicum* and *Teucrium polium* extracts, respectively, which were reduced to 70 and 15 nm respectively after incorporating montmorillonite to form nanosized composites. These nanocomposites exhibited effective antibacterial activity against *E. coli* and *S. aureus* bacterial pathogens, compared to nanosized silver particles [160]. These studies show that secondary metabolite extracts of plants can be widely utilized for the production of nanosized silver particles and composites with enhanced antibacterial efficacy.

### 7.4.2 ANTIFUNGAL AND ANTIALGAL PROPERTY

Nanosized silver particles possess effective antifungal and antialgal properties, similar to their antibacterial activity as shown in Figure 7.5. Jalal et al. [161] showed that the seed extracts of *Syzygium cumini* are beneficial for the formation of nanosized silver particles with effective antifungal activity against *Candida* species. The study revealed that these nanoparticles possess enhanced antifungal efficacy against *Candida parapsilosis*, *Candida tropicalis*, *Candida albicans*, *Ceriodaphnia dubliniensis* and *Candida krusei*, along with antibacterial activity, germ tube and biofilm inhibitory effect against *Candida albicans* [161]. Similarly, Bhagat et al. [162] demonstrated that the aqueous *Rosa brunonii Lindl* extract is useful for nanosized silver formation. The resultant nanoparticles showed enhanced antifungal activity against *Aspergillus niger*, *Curvularia lunata*, *Fusarium oxysporum* and *Bipolaris specifera*, along with antibacterial efficacy and enhanced photocatalytic activity to degrade Congo red dye via direct sunlight [162]. Likewise, Kumari et al. [163] emphasized that the filtrate of *Trichoderma viride*, that is free of cells, is able to act as a reducing agent to fabricate nanosized silver and stabilize the particles to avoid agglomeration. Further, the study stated that these silver nanoparticles are highly beneficial in inhibiting the proliferation of fungal pathogens such as *Alternaria brassicicola* and *Fusarium oxysporum*, compared to chemically synthesized silver nanoparticles. The findings also revealed that the osmotic balance disruption, reactive oxygen species (ROS) generation, oxidative enzyme, and antioxidant machinery downregulation and virulence loss are the possible mechanisms for the enhanced antifungal activity of biosynthesized silver nanoparticles [163]. Youssef et al. [164] reported that nanosized silver particles are fabricated via the culture isolates of *Bacillus subtilis* and are incorporated with chitosan to form novel nanosized composites. These nanocomposites are proven to possess enhanced antifungal property against *Aspergillus niger* and also inhibits the growth of *Candida albicans* yeast and gram-positive *Pseudomonas aeruginosa* bacteria [164]. Moreover, Roseline et al. [165] revealed that the aqueous extracts from carrageenan *Hypnea musciformis*, *Spyridia hypnoides*, agar *Gracilaria edulis,* and *Gracilaria coricata* seaweeds could be used for the synthesis of nanocomposites of silver with seaweed sulfated polysaccharides and proteins. The study showed that the particle size ranges from 36–55 nm with a spherical morphology, depending on the type of seaweed extracts used for the synthesis. These bio-nanocomposites proved to possess enhanced antifungal efficacy against *Ustilaginoidea virens*, along with antibacterial activity against *Xanthomonas oryzae* and *Xanthomonas axonopodis* [165]. All these studies show that the plant extract synthesized silver nanoparticles are exhibiting enhanced antifungal activity, followed by bacterial cell free extracts. In addition, there is little literature on biosynthesized silver-based nanocomposites with antifungal activity and it can be noted that only bacteria and seaweed extracts have been used to form nanosized antifungal silver composites.

Biosynthesized silver nanoparticles and nanosized composites are also proven to possess efficient antialgal properties. Kumari et al. [166] revealed that nanosized silver nanoparticles can be fabricated using the secondary metabolites of *Pseudomonas aeruginosa* DM1. The resultant nanoparticles are 45–100 nm-sized and spherical, exhibiting an enhanced, concentration-dependent antialgal property against *Chlorella pyenoidosa* and *Chlorella vulgaris* by inhibiting the chlorophyll content [166]. Similarly, marine plant extracts of *Nannochloropsis oculate* and *Tetraselmis tetrathele* are revealed to possess the ability to form smaller nanosized silver particles. In addition, these biosynthesized nanoparticles have shown an enhanced antialgal property against *Oscillatoria simplicissima cyanobacteria* that can inhibit the growth of aquatic organisms via neurotoxin release [167]. Further, nanosized silver particles are synthesized via bacterial chromophore sensing quorum named Violecein as a capping agent. The resultant nanoparticles are 34 nm in size with irregular shapes and agglomeration along with effective antialgal activity against *Dictyosphaerium* DHM1, DHM2 species and *Pectinodesmus* PHM3 species, along with antibacterial and antifungal property, compared to nanosized starch-capped silver particles [168]. Moreover, biocompatible chitosan is used to fabricate nanocomposites of silver, which are employed to exhibit antialgal activity by delivering nanosized particles at the target site. Natarajan et al. [169] showed that titanium dioxide-silver and its associated pristine films are formulated with chitosan to form biopolymeric nanocomposite with effective anti-algal properties. The resultant nanosized composite exhibited enhanced anti-algal and anti-fouling activity against marine *Dunaliella salina* algae via ROS generation [169]. Another study by the same group also mentioned that the pristine nanocomposite films with silver possess enhanced anti-algal property against algal species such as *Chlorella* and *Scenedesmus* [170].

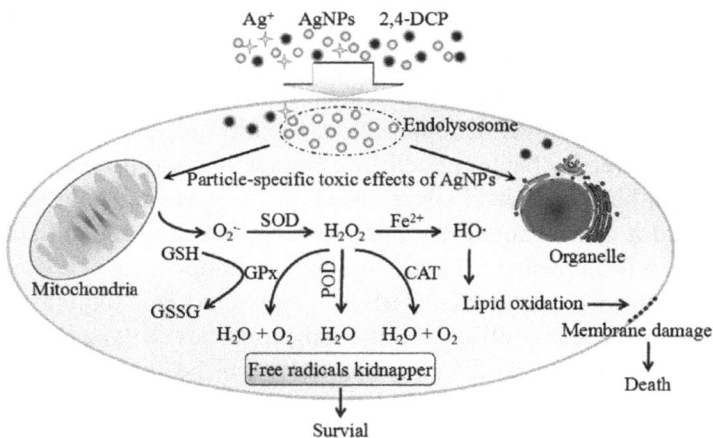

**FIGURE 7.5**　Antifungal mechanism of silver nanoparticles.
*Source:* Reprinted with permission from [171]. © 2018 Elsevier Ltd.

### 7.4.3  ANTIVIRAL PROPERTY

There are numerous reports in recent times, which have revealed the antiviral properties of nanosized silver particles and composites. Extracellular isolates of Bacillus species strains such as *Bacillus licheniformis, Bacillus pumilus* and *Bacillus persicus* were recently used as a potential reduction and stabilization agents for the formation of 77–92 nm-sized silver particles. The study further proposed that the hydroxyl peptide hydrolysate oxidation in the bacterial isolates is responsible for the reduction and nucleation of nanosized particles. These novel nanosized green synthesized silver particles are reported to be beneficial as a potential antiviral agent against Bean Yellow Mosaic Virus that can affect fava bean plant of Africa, along with effective antimicrobial activity against human pathogens [172]. Similarly, Yang et al. [173] showed that nanosized silver particles can be formed using the rhizome isolates of the *Curcuma longa* of the ginger family known as curcumin. The resultant nanoparticles are 11.95±0.23 nm in size with well-defined uniform spherical shapes and demonstrated to possess effective antiviral efficacy against respiratory syncytial viral infection without any significant toxicity towards normal human cells [173]. Likewise, secondary metabolites from plants such as *Phyllanthus niruri, Andrographis paniculata,* and *Tinospora cordifolia* are used for the fabrication of 50–70 nm-sized spherical silver clusters. These nanoparticles also exhibited potent antiviral activity against Chikungunya virus without any toxicity to normal and healthy human cells [174]. Further, silver nanoparticles that are synthesized using *Sargasum wightii* seaweed are proven to possess effective inhibition property against anti-Herpes Simplex Viral strains such as HSV-1 and HSV-2 [175]. Moreover, nanosized silver particles are fabricated via *Halodule uninervis* sea grasses to inhibit the proliferation of *Aedes aegypti*, which serves as a potential vector for dengue and Zika virus that cause deadly fevers in humans [176]. Furthermore, nanosized composites of GO and silver were also proven to possess enhanced antiviral property against porcine reproductive and respiratory syndrome virus [177], enveloped, and nonenveloped viruses [178]. These studies emphasized that nanosized silver particles are an effective antiviral agent as shown in Figure 7.6 that can mitigate several viral-mediated infections in plants, animals, and humans.

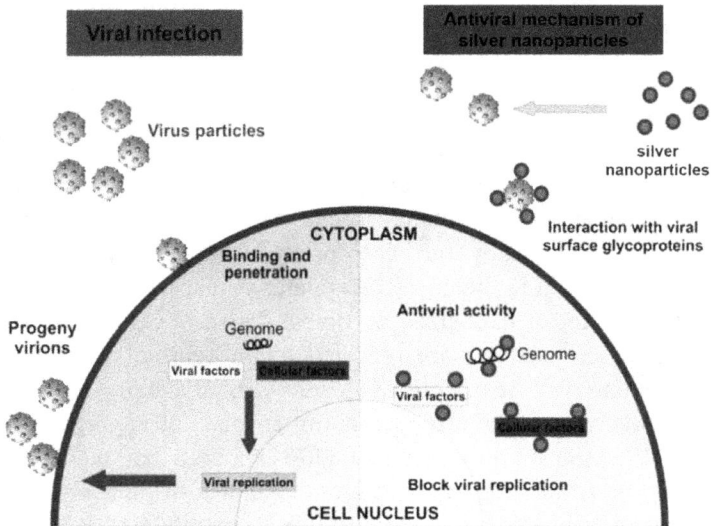

**FIGURE 7.6**    Antiviral mechanism of silver nanoparticles.
*Source:* Reproduced from [179], MDPI.

Table 7.2 is a summary of antimicrobial silver nanoparticles and nanocomposites that are fabricated from biological sources.

**TABLE 7.2**    Antimicrobial Property of Green Synthesized Silver Nanoparticles

| Biological Source for Silver Nanoparticle Synthesis | Antimicrobial Efficacy | References |
|---|---|---|
| **Antibacterial Activity** | | |
| Grass waste for 15 nm-sized silver nanoparticles | *Pseudomonas aeruginosa* and *Acinetobacter baumannii* | [180] |
| *Amorphophallus paeoniifolius* leaf extract for 20–30 nm-sized silver nanoparticles | *Bacillus subtilis* and *Klebsiella pneumoniae* | [152] |
| *Jasminum auriculatum* phytochemical extract for 10–20 nm-sized silver particles | *Pseudomonas aeruginosa, Enterococcus faecalis, Escherichia coli,* and *Staphylococcus aureus* | [153] |
| Filtered and fresh buttermilk for silver nanoparticle synthesis | *Xanthomonas axonopodis* plant pathogens, *Escherichia coli,* and *Staphylococcus aureus* | [154] |

**TABLE 7.2** *(Continued)*

| Biological Source for Silver Nanoparticle Synthesis | Antimicrobial Efficacy | References |
|---|---|---|
| *Neolamarckia cadamba* fruit and leaf extracts for silver nanoparticles | *Escherichia coli, Pseudomonas aeruginosa, Staphylococcus aureus,* and *Bacillus subtilis* | [155] |
| *Talaromyces purpureogenus* fungal extract for 25 nm-sized silver particles | *Staphylococcus aureus, Bacillus cereus, Salmonella enterica, Pseudomonas aeruginosa,* and *Escherichia coli* | [156] |
| Dextrin-poly (methyl methacrylate)-silver nanocomposites | *Staphylococcus aureus* resistant to methicillin (MRSA), *Klebsiella pneumoniae* ATCC 700603 and *Pseudomonas aeruginosa* PAO1 | [157] |
| Silver chloride-silver composite from *Arthrobacter* species | *Pseudomonas aeruginosa* KPC37 resistant to multiple drugs | [158] |
| Chitosan-silver nanocomposites | *Mycobacterium tuberculosis* | [159] |
| Silver-montmorillonite composites from *Teucrium polium* and *Ocimum basilicum* | *Escherichia coli* and *Staphylococcus aureus* | [160] |
| **Antifungal Activity** | | |
| Seed extracts of *Syzygium cumini* for silver nanoparticle synthesis | *Candida parapsilosis, Candida tropicalis, Candida albicans, Candida dubliniensis,* and *Candida krusei* | [161] |
| Aqueous *Rosa brunonii Lindl* extract for silver nanoparticle synthesis | *Aspergillus niger, Curvularia lunata, Fusarium oxysporum,* and *Bipolaris specifera* | [162] |
| *Trichoderma viride* extracts for silver nanoparticle synthesis | *Alternaria brassicicola,* and *Fusarium oxysporum* | [163] |
| Chitosan-silver nanocomposites using *B. subtilis* | *Aspergillus niger* | [164] |
| *Hypnea musciformis, Spyridia hypnoides,* agar *Gracilaria edulis* and *G. coricata* seaweed extract for silver nanocomposites | *Ustilaginoidea virens* | [165] |
| **Antialgal Activity** | | |
| *Pseudomonas aeruginosa* DM1 synthesized silver nanoparticles | *Chlorella pyenoidosa* and *Chlorella vulgaris* | [166] |

**TABLE 7.2**    *(Continued)*

| Biological Source for Silver Nanoparticle Synthesis | Antimicrobial Efficacy | References |
|---|---|---|
| Marine plant extracts of *Nannochloropsis oculate* and *Tetraselmis tetrathele* for silver nanoparticles | *Oscillatoria simplicissima* Cyanobacteria | [167] |
| Violecein bacterial extract for silver nanoparticles | *Dictyosphaerium* species strain DHM1, DHM2 and *Pectinodesmus* species strain PHM3 | [168] |
| Chitosan-titanium dioxide-silver nanocomposites | *Dunaliella salina* algae | [169] |
| Pristine-silver nanocomposites | *Chlorella* and *Scenedesmus* | [170] |
| **Antiviral Activity** | | |
| *B. licheniformis, B. pumilus* and *B. persicus* extracts for silver nanoparticles | Bean yellow mosaic virus | [172] |
| Rhizome isolates of *Curcuma longa* for silver nanoparticles | Respiratory syncytial viral infection | [173] |
| *Phyllanthus niruri, Andrographis paniculata* and *Tinospora cordifolia* extracts for silver nanoparticles | Chikungunya virus | [174] |
| *Sargasum wightii* seaweed | Anti-herpes simplex viral strains such as HSV-1 and HSV-2 | [175] |
| *Halodule uninervis* sea grasses | Dengue and zika virus | [176] |
| Graphene oxide-silver nanocomposite | porcine reproductive and respiratory syndrome virus | [177] |
| Graphene oxide-silver nanocomposite | Enveloped and nonenveloped viruses | [178] |

## 7.5    ANTIMICROBIAL MECHANISM OF SILVER NANOMATERIALS

The effective antimicrobial property of silver nanoparticles is due to characteristics such as size, shape, and surface charge. These properties of silver nanoparticles, along with secondary metabolites as capping agents and functional groups further facilitate their antimicrobial efficacy. The core mechanism that is extensively demonstrated to be the factor to inhibit broad spectrum microbial groups are the generation of ROS and lipid peroxidation, either directly by silver nanoparticles or via silver ions released from the nanoparticles [181]. Recently, it has been reported that cell membrane disruption, interaction with microbial nucleic acid, and ability to release, as well as concentration of, silver ions are the general mechanisms by which nanosized silver particles inhibit microbes [182]. However, the stages of the mechanism may be altered depending on the specific characteristics of the particular silver nanoparticles and the type of microbes in question. Further, Khadka et al. [183] revealed that silver nanoparticles cause DNA condensation of target microbes and damage them by enhancing the expression of histone-like nucleoid protein structures and its spatial recognition [183]. Further, it has been demonstrated that the addition of nanosized silver particles has led to the upregulation of alkyl hydroperoxide reductase, low oxygen regulating oxidases and organic hydroperoxide resistance protein, which eventually led to the ROS production and disruption of the morphology of the microbe, causing inhibition with its antioxidant property [184]. Moreover, it is noteworthy that nanosized silver particles can release silver ions under anoxic conditions or may transform into silver sulfide under anaerobic conditions, which may also lead to toxicity towards microbes. However, this mechanism is still under investigation to authenticate it as a crucial way to inhibit microbes by nanoparticles of silver [185]. Contrarily, most silver nano-composites exhibited antimicrobial efficacy via light irradiation. Viet et al. [186] showed that light irradiation will activate silver nanoparticles that are embedded with titanium dioxide nanotubes to release silver ions and oxide ions which will facilitate the formation of hydrogen peroxides to disrupt the microbial cell membrane or their internal organelles [186].

Figure 7.7 is the summary of various mechanisms that are stated in the literatures to be responsible for the antimicrobial potential of silver nanoparticles. There are four types of mechanisms that are widely proposed to be responsible for the antimicrobial property of silver nanoparticles in the literature. The first mechanism is the direct inhibition of the microbial cell membrane via the binding nature of the silver nanoparticle. The surface charges of the microbe and the nanoparticle will lead to an electrostatic attraction, upon which the nanoparticles bind to the cell membrane and inhibit microbial proliferation [187]. The second mechanism is similar; however, silver ions are released from the nanoparticles, which bind to the microbial cell membrane and causes damage to the cells. In this proposed mechanism, only negatively charged microbes will be targeted as silver ions are positively charged in nature [188]. However, surface charge in these mechanisms can be modified via biological functional groups to reduce their toxicity and increase antimicrobial efficacy, according to the desired application. The third mechanism involves the size and morphology-based properties of silver nanoparticles, allowing internalization in the microbial cells and subsequent binding with cell organelles such as mitochondria and DNA to cause disruption or damage the cell membrane and other cell organelles via ROS production, reducing microbial proliferation [189]. Similarly, silver nanoparticles can also disintegrate into its ionic state after internalization, and exhibit ROS mediated antimicrobial activity [190], as mentioned in the third mechanism. In all these conditions, it is noteworthy that ROS generation, lipid peroxidation and interruption of enzymatic pathways play a significant role in inhibiting the growth of pathogenic microbes.

## 7.6 FUTURE PERSPECTIVE, OUTLOOK, AND CONCLUSION

Nanoparticles of silver have been emphasized as an excellent antimicrobial agent to inhibit a wide range of microbes, compared to their bulk counterpart. The profound antimicrobial property has led to their incorporation in various commercial products such as antimicrobial paints, dresses, and socks. Numerous studies have shown that socks incorporating nanosized silver can be beneficial in inhibiting microbes and reducing odors [191, 192]. These antimicrobial socks are also helpful in inhibiting the growth of foot-borne pathogens and their associated diseases. Further, nanosized silver is incorporated in clinical dresses and gloves, which will control the growth of clinical pathogens to patients and doctors [193]. Antimicrobial silver nanoparticles are also incorporated in paints to protect building surfaces from microbial attack and to inhibit pathogenic microbes in rooms [194]. The release of these silver nanoparticles from the commercial products into the environment may cause toxic effects towards other organisms and may pollute the environmental entities such as soil, water, and air. Thus, biosynthesized silver nanoparticles are preferred to be included in these commercial applications, as it will enhance the antimicrobial efficacy by reducing toxicity towards the environment and other organisms.

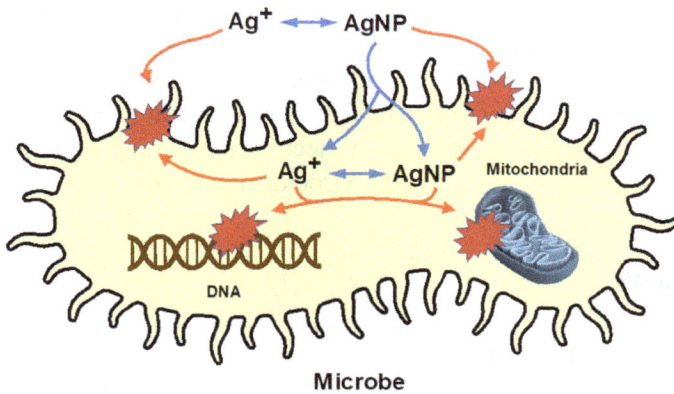

**FIGURE 7.7** Proposed antimicrobial mechanism of silver nanoparticles, AgNP-silver nanoparticles and Ag+-silver ions.

Multidrug resistance is another serious issue with the use of conventional antibiotics and antimicrobial agents for inhibiting their proliferation. The utilization of silver nanoparticles will inhibit microbes via increasing their ionic potential, without leading to any resistance mechanisms [194]. Thus, these nanoparticles are widely recommended for emerging outbreaks of diseases such as Nipah, SARS, and corona viral diseases. Moreover, these nanoparticles are beneficial in mitigating the proliferation of other pathogenic bacteria, algae, fungi, and viruses. In addition, nanoformulated or nanocomposites of silver nanoparticles will enhance their antimicrobial efficacy. In the future, it will be possible to design silver nanoparticles to detect pathogenic microbes via aptamers or peptides and exhibit specific antimicrobial treatment. Further, these nanosized particles are useful to trigger immunity against certain microbes in humans and animals [195]. Thus, biosynthesized silver nanoparticles encapsulated with vaccines will trigger an immune response by acting as a shield towards various microbial infections in plants, animals, and humans in the future.

This chapter is an overview of several nanosized silver particles that are synthesized by using the extracts of bacteria, fungi, algae, and plants. Further, the significance and need for fabricating silver nanocomposites was also discussed. The antimicrobial mechanism of silver nanoparticles denoted that oxidative stress and lipid peroxidation to disintegrate microbial cell membrane, organelles, and nucleic acid is responsible for their enhanced inhibition properties against pathogenic microbes. These novel green synthesized silver nanoparticles are extensively under research and few of them are currently employed in commercial applications. In future, green synthesized silver-based nanoparticles and nanocomposites will be potential antibiotic and antimicrobial agents in the future, as an alternative to conventional antimicrobials, to protect various living organisms from microbial pathogenic attack and its associated diseases.

## KEYWORDS

- **antimicrobial activity**
- **bio-degradibility**
- **green synthesis**
- **nanocomposites**
- **silver nanoparticles**
- **transmission electron microscope**

## REFERENCES

1. Ansari, M. A., et al., (2020). A current nanoparticles approaches in nose to brain drug delivery and anticancer therapy: A review. *Current Pharmaceutical Design.*
2. Gharpure, S., Akash, A., & Ankamwar, B., (2020). A review on antimicrobial properties of metal nanoparticles. *Journal of Nanoscience and Nanotechnology, 20*(6), 3303–3339.
3. Syafiuddin, A., et al., (2020). Silver nanoparticles adsorption by the synthetic and natural adsorbent materials: An exclusive review. *Nanotechnology for Environmental Engineering, 5*(1), 1.
4. Menazea, A. A., (2020). Femtosecond laser ablation-assisted synthesis of silver nanoparticles in organic and inorganic liquids medium and their antibacterial efficiency. *Radiation Physics and Chemistry, 168,* 108616.
5. Slepička, P., et al., (2020). Methods of gold and silver nanoparticles preparation. *Materials, 13*(1), 1.
6. Maddinedi, S. B., Mandal, B. K., & Anna, K. K., (2017). Tyrosine assisted size controlled synthesis of silver nanoparticles and their catalytic, *in-vitro* cytotoxicity evaluation. *Environmental Toxicology and Pharmacology, 51,* 23–29.
7. Jeevanandam, J., Chan, Y. S., & Danquah, M. K., (2016). Biosynthesis of metal and metal oxide nanoparticles. *Chem. Bio. Eng. Reviews, 3*(2), 55–67.
8. Kahnouji, Y. A., Mosaddegh, E., & Bolorizadeh, M. A., (2019). Detailed analysis of size-separation of silver nanoparticles by density gradient centrifugation method. *Materials Science and Engineering: C, 103,* 109817.

9. Jain, N., et al., (2019). Hydrothermal assisted biological synthesis of Silver nanoparticles by using honey and gomutra (cow urine) for qualitative determination of its antibacterial efficacy against *Pseudomonas* sp. isolated from contact lenses. *Eur. Asian Journal of BioSciences, 13*(1), 27–33.

10. Xu, G., et al. (2019). *Effects of Reaction Temperature on the Yield and Morphology of Silver Nanowires Prepared by Solvothermal Method*. Springer.

11. Maharjan, S., et al., (2019). Synthesis of stabilized silver nanoparticles in organosiloxane matrix via sol-gel method and its optical nonlinearity study. *Chemical Physics*, 110610.

12. Jeevanandam, J., et al., (2020). Sustainability of one-dimensional nanostructures: Fabrication and industrial applications. In: *Sustainable Nanoscale Engineering* (pp. 83–113). Elsevier.

13. Joshi, R. K., (2020). *Green Synthesis of Silver Nanoparticles Using Medicinal Plant Extracts and Assessment of its Antimicrobial Activity.*

14. Debnath, S., Swetha, D., & Babu, M. N., (2020). Green synthesis of nanoparticles using herbal extract. In: *Herbal Medicine in India* (pp. 205–213). Springer.

15. Anandaradje, A., et al., (2020). Microbial synthesis of silver nanoparticles and their biological potential. In: *Nanoparticles in Medicine* (pp. 99–133). Springer.

16. Ahmed, S., et al., (2016). A review on plants extract mediated synthesis of silver nanoparticles for antimicrobial applications: A green expertise. *Journal of Advanced Research, 7*(1), 17–28.

17. Pinto, M. N. (2019). *Design and Construction of Biocompatible Theranostic Carbon Monoxide and Silver Delivery Systems for Anticancer and Antibacterial Photochemotherapy* (Doctoral dissertation, UC Santa Cruz).

18. Handoko, C. T., Huda, A., & Gulo, F., (2019). Synthesis pathway and powerful antimicrobial properties of silver nanoparticle: A critical review. *Asian J. Sci. Res., 12*, 1–17.

19. Srikar, S. K., et al., (2016). Green synthesis of silver nanoparticles: A review. *Green and Sustainable Chemistry, 6*(01), 34.

20. Manivasagan, P., et al., (2013). Biosynthesis, antimicrobial and cytotoxic effect of silver nanoparticles using a novel *Nocardiopsis* sp. MBRC-1. *Bio Med Research International.*

21. Baltazar-Encarnación, E., et al., (2019). Silver nanoparticles synthesized through green methods using *Escherichia coli* top 10 (Ec-Ts) growth culture medium exhibit antimicrobial properties against nongrowing bacterial strains. *Journal of Nanomaterials.*

22. Rajeshkumar, S., et al., (2014). Algae mediated green fabrication of silver nanoparticles and examination of its antifungal activity against clinical pathogens. *International Journal of Metals.*

23. Sharma, G., et al., (2015). Biological synthesis of silver nanoparticles by cell-free extract of spirulina platensis. *Journal of Nanotechnology.*

24. Shahzad, A., et al., (2019). Size-controlled production of silver nanoparticles by *Aspergillus fumigatus* BTCB10: Likely antibacterial and cytotoxic effects. *Journal of Nanomaterials.*

25. Birla, S. S., et al., (2013). Rapid synthesis of silver nanoparticles from *Fusarium oxysporum* by optimizing physico cultural conditions. *The Scientific World Journal.*

26. Vo, T. T., et al., (2019). Biosynthesis of silver and gold nanoparticles using aqueous extract from *Crinum latifolium* leaf and their applications forward antibacterial effect and wastewater treatment. *Journal of Nanomaterials, 2019.*

27. Krithiga, N., Rajalakshmi, A., & Jayachitra, A., (2015). Green synthesis of silver nanoparticles using leaf extracts of *Clitoria ternatea* and *Solanum nigrum* and study of its antibacterial effect against common nosocomial pathogens. *Journal of Nanoscience.*

28. Siddiqi, K. S., Husen, A., & Rao, R. A. K., (2018). A review on biosynthesis of silver nanoparticles and their biocidal properties. *J. Nanobiotechnology, 16*(1), 14.

29. Ovais, M., et al., (2018). Biosynthesis of metal nanoparticles via microbial enzymes: A mechanistic approach. *Int. J. Mol. Sci., 19*(12).

30. Pugazhenthiran, N., et al., (2009). Microbial synthesis of silver nanoparticles by *Bacillus sp. Journal of Nanoparticle Research, 11.*

31. Shanthi, S., et al., (2016). Biosynthesis of silver nanoparticles using a probiotic *Bacillus licheniformis* Dahb1 and their antibiofilm activity and toxicity effects in *Ceriodaphnia Cornuta. Microb. Pathog., 93*, 70–77.

32. Ali, J., et al., (2019). Revisiting the mechanistic pathways for bacterial mediated synthesis of noble metal nanoparticles. *J. Microbiol. Methods, 159*, 18–25.

33. Shahverdi, A. R., et al., (2007). Rapid synthesis of silver nanoparticles using culture supernatants of enterobacteria: A novel biological approach. *Process Biochemistry. 42*, 919–923.

34. Ali, J., et al., (2017). Insight into eco-friendly fabrication of silver nanoparticles by *Pseudomonas aeruginosa* and its potential impacts. *Journal of Environmental Chemical Engineering, 5*(4), 3266–3272.

35. Ali, J., et al., (2016). Role of catalytic protein and stabilizing agents in the transformation of Ag ions to nanoparticles by *Pseudomonas aeruginosa. IET Nanobiotechnol., 10*(5), 295–300.

36. Huang, J., et al., (2015). Bio-inspired synthesis of metal nanomaterials and applications. *Chem. Soc. Rev., 44*(17), 6330–6374.

37. Sintubin, L., et al., (2009). Lactic acid bacteria as reducing and capping agent for the fast and efficient production of silver nanoparticles. *Appl. Microbiol. Biotechnol., 84*(4), 741–749.

38. Mokhtari, N., et al., (2009). Biological synthesis of very small silver nanoparticles by culture supernatant of *Klebsiella pneumonia*: The effects of visible-light irradiation and the liquid mixing process. *Materials Research Bulletin, 44*(6), 1415–1421.

39. Gurunathan, S., (2019). Rapid biological synthesis of silver nanoparticles and their enhanced antibacterial effects against *Escherichia fergusonii* and *Streptococcus mutans. Arabian Journal of Chemistry, 12*(2), 168–180.

40. Divya, M., et al., (2019). Biogenic synthesis and effect of silver nanoparticles (AgNPs) to combat catheter-related urinary tract infections. *Biocatalysis and Agricultural Biotechnology, 18*, 101037.

41. Almalki, M. A., & Khalifa, A. Y. Z., (2020). Silver nanoparticles synthesis from *Bacillus* sp. KFU36 and its anticancer effect in breast cancer MCF-7 cells via induction of apoptotic mechanism. *Journal of Photochemistry and Photobiology B: Biology., 204*, 111786.

42. Eswari, J. S., Dhagat, S., & Mishra, P., (2018). Biosurfactant assisted silver nanoparticle synthesis: A critical analysis of its drug design aspects. *Advances in Natural Sciences: Nanoscience and Nanotechnology, 9*(4), 045007.

43. Lengke, M. F., Fleet, M. E., & Southam, G., (2007). Biosynthesis of silver nanoparticles by filamentous cyanobacteria from a silver(I) nitrate complex. *Langmuir, 23*(5), 2694–2699.

44. Xie, J., et al., (2007). Silver nanoplates: From biological to biomimetic synthesis. *ACS Nano, 1*(5), 429–439.

45. Xie, J., et al., (2007). Identification of active biomolecules in the high-yield synthesis of single-crystalline gold nanoplates in algal solutions. *Small, 3*(4), 672–682.

46. Barwal, I., et al., (2011). Cellular oxido-reductive proteins of *Chlamydomonas reinhardtii* control the biosynthesis of silver nanoparticles. *J. Nanobiotechnology, 9*, 56.

47. Li, X., et al., (2015). Silver nanoparticle toxicity and association with the alga *Euglena gracilis*. *Environmental Science: Nano, 2*(6), 594–602.

48. Prasad, T. N., Kambala, V. S. R., & Naidu, R., (2013). Phyconanotechnology: Synthesis of silver nanoparticles using brown marine algae *Cystophora moniliformis* and their characterization. *Journal of Applied Phycology, 25*(1), 177–182.

49. Husain, S., et al., (2019). Cyanobacteria as a bioreactor for synthesis of silver nanoparticles-an effect of different reaction conditions on the size of nanoparticles and their dye decolorization ability. *J. Microbiol. Methods, 162*, 77–82.

50. Fatima, R., et al., (2020). Biosynthesis of silver nanoparticles using red algae *Portieria hornemannii* and its antibacterial activity against fish pathogens. *Microbial. Pathogenesis, 138*, 103780.

51. Bhuyar, P., et al., (2020). Synthesis of silver nanoparticles using marine macroalgae *Padina* sp. and its antibacterial activity towards pathogenic bacteria. *Beni-Suef University Journal of Basic and Applied Sciences, 9*(1), 3.

52. Hamida, R. S., et al., (2020). Synthesis of silver nanoparticles using a novel cyanobacteria *Desertifilum* sp. extract: Their antibacterial and cytotoxicity effects. *International Journal of Nanomedicine, 15*, 49–63.

53. Guilger-Casagrande, M., & De Lima, R., (2019). Synthesis of silver nanoparticles mediated by fungi: A review. *Front Bioeng. Biotechnol., 7*, 287.

54. Castro-Longoria, E., Vilchis-Nestor, A. R., & Avalos-Borja, M., (2011). Biosynthesis of silver, gold and bimetallic nanoparticles using the filamentous fungus *Neurospora crassa*. *Colloids Surf. B. Biointerfaces, 83*(1), 42–48.

55. Rajput, S., et al., (2016). Fungal isolate optimized for biogenesis of silver nanoparticles with enhanced colloidal stability. *Langmuir, 32*(34), 8688–8697.

56. Ashrafi, S. J., et al., (2013). Influence of external factors on the production and morphology of biogenic silver nanocrystallites. *J. Nanosci. Nanotechnol., 13*(3), 2295–2301.

57. Yahyaei, B., & Pourali, P., (2019). One step conjugation of some chemotherapeutic drugs to the biologically produced gold nanoparticles and assessment of their anticancer effects. *Sci. Rep., 9*(1), 10242.

58. Duran, N., et al., (2005). Mechanistic aspects of biosynthesis of silver nanoparticles by several *Fusarium oxysporum* strains. *J. Nanobiotechnology, 3*, 8.

59. Kumar, S. A., et al., (2007). Nitrate reductase-mediated synthesis of silver nanoparticles from AgNO$_3$. *Biotechnology Letters, 29*(3), 439–445.
60. Hietzschold, S., et al., (2019). Does nitrate reductase play a role in silver nanoparticle synthesis? Evidence for NADPH as the sole reducing agent. *ACS Sustainable Chemistry and Engineering, 7*(9), 8070–8076.
61. Lee, S. H., & Jun, B. H., (2019). Silver nanoparticles: Synthesis and application for nanomedicine. *Int. J. Mol. Sci., 20*(4).
62. Birla, S. S., et al., (2013). Rapid synthesis of silver nanoparticles from *Fusarium oxysporum* by optimizing physicocultural conditions. *Scientific World Journal, 2013,* 796018.
63. Saxena, J., et al., (2016). Process optimization for green synthesis of silver nanoparticles by *Sclerotinia sclerotiorum* MTCC 8785 and evaluation of its antibacterial properties. *Springer Plus, 5*(1), 861.
64. Ottoni, C. A., et al., (2017). Screening of filamentous fungi for antimicrobial silver nanoparticles synthesis. *AMB Express, 7*(1), 31.
65. Phanjom, P., & Ahmed, G., (2017). Effect of different physicochemical conditions on the synthesis of silver nanoparticles using fungal cell filtrate of *Aspergillus oryzae* (MTCC No. 1846 and their antibacterial effect. *Advances in Natural Sciences: Nanoscience and Nanotechnology, 8*(4).
66. Shahzad, A., et al., (2019). Size-controlled production of silver nanoparticles by *Aspergillus fumigatus* BTCB10: Likely antibacterial and cytotoxic effects. *Journal of Nanomaterials.*
67. Gade, A. K., et al., (2008). Exploitation of *Aspergillus niger* for synthesis of silver nanoparticles. *Journal of Biobased Materials and Bioenergy, 2*(3), 243–247.
68. Devi, L. S., & Joshi, S. R., (2015). Ultrastructures of silver nanoparticles biosynthesized using endophytic fungi. *J. Microsc. Ultrastruct., 3*(1), 29–37.
69. Azmath, P., et al., (2016). Mycosynthesis of silver nanoparticles bearing antibacterial activity. *Saudi Pharm. J., 24*(2), 140–146.
70. Costa, S. L. P., et al., (2017). Extracellular biosynthesis of silver nanoparticles using the cell-free filtrate of nematophagous fungus *Duddingtonia flagrans. Int. J. Nanomedicine, 12,* 6373–6381.
71. Qian, Y., et al., (2013). Biosynthesis of silver nanoparticles by the endophytic fungus *Epicoccum nigrum* and their activity against pathogenic fungi. *Bioprocess Biosyst Eng., 36*(11), 1613–1619.
72. Husseiny, S. M., Salah, T. A., & Anter, H. A., (2015). Biosynthesis of size controlled silver nanoparticles by *Fusarium oxysporum*, their antibacterial and antitumor activities. *Beni-Suef University Journal of Basic and Applied Sciences, 4*(3), 225–231.
73. Hamedi, S., et al., (2017). Controlled biosynthesis of silver nanoparticles using nitrate reductase enzyme induction of filamentous fungus and their antibacterial evaluation. *Artif. Cells Nanomed. Biotechnol., 45*(8), (1588). –1596.
74. Balakumaran, M. D., Ramachandran, R., & Kalaichelvan, P. T., (2015). Exploitation of endophytic fungus, *Guignardia mangiferae* for extracellular synthesis of silver nanoparticles and their *in vitro* biological activities. *Microbiol. Res., 178,* 9–17.
75. Banu, A. N., & Balasubramanian, C., (2014). Optimization and synthesis of silver nanoparticles using *Isaria fumosorosea* against human vector mosquitoes. *Parasitol Res., 113*(10), 3843–3851.

76. Nayak, R. R., et al., (2011). Green synthesis of silver nanoparticle by *Penicillium purpurogenum* NPMF: The process and optimization. *Journal of Nanoparticle Research, 13*(8), 3129–3137.

77. Rose, G. K., et al., (2019). Optimization of the biological synthesis of silver nanoparticles using *Penicillium oxalicum* GRS-1 and their antimicrobial effects against common food-borne pathogens. *Green Processing and Synthesis, 8*(1), 144–156.

78. Abdel-Rahim, K., et al., (2017). Extracellular biosynthesis of silver nanoparticles using *Rhizopus stolonifer*. *Saudi J. Biol. Sci., 24*(1), 208–216.

79. Ahluwalia, V., et al., (2014). Green synthesis of silver nanoparticles by *Trichoderma harzianum* and their bio-efficacy evaluation against *Staphylococcus aureus* and *Klebsiella pneumonia*. *Industrial Crops and Products, 55*, 202–206.

80. Gherbawy, Y. A., et al., (2013). The anti-fasciolasis properties of silver nanoparticles produced by *Trichoderma harzianum* and their improvement of the anti-fasciolasis drug triclabendazole. *Int. J. Mol. Sci., 14*(11), 21887–21898.

81. Elamawi, R. M., Al-Harbi, R. E., & Hendi, A. A., (2018). Biosynthesis and characterization of silver nanoparticles using *Trichoderma longibrachiatum* and their effect on phytopathogenic fungi. *Egyptian Journal of Biological Pest Control, 28*(1), 28.

82. Feroze, N., et al., (2020). Fungal mediated synthesis of silver nanoparticles and evaluation of antibacterial activity. *Microscopy Research and Technique, 83*(1), 72–80.

83. Yousef, S., et al., (2020). Mycosynthesis of silver nanoparticles by the endophytic fungus *Alternaria tenuissima* AUMC 13621 and evaluation of their antimicrobial, antioxidant effect. *Egyptian Journal of Microbiology, 54*(1), 63–76.

84. Kobashigawa, J. M., et al., (2019). Influence of strong bases on the synthesis of silver nanoparticles (AgNPs) using the ligninolytic fungi *Trametes trogii*. *Saudi Journal of Biological Sciences, 26*(7), 1331–1337.

85. Manjunath, H. M., & Joshi, C. G., (2019). Characterization, antioxidant and antimicrobial activity of silver nanoparticles synthesized using marine endophytic fungus-*Cladosporium cladosporioides*. *Process Biochemistry, 82*, 199–204.

86. Ahmed, S., et al., (2016). A review on plants extract mediated synthesis of silver nanoparticles for antimicrobial applications: A green expertise. *J. Adv. Res., 7*(1), 17–28.

87. Singh, P., et al., (2016). Biological synthesis of nanoparticles from plants and microorganisms. *Trends Biotechnol., 34*(7), 588–599.

88. Sadeghi, B., & Gholamhoseinpoor, F., (2015). A study on the stability and green synthesis of silver nanoparticles using *Ziziphora tenuior* (Zt) extract at room temperature. *Spectrochimica Acta Part A: Molecular and Biomolecular Spectroscopy, 134*, 310–315.

89. Ghaseminezhad, S. M., Hamedi, S., & Shojaosadati, S. A., (2012). Green synthesis of silver nanoparticles by a novel method: Comparative study of their properties. *Carbohydrate Polymers, 89*(2), 467–472.

90. Banasiuk, R., et al., (2020). Carnivorous plants used for green synthesis of silver nanoparticles with broad-spectrum antimicrobial activity. *Arabian Journal of Chemistry, 13*(1), 1415–1428.

91. Nasr, H. A., et al., (2020). Characterization and antimicrobial activity of lemon peel mediated green synthesis of silver nanoparticles. *International Journal of Biology and Chemistry, 12*(2).

92. Balu, S., et al., (2020). Facile synthesis of silver nanoparticles with medicinal grass and its biological assessment. *Materials Letters, 259*, 126900.

93. Aygün, A., et al., (2020). Synthesis and characterization of Reishi mushroom-mediated green synthesis of silver nanoparticles for the biochemical applications. *Journal of Pharmaceutical and Biomedical Analysis, 178*, 112970.

94. Chinyerenwa, A. C., et al., (2018). Ecofriendly sweet scented *Osmanthus* leaf extract mediated synthesis of silver nanoparticles (SNPs). *Int. J. Text. Sci., 7*, 35–42.

95. Athreya, A. G., Shareef, M. I., & Gopinath, S. M., (2019). Antibacterial activity of silver nanoparticles isolated from cow's milk, hen's egg white and lysozyme: A comparative study. *Arabian Journal for Science and Engineering, 44*(7), 6231–6240.

96. Parmar, K., & Jangir, O. P., (2017). Evaluation and efficacy of the antibacterial activity of silver and gold nanoparticles synthesize from camelus dromedarius (Camel) milk against oral pathogenic bacteria. *Int. J. Curr. Microbiol. App. Sci., 6*(4), 600–605.

97. Lateef, A., et al., (2016). Cobweb as novel biomaterial for the green and eco-friendly synthesis of silver nanoparticles. *Applied Nanoscience, 6*(6), 863–874.

98. Phongtongpasuk, S., Poadang, S., & Yongvanich, N., (2016). Environmental-friendly method for synthesis of silver nanoparticles from dragon fruit peel extract and their antibacterial activities. *Energy Procedia, 89*, 239–247.

99. Mythili, R., et al., (2018). Utilization of market vegetable waste for silver nanoparticle synthesis and its antibacterial activity. *Materials Letters, 225*, 101–104.

100. Devadiga, A., Shetty, K. V., & Saidutta, M. B., (2015). Timber industry waste-teak (*Tectona grandis* Linn.) leaf extract mediated synthesis of antibacterial silver nanoparticles. *International Nano Letters, 5*(4), 205–214.

101. Kumar, R., et al., (2012). Agricultural waste *Annona squamosa* peel extract: Biosynthesis of silver nanoparticles. *Spectrochimica Acta Part A: Molecular and Biomolecular Spectroscopy, 90*, 173–176.

102. Baruwati, B., & Varma, R. S., (2009). High value products from waste: Grape pomace extract—a three-in-one package for the synthesis of metal nanoparticles. *Chem. Sus. Chem: Chemistry and Sustainability Energy and Materials, 2*(11), 1041–1044.

103. Anup Bajracharya, Dnyaneshwar Pawar, Priya Mourya, & Aniket Patil, (2018). Bacterial synthesis of silver nanoparticles (AGNPS), *World Journal of Pharmaceutical Research, 7*(6), 872–887.

104. Saravanan, M., et al., (2018). Synthesis of silver nanoparticles from *Bacillus brevis* (NCIM 2533) and their antibacterial activity against pathogenic bacteria. *Microbial Pathogenesis, 116*, 221–226.

105. Peiris, M. M. K., Gunasekara, T. D. C. P., Jayaweera, P. M., & Fernando, S. S. N. (2019). Bacterial enzyme-mediated synthesis of silver nanoparticles and antimicrobial activity. *4th International Research Symposium on Pure and Applied Sciences*, Faculty of Science, University of Kelaniya, Sri Lanka. p20

106. Saravanan, C., et al., (2017). Synthesis of silver nanoparticles using bacterial exopolysaccharide and its application for degradation of azo-dyes. *Biotechnology Reports, 15*, 33–40.

107. Agrawal, P., & Kulkarni, N., (2018). Studies on bacterial synthesis of silver nanoparticles and its synergistic antibacterial effect with antibiotics against selected MDR enteric bacteria. *Int. J. Life. Sci. Scienti. Res. eISSN: 2455*(1716), 1716.

108. Sani, N. J., Aminu, B. M., & Mukhtar, M. D., (2017). Eco-friendly synthesis of silver nanoparticles using *Lactobacillus delbrueckii* subsp. bulgaricus isolated from kindrimo (locally fermented milk) in Kano State, Nigeria. *Bayero Journal of Pure and Applied Sciences, 10*(1), 481–488.

109. Wang, C., et al., (2016). Green synthesis of silver nanoparticles by *Bacillus methylotrophicus*, and their antimicrobial activity. *Artificial Cells, Nanomedicine, and Biotechnology, 44*(4), 1127–1132.

110. Aboelfetoh, E. F., El-Shenody, R. A., & Ghobara, M. M., (2017). Eco-friendly synthesis of silver nanoparticles using green algae (*Caulerpa serrulata*): Reaction optimization, catalytic and antibacterial activities. *Environmental Monitoring and Assessment, 189*(7), 349.

111. Edison, T. N. J. I., et al., (2016). *Caulerpa racemosa*: A marine green alga for eco-friendly synthesis of silver nanoparticles and its catalytic degradation of methylene blue. *Bioprocess and Biosystems Engineering, 39*(9), 1401–1408.

112. Massironi, A., et al., (2019). Ulvan as novel reducing and stabilizing agent from renewable algal biomass: Application to green synthesis of silver nanoparticles. *Carbohydrate Polymers, 203*, 310–321.

113. Murugesan, S., Bhuvaneswari, S., & Sivamurugan, V., (2017). Green synthesis, characterization of silver nanoparticles of a marine red alga *Spyridia fusiformis* and their antibacterial activity. *Int. J. Pharm. Pharm. Sci., 9*(5), 192–197.

114. Moshfegh, A., et al., (2019). Biological synthesis of silver nanoparticles by cell-free extract of *Polysiphonia* algae and their anticancer activity against breast cancer MCF-7 cell lines. *Micro and Amp. Nano Letters, 14*, 581–584.

115. Arya, A., Mishra, V., & Chundawat, T. S., (2019). Green synthesis of silver nanoparticles from green algae (*Botryococcus braunii*) and its catalytic behavior for the synthesis of benzimidazoles. *Chemical Data Collections, 20*, 100190.

116. Vadlapudi, V., & Amanchy, R., (2017). Synthesis, characterization and antibacterial activity of silver nanoparticles from red algae, *Hypnea musciformis*. *Advances in Biological Research, 11*(5), 242–249.

117. Gudikandula, K., Vadapally, P., & Singara, C. M. A., (2017). Biogenic synthesis of silver nanoparticles from white rot fungi: Their characterization and antibacterial studies. *Open Nano, 2*, 64–78.

118. Elegbede, J. A., et al., (2018). Fungal xylanases-mediated synthesis of silver nanoparticles for catalytic and biomedical applications. *IET Nanobiotechnology, 12*(6), 857–863.

119. Qamandar, M. A., & Shafeeq, M. A. A., (2017). Biosynthesis and properties of silver nanoparticles of fungus *Beauveria bassiana*. *Int. J. Chem. Tech. Res., 10*(9), 1073–1083.

120. Shende, S., Gade, A., & Rai, M., (2017). Large-scale synthesis and antibacterial activity of fungal-derived silver nanoparticles. *Environmental Chemistry Letters, 15*(3), 427–434.

121. Popli, D., et al., (2018). Endophyte fungi, Cladosporium species-mediated synthesis of silver nanoparticles possessing *in vitro* antioxidant, anti-diabetic and anti-Alzheimer activity. *Artificial Cells, Nanomedicine, and Biotechnology, 46*, 676–683.

122. Singh, T., et al., (2017). Biosynthesis, characterization and antibacterial activity of silver nanoparticles using an endophytic fungal supernatant of *Raphanus sativus*. *Journal of Genetic Engineering and Biotechnology, 15*(1), 31–39.

123. Xue, B., et al., (2016). Biosynthesis of silver nanoparticles by the fungus *Arthroderma fulvum* and its antifungal activity against genera of candida, *Aspergillus* and *Fusarium*. *International Journal of Nanomedicine, 11*, 1899–1906.

124. Quester, K. , Avalos-Borja, M., & Castro-Longoria, E. (2016). Controllable Biosynthesis of Small Silver Nanoparticles Using Fungal Extract. *Journal of Biomaterials and Nanobiotechnology, 7*, 118–125. doi: 10.4236/jbnb.2016.72013.

125. Rani, R., et al., (2017). Green synthesis, characterization and antibacterial activity of silver nanoparticles of endophytic fungi *Aspergillus terreus*. *J. Nanomed. Nanotechnol., 8*(4).

126. Ahmed, S., et al., (2016). Green synthesis of silver nanoparticles using *Azadirachta indica* aqueous leaf extract. *Journal of Radiation Research and Applied Sciences, 9*(1), 1–7.

127. Tippayawat, P., et al., (2016). Green synthesis of silver nanoparticles in aloe vera plant extract prepared by a hydrothermal method and their synergistic antibacterial activity. *Peer J., 4*, e2589.

128. Bagherzade, G., Tavakoli, M. M., & Namaei, M. H., (2017). Green synthesis of silver nanoparticles using aqueous extract of saffron (*Crocus sativus* L.) wastages and its antibacterial activity against six bacteria. *Asian Pacific Journal of Tropical Biomedicine, 7*(3), 227–233.

129. Shaik, M. R., et al., (2018). Plant-extract-assisted green synthesis of silver nanoparticles using *Origanum vulgare* L. extract and their microbicidal activities. *Sustainability, 10*(4), 913.

130. Allafchian, A. R., et al., (2016). Green synthesis of silver nanoparticles using phlomis leaf extract and investigation of their antibacterial activity. *Journal of Nanostructure in Chemistry, 6*(2), 129–135.

131. Pirtarighat, S., Ghannadnia, M., & Baghshahi, S., (2019). Green synthesis of silver nanoparticles using the plant extract of Salvia spinosa grown in vitro and their antibacterial activity assessment. *Journal of Nanostructure in Chemistry, 9*(1), 1–9.

132. Jeevanandam, J., et al., (2019). Metal oxide nanocomposites: Cytotoxicity and targeted drug delivery applications. In: *Hybrid Nanocomposites: Fundamentals, Synthesis and Applications* (pp. 111–147). Pan Stanford Publishing.

133. Egger, S., et al., (2009). Antimicrobial properties of a novel silver-silica nanocomposite material. *Appl. Environ. Microbiol., 75*(9), 2973–2976.

134. Adepu, S., & Khandelwal, M., (2018). Broad-spectrum antimicrobial activity of bacterial cellulose silver nanocomposites with sustained release. *Journal of Materials Science, 53*(3), 1596–1609.

135. Pinto, R. J. B., et al., (2009). Antibacterial activity of nanocomposites of silver and bacterial or vegetable cellulosic fibers. *Acta Biomaterialia, 5*(6), 2279–2289.

136. Sureshkumar, M., Siswanto, D. Y., & Lee, C. K., (2010). Magnetic antimicrobial nanocomposite based on bacterial cellulose and silver nanoparticles. *Journal of Materials Chemistry, 20*(33), 6948–6955.

137. Liu, C., et al., (2012). Fabrication of antimicrobial bacterial cellulose-Ag/AgCl nanocomposite using bacteria as versatile biofactory. *Journal of Nanoparticle Research, 14*(8), 1084.

138. Satheeshkumar, M. K., et al., (2020). Structural, morphological and magnetic properties of algae/CoFe$_2$O$_4$ and algae/Ag-Fe-O nanocomposites and their biomedical applications. *Inorganic Chemistry Communications, 111,* 107578.

139. Madhusudhan, K. N., (2017). Extraction and characterization of chitin and chitosan from *Aspergillus niger*, synthesis of silver-chitosan nanocomposites and evaluation of their antimicrobial potential. *Journal of Advances in Biotechnology, 6*(3), 939–945.

140. Majumder, D. R., et al., (2018). Eco-friendly synthesis of Chitosan-PVA-Silver nanocomposite for sustained release of aspirin. *World Journal of Pharmaceutical Research, 7*(4), 71–88.

141. Baskar, G., Bikku, G. G., & Chamundeeswari, M., (2017). Synthesis and characterization of asparaginase bound silver nanocomposite against ovarian cancer cell line A2780 and lung cancer cell line A549. *Journal of Inorganic and Organometallic Polymers and Materials, 27*(1), 87–94.

142. Sathiyaseelan, A., et al., (2017). Fungal chitosan based nanocomposites sponges: An alternative medicine for wound dressing. *International Journal of Biological Macromolecules, 104,* 1905–1915.

143. Batool, S., et al., (2019). Biogenic synthesis of silver nanoparticles and evaluation of physical and antimicrobial properties of Ag/PVA/starch nanocomposites hydrogel membranes for wound dressing application. *Journal of Drug Delivery Science and Technology, 52,* 403–414.

144. Omidi, S., et al., (2018). Biosynthesis of silver nanocomposite with Tarragon leaf extract and assessment of antibacterial activity. *Journal of Nanostructure in Chemistry, 8*(2), 171–178.

145. Ghiassi, S., et al., (2018). Plant-mediated bio-synthesis of silver-montmorillonite nanocomposite and antibacterial effects on gram-positive and -negative bacteria. *Journal of Nanostructure in Chemistry, 8*(3), 353–357.

146. Naeimi, A., Amiri, A., & Ghasemi, Z., (2017). A novel strategy for green synthesis of colloidal porphyrins/silver nanocomposites by *Sesbania sesban* plant and their catalytic application in the clean oxidation of alcohols. *Journal of the Taiwan Institute of Chemical Engineers, 80,* 107–113.

147. Zheng, Y., et al., (2016). Hydrothermal preparation of reduced graphene oxide-silver nanocomposite using *Plectranthus amboinicus* leaf extract and its electrochemical performance. *Enzyme and Microbial Technology, 95,* 112–117.

148. Song, C., et al., (2019). Thorough utilization of rice husk: Metabolite extracts for silver nanocomposite biosynthesis and residues for silica nanomaterials fabrication. *New Journal of Chemistry, 43*(23), 9201–9209.

149. Bordbar, M., & Mortazavimanesh, N., (2018). Biosynthesis of waste pistachio shell supported silver nanoparticles for the catalytic reduction processes. *IET Nanobiotechnology, 12,* 939–945.

150. Patil, P. O., et al., (2017). Green fabrication of graphene-based silver nanocomposites using agro-waste for sensing of heavy metals. *Research on Chemical Intermediates, 43*(7), 3757–3773.

151. Sportelli, C. M., et al., (2018). The pros and cons of the use of laser ablation synthesis for the production of silver nano-antimicrobials. *Antibiotics, 7*(3).

152. Gomathi, M., Prakasam, A., & Rajkumar, P. V., (2019). Green synthesis, characterization and antibacterial activity of silver nanoparticles using *Amorphophallus paeoniifolius* leaf extract. *Journal of Cluster Science, 30*(4), 995–1001.

153. Balasubramanian, S., Jeyapaul, U., & Kala, S. M. J., (2017). Antibacterial activity of silver nanoparticles using *Jasminum auriculatum* stem extract. *International Journal of Nanoscience, 18*(01), 1850011.

154. Agnihotri, S., et al., (2019). Antibacterial activity of silver nanoparticles synthesized from buttermilk. *Drug Invention Today, 11*(10).

155. Kirtiwar, S., Gharpure, S., & Balaprasad, A., (2019). Effect of nutrient media on antibacterial activity of silver nanoparticles synthesized using *Neolamarckia cadamba*. *Journal of Nanoscience and Nanotechnology, 19*(4), 1923–1933.

156. Hu, X., et al., (2019). Mycosynthesis, characterization, anticancer and antibacterial activity of silver nanoparticles from endophytic fungus *Talaromyces purpureogenus*. *International Journal of Nanomedicine, 14*, 3427–3438.

157. Hasan, I., et al., (2019). Eco-friendly green synthesis of dextrin based poly (methyl methacrylate) grafted silver nanocomposites and their antibacterial and antibiofilm efficacy against multi-drug resistance pathogens. *Journal of Cleaner Production, 230*, 1148–1155.

158. Rolim, W. R., et al., (2019). Antibacterial activity and cytotoxicity of silver chloride/ silver nanocomposite synthesized by a bacterium isolated from Antarctic soil. *Bio. Nano Science*.

159. Abdel-Aziz, M. M., Elella, M. H. A., & Mohamed, R. R., (2020). Green synthesis of quaternized chitosan/silver nanocomposites for targeting mycobacterium tuberculosis and lung carcinoma cells (A-549*). International Journal of Biological Macromolecules, 142*, 244–253.

160. Moradi, F., et al., (2019). Biosynthesis of silver-montmorillonite nanocomposites using *Ocimum basilicum* and *Teucrium polium*; a comparative study. *Materials Research Express, 6*(12), 125008.

161. Jalal, M., et al., (2019). Anticandidal activity of biosynthesized silver nanoparticles: Effect on growth, cell morphology, and key virulence attributes of candida species. *International Journal of Nanomedicine, 14*, 4667–4679.

162. Bhagat, M., et al., (2019). Green synthesis of silver nanoparticles using aqueous extract of rosa *Brunonii lindl* and their morphological, biological and photocatalytic characterizations. *Journal of Inorganic and Organometallic Polymers and Materials, 29*(3), 1039–1047.

163. Kumari, M., et al., (2019). An insight into the mechanism of antifungal activity of biogenic nanoparticles than their chemical counterparts. *Pesticide Biochemistry and Physiology, 157*, 45–52.

164. Youssef, A. M., Abdel-Aziz, M. S., & El-Sayed, S. M., (2014). Chitosan nanocomposite films based on Ag-NP and Au-NP biosynthesis by *Bacillus subtilis* as packaging materials. *International Journal of Biological Macromolecules, 69*, 185–191.

165. Roseline, T. A., et al., (2019). Nanopesticidal potential of silver nanocomposites synthesized from the aqueous extracts of red seaweeds. *Environmental Technology and Innovation, 13*, 82–93.

166. Kumari, R., Barsainya, M., & Singh, D. P., (2017). Biogenic synthesis of silver nanoparticle by using secondary metabolites from *Pseudomonas aeruginosa* DM1 and its anti-algal effect on chlorella vulgaris and chlorella pyrenoidosa. *Environmental Science and Pollution Research, 24*(5), 4645–4654.

167. El-Kassas, H. Y., & Ghobrial, M. G., (2017). Biosynthesis of metal nanoparticles using three marine plant species: Anti-algal efficiencies against "*Oscillatoria simplicissima*". *Environmental Science and Pollution Research, 24*(8), 7837–7849.

168. Arif, S., et al., (2017). Comparative analysis of stability and biological activities of violacein and starch capped silver nanoparticles. *RSC Advances, 7*(8), 4468–4478.

169. Natarajan, S., et al., (2018). Antifouling and anti-algal effects of chitosan nanocomposite (TiO$_2$/Ag) and pristine (TiO$_2$ and Ag) films on marine microalgae *Dunaliella salina*. *Journal of Environmental Chemical Engineering, 6*(6), 6870–6880.

170. Natarajan, S., et al., (2017). Antifouling activities of pristine and nanocomposite chitosan/TiO$_2$/Ag films against freshwater algae. *RSC Advances, 7*(44), 27645–27655.

171. Huang, Z., et al., (2018). Antioxidative response of *Phanerochaete chrysosporium* against silver nanoparticle-induced toxicity and its potential mechanism. *Chemosphere, 211*, 573–583.

172. Elbeshehy, E. K. F., Elazzazy, A. M., & Aggelis, G., (2015). Silver nanoparticles synthesis mediated by new isolates of *Bacillus* spp., nanoparticle characterization and their activity against bean yellow mosaic virus and human pathogens. *Frontiers in Microbiology, 6*, 453.

173. Yang, X. X., Li, C. M., & Huang, C. Z., (2016). Curcumin modified silver nanoparticles for highly efficient inhibition of respiratory syncytial virus infection. *Nanoscale, 8*(5), 3040–3048.

174. Sharma, V., et al., (2019). Green synthesis of silver nanoparticles from medicinal plants and evaluation of their antiviral potential against chikungunya virus. *Applied Microbiology and Biotechnology, 103*(2), 881–891.

175. Dhanasezhian, A., et al., (2019). Anti-herpes simplex virus (HSV-1 and HSV-2) activity of biogenic gold and silver nanoparticles using seaweed *Sargassum wightii*. *Indian Journal of Geo-Marine Sciences, 48*(8), 1252–1257.

176. Mahyoub, J. A., et al., (2017). Seagrasses as sources of mosquito nano-larvicides? Toxicity and uptake of *Halodule uninervis-biofabricated* silver nanoparticles in dengue and zika virus vector aedes aegypti. *Journal of Cluster Science, 28*(1), 565–580.

177. Du, T., et al., (2018). Antiviral activity of graphene oxide-silver nanocomposites by preventing viral entry and activation of the antiviral innate immune response. *ACS Applied Bio. Materials, 1*(5), 1286–1293.

178. Chen, Y. N., et al., (2016). Antiviral activity of graphene-silver nanocomposites against non-enveloped and enveloped viruses. *International Journal of Environmental Research and Public Health. 13*(4), 430.

179. Galdiero, S., et al., (2011). Silver nanoparticles as potential antiviral agents. *Molecules. 16*(10).

180. Khatami, M., et al., (2018). Waste-grass-mediated green synthesis of silver nanoparticles and evaluation of their anticancer, antifungal and antibacterial activity. *Green Chemistry Letters and Reviews, 11*(2), 125–134.

181. Yan, X., et al., (2018). Antibacterial mechanism of silver nanoparticles in Pseudomonas aeruginosa: Proteomics approach. *Metallomics, 10*(4), 557–564.

182. Durán, N., et al., (2016). Silver nanoparticles: A new view on mechanistic aspects on antimicrobial activity. *Nanomedicine: Nanotechnology, Biology and Medicine, 12*(3), 789–799.

183. Khadka, P., et al., (2018). Quantitative investigations reveal new antimicrobial mechanism of silver nanoparticles and ions. *Biophysical Journal, 114*(3), 690a.

184. Liao, S., et al., (2019). Antibacterial activity and mechanism of silver nanoparticles against multidrug-resistant Pseudomonas aeruginosa. *International Journal of Nanomedicine, 14*, 1469–1487.

185. Zhang, C., Hu, Z., & Deng, B., (2016). Silver nanoparticles in aquatic environments: Physiochemical behavior and antimicrobial mechanisms. *Water Research, 88*, 403–427.

186. Viet, P. V., et al., (2018). Silver nanoparticle loaded $TiO_2$ nanotubes with high photocatalytic and antibacterial activity synthesized by photoreduction method. *Journal of Photochemistry and Photobiology A: Chemistry, 352*, 106–112.

187. Abbaszadegan, A., et al., (2015). The effect of charge at the surface of silver nanoparticles on antimicrobial activity against gram-positive and gram-negative bacteria: A preliminary study. *Journal of Nanomaterials, 2015*.

188. Xiu, Z. M., Ma, J., & Alvarez, P. J. J., (2011). Differential effect of common ligands and molecular oxygen on antimicrobial activity of silver nanoparticles versus silver ions. *Environmental Science and Technology, 45*(20), 9003–9008.

189. Meyer, J. N., et al., (2010). Intracellular uptake and associated toxicity of silver nanoparticles in *Caenorhabditis elegans*. Aquatic *Toxicology, 100*(2), 140–150.

190. Choi, O., et al., (2008). The inhibitory effects of silver nanoparticles, silver ions, and silver chloride colloids on microbial growth. *Water Research, 42*(12), 3066–3074.

191. Benn, T. M., & Westerhoff, P., (2008). Nanoparticle silver released into water from commercially available sock fabrics. *Environmental Science and Technology, 42*(11), 4133–4139.

192. Shastri, J. P., Rupani, M. G., & Jain, R. L., (2012). Antimicrobial activity of nanosilver-coated socks fabrics against foot pathogens. *Journal of the Textile Institute, 103*(11), 1234–1243.

193. Zhang, F., et al., (2009). Application of silver nanoparticles to cotton fabric as an antibacterial textile finish. *Fibers and Polymers, 10*(4), 496–501.

194. Lateef, A., et al., (2016). Biogenic synthesis of silver nanoparticles using a pod extract of *Cola nitida*: Antibacterial and antioxidant activities and application as a paint additive. *Journal of Taibah University for Science, 10*(4), 551–562.

195. Shi, G., et al., (2018). An antifouling hydrogel containing silver nanoparticles for modulating the therapeutic immune response in chronic wound healing. *Langmuir, 35*(5), 1837–1845.

# CHAPTER 8

# Plant Extract: Isolation, Purification, and Applications of Green Nanomaterials Stabilization

S. SREEVIDYA,[1] KIRTANA SANKARA SUBRAMANIAN,[2]
YOKRAJ KATRE,[1] ANIL KUMAR,[3] and AJAYA KUMAR SINGH[4]

[1]*Department of Chemistry, Kalyan PG College, Bhilai Nagar, Durg – 490006, Chhattisgarh, India*

[2]*Department of Food Science, Faculty of Veterinary and Agriculture Science, University of Melbourne, Melbourne, Australia*

[3]*Department of Biotechnology, Government V.Y.T. PG. Autonomous College, Durg – 491001, Chhattisgarh, India*

[4]*Department of Chemistry, Government V.Y.T. PG. Autonomous College, Durg – 491001, Chhattisgarh, India, E-mail: ajayaksingh_au@yahoo.co.in*

## ABSTRACT

The wonderful precious gift of nature, beckoned as the Sec-Met has an impending versatility in all avenues. As a bio-consumable one, these are the most sorted organics, in the flowering field of green nano-trend, that adopt the flora and fauna kingdom as their source. Extraction is a powerful media to hunt these PC's. The reservoir of functionable extracting tools for extractables enhances the active separation of these Sec-Met. This can be individually segregated and purified as per applicational needs. With the uniqueness of bio-degradability, these protecting Sec-Met from the plant kingdom, function for an operative bio-reductant and bio-stabilization procedures, commanding non-toxicities and non-expensive etiquettes. The routes for the green nano-trend, harvest the NP's, to bargain their application in distinct pitches. Here, we have narrated a trail to interpret these assorted segments involved in operational, stabilization, and applicational forums of NP's by green nano-trend.

## 8.1  INTRODUCTION

A huge variation of 3,00,000 plant species [1] is found in our nature, but only 15% are effectively noticed to be of utility as medicinal herbs. Potent medicinal species were identified and recognized as valuable reserves by WHO [2], of which, many may disappear, are essentially needed to be protected for the future. The reserve of secondary metabolite (Sec-Met), with many phyto-constituents (PCs) in it, varying in accordance with their origin, undergo phytoremediation, has a noteworthy contribution, in protecting nature as a whole, though not in reproducing and in growing [3].

While the use of botanical extracts, as a welcome drink, shows the acceptance of organics culturally, it is noteworthy that it is also appreciated scientifically in the area of nanoparticle syntheses [4]. It drives well from folklore to scientific forums as in Nanotechnology to genomics and bio-informatics, works out well as a strong reducing, capping or stabilizing agent, with a clinch to attract and adsorb the particles during NP fabrication [5]. With domains center for effective resource, as plant's botanical filtrate, where it is utilized as stabilizers, focuses on the shape morphology and inter-dimensions of size, can be altered physically by varying kinetics. With a crucial part in the fabricating nanoparticle(s) (NP), together with reduced toxic effects to the external system, they find their application with diversity. They find their place in water treatment [6], bio-sensing [7], textiles [8], pharmaceutical, and medical industries [9], photo-catalysis [10], opto-electronics [11], space, and defense wing [12], oil-recovery [13], pesticide-insecticide [14] and many, witness broad venues commercially [15], with various hues of bio-chemical and bio-physical properties, as a day-to-day tool [16]. The green nano-trend that protects the reserves and resources is the most sought-after platform, being simple, non-toxic, and economical, with eco-friendly protocols [17]. Cellular fragments with PCs in them, effectively used as probes, form a reserve for NP synthesis in the green nano-fields. As a user friendly one, effectively works with water, obviating the requirement for additional hazardous external chemical agents [18]. Distinct electrostatic interactions among the bio-molecular organic templates and inorganic ones control the size and shape dimensions while stabilizing the NP's engineered by the biosynthetic approach [19].

In spite of the voluminous work in green nano-block as per [20], the potential reserve of the voluminous biodegradables, with a sack full of PCs, from various plant species are utilized only in a limited way for NP synthesis. They are to be tapped efficiently and economically from the nature, delivered to the nature, for the nature in a simple way [21]. Phyto-molecules as a Sec-Met [22] work as a health benefiter in the form of antioxidants, cholesterol inhibitors [23], antibacterial, insecticide, and anticancer agents and thus find their way into drug, flavor, dye, fragrance, food, and other industries, as supporters in the nano-block [24].

## 8.2   BOUNDARIES: AN OPERATIVE ENTITY

Plant extract, a remarkable source for natural products, with diversified bioactive (BA) components, serves as a supplement and a protectant [25]. Figure 8.1 portrays various extraction modules generally used to get potent BAs.

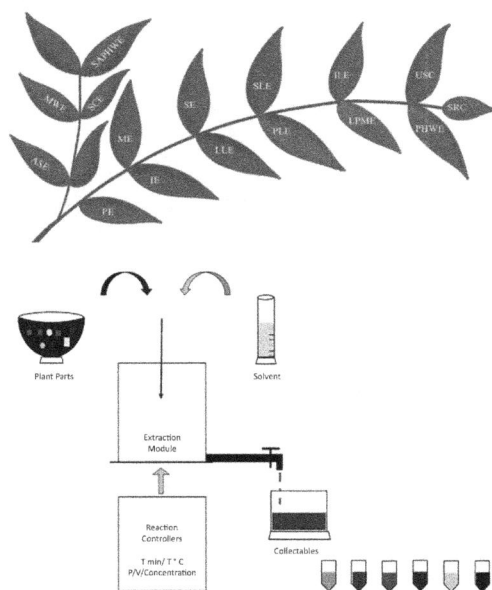

**FIGURE 8.1**   Extraction modules used to get BAs from plants.

Extraction is a preliminary wing prior to isolation for separation and purification and is an important step for retrieval of BA's. Pre-concentration of extracts ensures no alterations of the constituents and would reduce 30% of errors associated analytically [26]. Bio-molecules are extracted effectively with a higher degree of proximity, with the use of solvent in single or in combination, in different rates, to give better achievements of phytocomponents.

## 8.3  AUTOMATED APPROACHES FOR BA'S: ISOLATION AND PURIFICATION

The unavoidable essential markers are to be pinned down, from a complex extract to identify targets by physical, chemical or biological evaluates, for its quick recovery of isolates [27], where the new technical approaches provide a platform for parallel development and applicability [28]. The extracts with different BAs, of varying polarities need to be isolated and purified, undergo various technical requirements depending upon the new emerging establishments [29]. Different technical attempts vary from classical to new novel approaches, where the next generation of technology incorporates different spectroscopic methods for accurateness.

The high end of chromatographic versions like HPLC, HP-TLC, HSCCC, enhance the purification process of isolates, along with spectroscopic searches of UV, FTIR, NMR, MS. It would assist in the identification of BA's from economical to expensive. The versions can be associated with hyphenated ones like HPLC-DAD, LC-MS, GC-MS [30, 31]. The choices vary with the nature and functions of stability, solubility, polarity, particle size, charge, and pH value with an organic or aqueous segment as a terrain for mobility, supported by Silica/C-18/Alumina as a stationary platform, from unknown to known of various classes for Isolation, Identification, Separation, and Purification [32–34]. Purification of active ingredients, an important one, finds a suitable place in food, medicinal, pharmaceutical, and other industries, where the quality of these components is incessantly expanding. Purification of flavonoids of quercetin and rutin was successfully portrayed by [35] using HPLC-DAD followed by adsorption and desorption practices, to quantify the content. SCF-$CO_2$ has been successfully employed in many isolation and purification using modifiers to assist the process [36]. A simple schematic description of the isolation and purification of green nanomaterials stabilization process is represented in Figure 8.2.

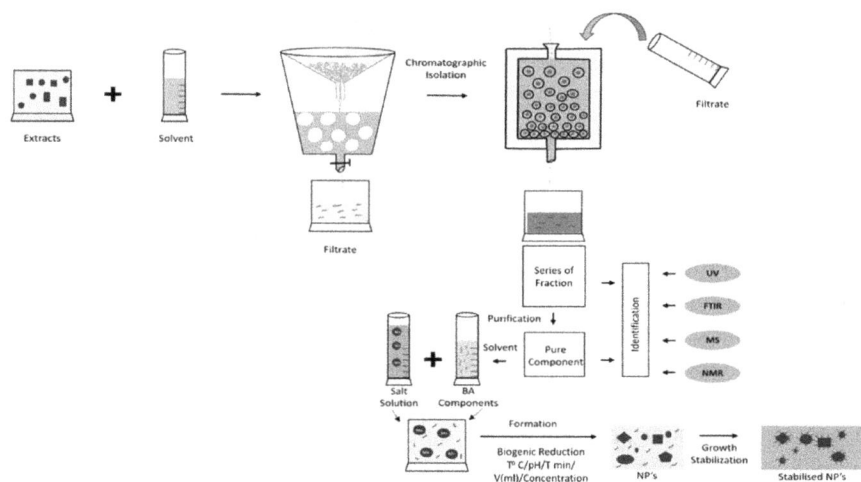

**FIGURE 8.2** A simple schematic description of isolation and purification of green nanomaterial's stabilization.

Floral petal extract of *Begonia semperflorens* of various hues packed with flavonoids and anthocyanins, discussed by [37] had silica platform as adsorbent, with n-$C_6C_{14}$-EtOAc, and had been analyzed using CC. Curcumin and Xanthones from *Curcuma zanthorrhiza*, Tanshinones from *Salvia miltiorrhiza* and amides from *Piper nigrum* have been reported as isolates using RP-18 cartridges [38]. Quercetin, a flavonoid, was successfully isolated by FC method [39], was supported by hi-tech spectrophotometric methods of FTIR, $^1$H-NMR, and $^1$C-NMR to give accurate and reliable outcomes. Isolates of polyphenolics from EtOAc of *Eucalyptus camaldulensis* known for potent antimicrobial activity was reported by [40], where the plant extract subjected to fractionation by VLC, validated the presence of six components when recorded by (proton) $^1$H-NMR and $^1$C-NMR and as flavonoids-glycosides from *Genipa Americana* by employing HPLC/ESI/IT/MS/MS [41] philosophies. TLC was used to judge the presence of the molecular structures of phenolic acids, flavonoids, glycosides, and flavanols in *Citrus sinensis* and *Artocarpus heterophyllus* V. [42]. Complex constituents to be separated are governed by hydrophobic and hydrophilic that balance the interaction between the

BA analyte in both phases. *Passifloraalata* studied by [43] showed unique fingerprints of flavonoids using ethanolic extracts. The poly phenols from *Aspalathus linear* are from different geographical zones and were found to have aspalathin, a rare rooibos compounds (polyphenolic), as reported by [44], using mobile phase (MP) as $CH_3COCH_3$-$CHCl_3$-$H_2O$ mixtures, and Silica/Alumina as stationary phase (SP).

A rapid extraction using carbon nanotubes [45] as adsorbent was used to analyze the stability in different conditions with selectivity. Claude et al. [46] achieved a good yield of extraction (98%) by SPE-MIP, using *Glycirrhiza glabra* roots, found to be anti-inflammatory and anti-allergic, had 18-α glycyrrhetinic acid in it. Awouafack, Tane, and Morita [47] isolated Lachnoisoflavones (a polyphenolic Sec-Met) from *Crotalaria lachnophora* using $H_2O$-MeOH as mobiles by MPLC tunes. In another situation, Liang et al. [48] separated and purified target compounds by MPLC followed by HSCCC to get indole derivatives from *Radix isatidisa*, a potent anticancer and anti-virus, commonly used as an herbal tonic by people of traditional China, was characterized and later ascertained by spectroscopic techniques of (functional) FT-IR, (proton) $^1$H-NMR, and (electrospray) ESI-MS. Natural products of cinnamic acid, rutin, piperine, phenol, p-coumarinic acid, phloroglucinol, anthracene, and caffeic acid were identified by MPLC-HPLC-/UV-MS technique using Al Column in reverse phase (RP) modes, were monitored at $\lambda_{max}$ 280 nm [49].

HPLC plays an important part in identification and purification of raw extract of a multiplex mixture and are used to isolate the contents [50]. The degree of separation is controlled by Stationary (SP) and Mobile (MP) Phases, with mobiles as isocratic or gradient [51]. Purification by HPLC, with an optimized flow rate, enhances the movement of BA component in the analyte, when the non-polar part of the mobile firmly binds with the SP (low as 2–5 μm). It assists the speed of eluting the components [52], and delivers clean-ups in the columns to enable successive application. Right optimizing detectors such as UV, IR, Mass (LC/GC) and NMR ensure specific peak characteristics for each one. Potentials of anti-diabetic activity in *Costusigneus* were studied by [53], where the methanolic leaf extract, showed the validation of flavonoids, like kaempferol, roseoside, quercetin, and epicatechin. Phenolic acid, in free state, was isolated with $CH_3OH$:$H_2O$:$CH_3COOH$ as mobiles, using EtOH extracts of *Eleutherococcus senticosus* and *Acanthopanax senticosus* plant roots by [54].

A potent advanced analytical tool for multidimensional work augmented with optimization, automation, and hyphenation, demands a optimized amount of mobiles, for a quick and easy separation in a single run [55]. It has an advantage, for combinatorial BA's to be resolved simultaneously with the same MP and to lower the disposal snags [56]. HP-TLC delivers economic non-toxicity, with high yields of resolution, with great sensitivity, where the output of fingerprint data is retrieved from the electronic metaphors. HP-TLCs are governed by zones of thickness, types, and binders in SP, solvents in MP, T°C, and flow rate. The protocol maintained by [57] for phenolics and flavonoids by HP-TLC certification was silica gel $60F_{254}$ in SP and $CH_3COOC_2H_5$/$CH_3OH/H_2O$ (10:1.65:1.35) v/v in MP, were documented by UV at 254 and 366 nm.

The two important diagnostic tools to understand the metabolites are chromatography and spectroscopy. The former separates the metabolite isolates, while the latter gives quantity and identity to the isolates. Hyphenation of an online linking of various isolating techniques associated with spectroscopic detection is a potentially valuable tool in science that offers separation and molecular information in depth. Chromatographic fingerprints, mainly LC and GC coupled with associated detectors of NMR, MS/MS, DAD, are fruitfully addressed for isolating and purifying the natural Sec-Met. LC-MS/MS, whose signal noise is very high, along with sensitivity and selectivity, has been employed by many workers as an utmost dependable technique [58]. For the targeted and untargeted approaches of MS and NMR, benefits, and limitations are complementary to each other [59], with a little difference between them in preparation and sample handling techniques. Distinct selectivity and unique sensitivity are principal features achieved in GC-MS analysis and profiling [60], where the thermal stability and volatility of polar components are to be taken care of while using SPs with variation. Carrier gas in GC port allows the sample to be vaporized, separated, analyzed, and detected in interface modes. A thumbprint input is represented in Table 8.1.

A simple, versatile hyphenated method of chromatography, coupled with spectroscopic units as HPLC/UV/IR/[1]H NMR/[13]C NMR was bio-autographed by [72] to isolate quercetin, from the methanolic extracts of the leaves of *Lagerstroemia speciose*. $\lambda_{Max}$ at 254 nm, with Rf of 3.59 (HPLC), showed 91.39% purity of the samples isolated as flavonoids.

**TABLE 8.1**　A Thumbprint Input about the BAs Present, with Various Modes of Hyphenated Fingerprints

| Plant Source/Extraction | Bio-Actives/No. Identified | Reaction Profiles SP/Flow Rate/MP | Analytical Models | UV $\lambda_{Max}$ nm | References |
|---|---|---|---|---|---|
| *Gossypium herbaceam*/EtOH | Flavonoid glycosides/12 | C18-5 μm/5 mL min⁻¹ MeO-H₂O | FC/NMR/LC-MS PDS | 370 | [61] |
| *Calycotome villosa*/MeOH | Flavonols/2 | Silica gel/CH₂Cl₂-MeOH | CC/IR/MS/¹H NMR,¹³C NMR | 255, 370 | [62] |
| *Juniperus phoenicea*/MeOH | Flavonoids/32 | C18-5 μm/CH₃COOH-H₂O/ MeOH | HPLC-DAD-ESI/MS, GC/MS | 320–370 250–280 | [63] |
| *Anoectochilus roxburghii*/ EtOH | Flavonoids/13 | C18-5 μm/10 mL min⁻¹/ H₂O-ACN/ | HPLC-UV, ¹H NMR/ RRLC-MS PDS | 345 | [64] |
| *Euphorbia neriifolia*/EtOH/H₂O | Flavonoids | Silica gel 60 F254/ BuOH-AcH-H₂O/ | TLC/HPTLC/IR, ¹H NMR/MS | 254, 366 | [65] |
| *Sambucus nigra, Calluna vulgaris, C. aurantium, C. limon* / MeOH | Flavones, Flavanones/46 | C18-3.5 μm/RP-18, 5 μm/H₂O/MeOH/MeCN/ HCOOH | HPLC/UHPLC/ ¹H NMR/¹³CNMR | – | [66] |
| *E. giganteum, E. bogotense, E. arvense, E. hyemale*/ EtOH | Flavonoids, Styrylpyrones/4 | C18-5 μm/0.9 mL min⁻¹/ HCOOH/H₂O/ACN/MeOH | LC-DAD/LC-UV/ LC-ESI-MS/MS | 254, 370 | [67] |
| *Murraya koenegii*/MeOH, EtOH, CH₃COCH₃ | Flavonols/10 | C18/1 mL min⁻¹/MeOH / H₂O/HCOOH/ACN/ | HPLC / LC/MS/MS, HPLC/DAD/MS/MS/ HPLC/APCI/MS/MS | 366 | [68] |
| *Launeae arboescens*/BuOH, H₂O, CH₃COCH₃ | Flavanone/8 | silica gel/CH₃COCH₃-C₆H₅CH₃-HCOOH | LC-UV/ ¹H NMR /¹³C NMR | 203–254, 286, 330, | [69] |
| *Cytisus multiflorus*/EtOH | Flavones/12 | C18-5 μm/1.0 mL min⁻¹/ HCOOH/ H₂O/CAN | HPLC-DAD/ HPLC-ESI-MS-NMR | 280 | [70] |
| *Scutellaria baicalensis*/EtOH | Flavonoids/21 | C18-5 μm/1.0 mL min⁻¹/ AcH/CAN | HPLC-UV/MS/MSn, LC-UV/MS, 1D-2D NMR | 276 | [71] |

The FT-IR studies, with representative broad peaks, focused at 3334.92 cm$^{-1}$ for (hydroxyl) OH $_{stretch}$ and 1724.36 cm$^{-1}$ (C=O) for carbonyls, along with proton NMR and $^{13}$C NMR were characteristics of the study. The molecular formula was proven to be $C_{15}H_{10}O_{7,}$ form its molecular ion, with m/z 302 [M$^{+}$H]$^{+}$ by EIMS spectral studies.

## 8.4  NANOSTABILIZATION

Ecological catastrophies to balance the bio-diversity attract the scientific commutators to supersede the older innovations. Nanotechnology, redefined with scientific burgeoning endeavors, marches towards green trend with wide frontiers of sustainability, fabricating veritable positive centers to reframe (i.e., to present new ideas or beliefs in a different way), so as to bring positive changes to our earth [73]. Nano-structures, produced in a wide array of ways, use bio-organics, chemical, and mechanical approaches [74]. Nanomaterials fit as a perfect candidate for scientific break-up, from environmental to medicine, as in pollution reduction (water, soil, and air). They are also fit for unique applications such as labeling, biosensing, optical, pesticidal, antimicrobial, defense, space sectors, electronics, textiles, and drug delivery [18]. A voluminous input about size, crystal structure, shape, elemental-composition, binding, surface area, charge, stability, and many more can be precisely drawn from measures like TEM, FTIR, XPS, NMR, EDX-SEM, DLS, Zeta potential, XRD, UV-Vis, and others [75].

A herculean task is to synthesize the NP's with required physio-chemical properties like chemical, catalytic, electrical, electronic, mechanical, magnetic, and optical, governed by targeted shape, fixed size, and specific orderliness of the crystal structure [76]. In the green nano-trend [77], nature's botanical sources serve as a reductant, stabilize, or cap the particles in the system to evade aggregation by developing electrostatic forces of attraction between them in the formation, thereby enforcing no toxicity, to assure a threat-free zone [78]. Utilization of fungi [79], bacteria [80] as microorganisms, algae [81], yeast [79], enzymes [82], animal, and human wastes [83], plant parts [84], and agri wastes [85] help to attain this goal in a short scale of time.

## 8.5   PLANT BIO-REDUCTANTS AND BIO-STABILIZERS: MAIN FOCUS IN GREEN SYNTHESIS

Secondary metabolites (Sec-Met) like flavonoids [86], terpenoids [87], alkaloids [88], saponins [43], steroids [89], and glycosides [90] from different literatures are capable of forming nano-associates with inorganic templates. Sorted out into three sectors as prime-activation (reduction of metallic ions by BAs), middle-growth (nucleation), final-termination (stabilization of nucleated NPs by BAs), ultimately leading to a stable morphological structure. A simple representation of bio-stabilizers with purposeful proposal in stabilizing NP's is depicted in Figure 8.3.

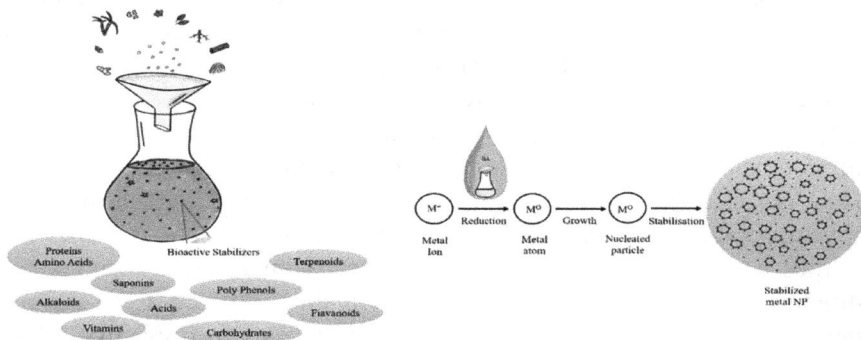

**FIGURE 8.3**   BAs from different sources and a pictorial representation of NP's stabilization.

A protective layer is formed by the stabilizing agents to prevent agglomeration of the metals, as boundary coating to avoid oxidation [91]. Electrostatic stabilization deals with formation of an electrical double layer [92] with electrical repulsive forces, whereas steric stabilization deals with sterically hindered repulsion amongst the molecules or ions. In the biogenic reaction, some metabolites of polyphenols and flavonoids that are water (aqua) soluble, functions with a potential of a works like a reducer and a stabilizer (R&S) [93] to assist in NP's materialization. In a classical work [94], it is reported that $Fe^{3+}$ ions are chelated by organic polyphenols. Fresh fruit juice of *pomegranate* and liquid red wine [95], potential sources of polyphenol, [96, 97] inferred that flavonoids, amaranthine, and amino acids were found to host NP's formation and FTIR studies of [98] revealed that polyphenols were responsible for capping.

## 8.6    REACTION PROTOCOLS FOR EFFECTIVE BIOGENIC SYNTHESIS AND THEIR UTILITY

Physicochemical features of the NP's formed are solely governed by a number of reaction parameters with a key note for plant extraction, temperature, time, methods employed, strength of extract, pH, metallic ion's strength and quantity of extract used, of the ongoing reaction. Plant juices from different or same species would vary with the pH values [99]. Kinetics of the reaction eluted by the pH [100] affects the morphological shape, identity, and size dimensions of the NP's, even over a small narrow variation [101], while [102] needed an alkaline one. pH affects the toxicity of nanoscale products formed, as per [103] report, when FeO NP's formed by the bio-genic synthetic reduction using husk filtrate of Juglans regia, was proven to be cytotoxic for medico-biological lines. Change in catalytic activity was influenced when pH was altered in the system, in the selective formation of Cu NP's by [104] as an antioxidant, a sensor and with non-toxic zones on prostate cancer cells. Generally, acidic pH inhibits the formation of NPs. Nevertheless, as per the counter-statement of [105], NPs had a powerful bactericidal property on cloth and [106] inferred that at acidic values of pH provided a large-sized particle, while neutral and basic [107] conditions aids in crystalline shape and size, if the pH is increased.

Increase of T°C diminishes the size of the NP's, synthesized from *Pinus eldarica* tree bark is proven by [108], while [109] reported that T°C alters the rate of nano-formation in a direct proportionality. High magnitude of reaction T°C resulted in spherical, while lower ones gave triangular shape using *Cymbopogon flexosus*, later used efficiently to remove the noxious metal As(V) [110]. At higher temperatures, no degradation of antioxidant properties was observed [96], and the enhancement of it was noticed on increasing the action T°C to 80°C, while [97] reported a temperature between 40–50°C. The intensity in color increases with raise in T°C from 30°C–95°C, with a maximum absorbance at 95C was noticed by [111], in Ag NP synthesis from *Melia azedarach* to eliminate MCB's in wastewater.

Strength of decoction from plant, determines the rate of stabilization, shape, volume, temperature, and required size formation of NPs. NP size reduction and decrease in SPR bandwidth, with rise in concentration of plant juice, was noticed by [112], who later confirmed it by HR-TEM when using leaves of *Coleus amboinicus Lour*. Destabilization at a very high limit of plant juice with modification in shape and size was observed by [113] in Ag NP synthesis using *Caricapapya*, which showed the decrease in absorbance too. Ag NPs are proved to have more impact against human and pest pathogens (bacterial and fungal). A direct proportionality between the concentration of salt solution and the absorbance peak was observed by [106] for Ag NP formation, while an indirect one was offered for Au NPs under the same reaction condition. In a similar experiment, [109] reported that the particle size varied directly with concentration and inversely with reaction rate. Yallappa et al. [114] reported that 8 minutes of incubation time was sufficient to get a sharp highest point with *Terminalia arjuna* botanical extracts, a powerful antioxidant, while [115] required 5 h, 9 h, and 13 h to get a different size, with varying shapes of spherical and polycrystalline, in a different set up using *Capsicum annum*. Jinu et al. [116] used *Prosopis cineraria* that required 1 h duration for nucleation and complete stabilization and was proven for its antimicrobial and cytotoxicity on cancerous cells in breast. To achieve the final nanoproduct with an efficient property of light sensitivity, stabilization, storage, and durability, a sufficient length of time is an utmost requirement.

## 8.7  BIOGENIC-STABILIZERS IN NP MATERIALIZATION, WITH ITS UTILIZATION

Plants juice with a broad spectrum of PCs, with BAs isolated and identified, function as a powerful biogenic reductant and a potent natural biostabilizer, find their utility in a wide array of platforms, were reported by [117, 118]. A polyphenol-Fe complex using *Eucalyptus Robusta* Sm (aq) [119], (antimicrobial/antioxidant), *Calotropis gigantea* [120] (eliminates aniline and methylene blue (MB) from polluted water source), *Rosmarinus officinalis, Eucalyptus tereticornis, and Melaleuca nesophila* [121] (a Fenton-catalyst to eliminate dye), *Lagenaria siceraria* [122] (antimicrobial), were applied as a R&S. Nevertheless, these Metal-polyphenols using natural sources work out as good antioxidants, with a high phenolic content, in some vectors like in the *hulls of Pistachio* and *Shirazi thyme* [123] (eliminates P from polluted water).

In the past few years, many progressive works have been done to get Cu or CuO NPs, that use polyphenolic acids and polyphenols-flavonoids, a potent antioxidant, present in plant decoction, to donate its Sec-Met for an effective reduction and stabilization. The phenolic group, with its antioxidant capacity, found by DPPH [104], and other organic moieties, are responsible for bridging and capping, as depicted in Figure 8.4. For instance, the -OH moiety aids as a reductant, to convert Cu salts into CuO (nm range) NPs [124], are found to be very useful for germination and growth of seeds.

Some representatives of plant species as nanoparticle stabilizers with different functionalities like *Tilia plant* [125] find its place in electronic, together as energy storing ones, with antibacterial and anticancer functionalities, *Eclipta prostrata [126] as a* therapeutic applicant, with antioxidant and cytotoxic property, *Tabernaemontana divaricate* [127] effective against pathogen of urinary tract, *Ziziphus spina-christi [128], an* effective nanomaterial adsorbent for crystal violet removal. Nazar *et al. [129] established that P. granatum shows* photocatalytic action. Some useful medicinal species (*Murraya koenigii, Azadirachta indica, Moringa oleifera, Hibiscus rosa-sinensis,* and *Tamarindus indica*), show cytotoxicity against cancerous cells [130]. The organic group present caps the metallic ions for stabilization.

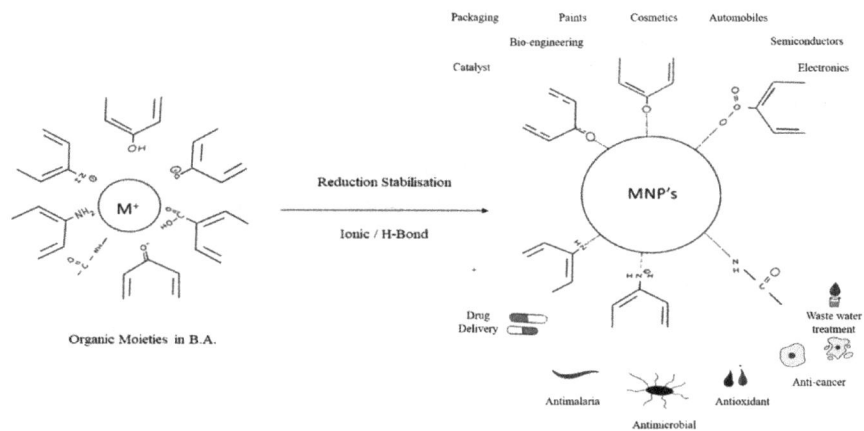

**FIGURE 8.4** Organic platforms for bio-reduction and stabilized NP's application in different arenas.

## 8.8   PLAUSIBLE MECHANISTIC APPROACH FOR NPS FORMATION WITH BAS FROM BOTANICAL EXTRACTS

Scientific platforms are dealing with this development to find the possible path for the stabilization. The main functional moieties of organic templates in plant source, govern the dimensions of size and shape, together with their potential application. Justified mechanistic routes have been reported using plant sources like *Impatiens balsamina* and *Lantana camara* [131], *Premna integrifolia* [132], *Ocimum Sanctum* [133], *Vitex negundo* [134], *Azadirachta indica* [135], *Ziziphora tenuior* [136], *Hubertia ambavilla*, and *Hypericum lanceolatum* [137], *Anthemis xylopoda* [138], *Barberry fruit* [139], *Plantago asiatica* [140], *Euphorbia bungei* [141], *Camellia Sinensis* [142], *Grape leaf* [143], *Juglans Regia* [103], *Eucalyptus tereticornis, Melaleuca nesophila,* and *Rosemarinus officinalis* [121]. Pragmatic utilization of NPs as anti-microbial, anti-bacterial [131–135], as an anti-oxidant [132, 137], for photocatalysis [135, 143], with catalytic action [138–141] has been reported.

FTIR spectroscopic studies infer that Sec-Met are characteristics for the stabilization of the metallic NPs formed. The presence of polyphenols responsible for capping, are quantified by DDPH and FRAP analysis. PCs present on the outer surface of the nucleated particle give protection and stability to them. Table 8.2 interprets the factors that govern the fabrication and characterization with utilities.

## 8.9   CONCLUSIONS AND OUTLOOK

Versatile approaches for the isolation and purification of Sec-Met and an eco-friendly; simple biogenic synthesis and application of NPs are delivered in a segmented manner. A single-step synthesis of reduction of inorganic metallic salt ions to NPs, by the organic PCs from the plant source is efficiently used in a user-friendly way. Here, a shortlist with technical approaches for isolation and purification in the former and reaction parameters and the functionalities of NPs formed in the latter is provided. The green nano-based formulation, with resourceful applications in an extensive mapping area, as documented in Table 8.2, delivers an excellent contribution to primary research segments in various zones. In a perspective view, we consider that the research advances in green nano-stabilization

**TABLE 8.2** Fabrication, Stabilization, and Characterization with Utilities

| Plant Species/ Concentration Salt (M) | Parameters T-°C/Time/ pH/Calc.-T | $\lambda_{max}$ (nm)/ζ-Potential/ DLS | FTIR-cm⁻¹ | Reducer-Stabilizer/ Groups | Pragmatic Utility | References |
|---|---|---|---|---|---|---|
| *Syzygium alternifo-lium*/Cu²⁺ (5 mM) | 50°C/2 h/8.2–9.0/ | 285/–49.2 mV/61.1 nm | O-H stretch -3253, N-H-1461 | Phenols, 1° amines | Antiviral | [144] |
| *Aloe barbadensis* Miller/Cu²⁺ (10 mM) | –/24 h/–/100–120°C/5 h | 265–285, 670, /–/ | O-H stretch -3450 | Hydroxyls, alkenes and other PC's | Antibacterial | [145] |
| *Tinospora cordifolia*/Cu²⁺ (0.25 mM) | 87°C/–/–/ | 248/–33.98 mV/–/ | O-H stretch -3329 | Alkaloids, steroids | Antimicrobial | [146] |
| *C. occidental*/Ag⁺ (1 mM), Cu²⁺ (5 mM) | Room T°C/5, 10,15.30 min, 1, 2, 3, 4, 24 h | 461.02, 544.89 /–/ | O-H 3186, 3341 | Polyphenols or Proteins | Antibacterial, antioxidant | [147] |
| *Pisidium guvajava, Aloe vera*/Mg²⁺ (1 mM) | 80°C /–/–/ 600°C-2 h | 221 /–/–/ | O-H stretch -3433 | Alcoholics | Antibacterial | [148] |
| *Solanum nigrum*/Zn²⁺ | 60°C/–/–/400C / 2 h | 358/–/–/ | N-H stretch -1450–1500, O-H stretch -3429 | Proteins, terpenoids | Antibacterial | [149] |
| *Calotropis gigantea*/Zn²⁺ (200 mM) | 60°C/6 h/11–12/ | –/–20.7 mV/11 nm | O-H stretch -3390 | Phytol, Flavanoids | Seedling-growth | [150] |
| *Polygala tenuifolia*/Zn²⁺ | 150°C/5 h/11–12/80°C/7–8 h | 314/–/–/ | O-H stretch -3380 | Polyphenolics Flavonoid-Quercetin | Anti-inflammatory, antioxidant | [151] |
| *Ceropegia candelabrum*/Zn²⁺ | 60°C/–/–/400°C/2 h | 320/–12.3 mV/76.5 nm | N-H-3273 | Amine | Antibacterial, antioxidant | [152] |

**TABLE 8.2** (Continued)

| Plant Species/ Concentration Salt (M) | Parameters T-°C/Time/ pH/Calc.-T | $\lambda_{max}$ (nm)/ζ-Potential/ DLS | FTIR-cm$^{-1}$ | Reducer-Stabilizer/ Groups | Pragmatic Utility | References |
|---|---|---|---|---|---|---|
| *Passiflora caerulea*/ $Zn^{2+}$ (1.0 M) | 60°C/1 h/–/80°C/2 h | 380/–/– | O-H$_{stretch}$-3321.42, C-O$_{stretch}$-1083.99, | Amino acid, terpenoids, alkaloid, flavonoids | Antimicrobial | [153] |
| *Terminalia chebula*/ $Fe^{2+}$, $Pd^{2+}$ (0.01 M) | Room T°C/40 min/2.18/ | 425/–/– | O-H$_{stretch}$-3400 | Polyphenols | – | [154] |
| *Azardirachta Indica*/ $Fe^{2+}$ (0.1 M) | 80°C/–/–/ | 325, 296/–/– | OH-3550, 3200 | Polyphenols | Antibacterial | [155] |
| *Musa ornata* flower sheath/$Fe^{2+}$ (5 mM) | 70–80°/8 h/9.0 | 310/±35 mV/– | O-H$_{stretch}$-3254.05 | Phenol groups | Antibacterial | [156] |
| *Trigonella foenum- graecum*/$Fe^{3+}$ (0.01 M) | 30°C/15 min/–/ | 229, 314/–/– | O-H$_{stretch}$-3428, N-H$_{stretch}$ | Polyphenol, flavonoids, proteins | Photocatalytic | [157] |
| *Acacia nilotica*/$Fe^{2+}$ (0.1 M) | Room T°C/–/6/ | 217 nm, 283 nm | O-H$_{stretch}$-3420 | Phenolic group | Catalytic, antibacterial | [158] |
| *Azadirachta indica*/ $Fe^{2+}$: $Fe^{3+}$ (2:1) | 60°C/5 min/5.29 to 2.21/ | 250, 390/–38.62 mV/– | O-H$_{stretch}$-3441.6 | Polyphenols | Water treatment, x-ray imaging | [159] |
| *Eichhornia crassipes*/$Fe^{2+}$ (0.1 M) | 55°C/2 h/–/ | 379/–/– | N-H$_{bond}$-1500–1514 | Amides | Antibacterial | [160] |

of different NPs, got by using botanical BAs, by employing green nano-trend technology, with enhanced biocompatibility, elevated sensitivity, beneficial specificity, reliability, and safety, would greatly stimulate the advancement of clinical analysis, new drug innovation, biomedical exploration. Similarly, this trend may be effectively applied to environmental management of water and soil; biosensing of pesticides, dyes, and drugs. This can be used to control or remove toxicity from effluents delivered by colored dyes, pesticides, and narcotics or therapeutics drug by an efficient bio-degradation, to control pest pathogens and other well-designed applications in the near future. In the current scenario, highlighted keynotes promoting the biogenic synthesis of NPs would deliver a promising note, so as to overcome the unwanted fronts, in various fields for a day-to-day implication, by green nano-trend using botanicals.

## KEYWORDS

- **isolation**
- **methylene blue**
- **phytoconstituents**
- **reverse phase**
- **Sec-Met**

## REFERENCES

1. De Luca, V., Salim, V., Atsumi, S. M., & Yu, F., (2012). Mining the biodiversity of plants: A revolution in the making. *Science, 336*(6089), 1658–1661. doi: 10.1126/science.1217410.
2. Palhares, R. M., Gonçalves, D. M., Dos, S. A. F. B. B., Pereira, C. G., Das, G. L. B. M., & Oliveira, G., (2015). Medicinal plants recommended by the world health organization: DNA barcode identification associated with chemical analyses guarantees their quality. *Plos One, 10*(5), e0127866. doi: 10.1371/journal.pone.0127866.
3. Ali, H., Khan, E., & Sajad, M. A., (2013). Phytoremediation of heavy metals: Concepts and applications. *Chemosphere, 91*, 869–881. doi: 10.1016/j.chemosphere.2013.01.075.
4. Aslanargun, P., Cuvas, O., Dikmen, B., Aslan, E., & Yuksel, M. U., (2012). *Passiflora incarnata* Linneaus as an anxiolytic before spinal anesthesia. *Journal of Anesthesia, 26*, 39–44. doi: 10.1007/s00540-011-1265-6.

5. Marslin, G., Siram, K., Maqbool, Q., Selvakesavan, R., Kruszka, D., Kachlicki, P., & Franklin, G., (2018). Secondary metabolites in the green synthesis of metallic nanoparticles. *Materials, 11*, 940. doi: 10.3390/ma11060940.

6. Das, P., Ghosh, S., Ghosh, R., Dam, S., & Baskey, M., (2018). *Madhuca longifolia* plant mediated green synthesis of cupric oxide nanoparticles: A promising environmentally sustainable material for wastewater treatment and efficient antibacterial agent. *Journal of Photochemistry and Photobiology B: Biology.* doi: 10.1016/j.jphotobiol.2018.09.023.

7. Gayda, G., Demkiv, O., Stasyuk, N., Serkiz, R., Lootsik, M., Errachid, A., & Nisnevitch, M., (2019). Metallic nanoparticles obtained via "green" synthesis as a platform for biosensor construction. *Applied Sciences, 9*, 720. doi: 10.3390/app9040720.

8. Vasantharaj, S., Sathiyavimal, S., Saravanan, M., Senthilkumar, P., Kavitha, G., Shanmugavel, M., & Pugazhendhi, A., (2019). Synthesis of ecofriendly copper oxide nanoparticles for fabrication over textile fabrics: Characterization of antibacterial activity and dye degradation potential. *Journal of Photochemistry and Photobiology B: Biology, 191*, 143–149. doi: 10.1016/j.jphotobiol.2018.12.026.

9. Chokkareddy, R., & Redhi, G. G., (2018). Green synthesis of metal nanoparticles and its reaction mechanisms. *Green Metal Nanoparticles*, 113–139. doi: 10.1002/9781119418900.ch4.

10. Ravichandran, V., Vasanthi, S., Shalini, S., Shah, S. A. A., Tripathy, M., & Paliwal, N., (2019). Green synthesis, characterization, antibacterial, antioxidant, and photocatalytic activity of *Parkia speciosa* leaves extract mediated silver nanoparticles. *Results in Physics, 15*, 102565. doi: 10.1016/j.rinp.2019.102565.

11. Gour, A., & Jain, N. K., (2019). Advances in green synthesis of nanoparticles. *Artificial Cells, Nanomedicine, and Biotechnology, 47*(1), 844–851. doi: 10.1080/21691401.2019.1577878.

12. Yadi, M., Mostafavi, E., Saleh, B., Davaran, S., Aliyeva, I., Khalilov, R., & Milani, M., (2018). Current developments in green synthesis of metallic nanoparticles using plant extracts: A review. *Artificial Cells, Nanomedicine, and Biotechnology.* doi: 10.1080/21691401.2018.1492931.

13. Abdullah, M., Atta, A., Allohedan, H., Alkhathlan, H., Khan, M., & Ezzat, A., (2018). Green synthesis of hydrophobic magnetite nanoparticles coated with plant extract and their application as petroleum oil spill collectors. *Nanomaterials, 8*, 855. doi: 10.3390/nano8100855.

14. Pilaquinga, F., Morejón, B., Ganchala, D., Morey, J., Piña, N., Debut, A., & Neira, M., (2019). Green synthesis of silver nanoparticles using *Solanum mammosum* L. (Solanaceae) fruit extract and their larvicidal activity against *Aedes aegypti* L. (Diptera: Culicidae). *Plos One, 14*(10), e0224109. doi: 10.1371/journal.pone.0224109.

15. Shapira, P., & Youtie, J., (2015). The economic contributions of nanotechnology to green and sustainable growth. *Green Processes for Nanotechnology*, 409–434. doi: 10.1007/978-3-319-15461-9_15.

16. Mody, V. V., Nounou, M. I., & Bikram, M., (2009). Novel nanomedicine-based MRI contrast agents for gynecological malignancies. *Advanced Drug Delivery Reviews, 61*, 795–807. doi: 10.1016/j.addr.2009.04.020.

17. El-Seedi, H. R., El-Shabasy, R. M., Khalifa, S. A. M., Saeed, A., Shah, A., Shah, R., & Guo, W., (2019). Metal nanoparticles fabricated by green chemistry using natural extracts: Biosynthesis, mechanisms, and applications. *RSC Advances, 9*, 24539–24559. doi: 10.1039/c9ra02225b.

18. Peralta-Videa, J. R., Huang, Y., Parsons, J. G., Zhao, L., Lopez-Moreno, L., Hernandez-Viezcas, J. A., & Gardea-Torresdey, J. L., (2016). Plant-based green synthesis of metallic nanoparticles: Scientific curiosity or a realistic alternative to chemical synthesis? *Nanotechnology for Environmental Engineering, 1*, 4. doi: 10.1007/s41204–016–0004–5.

19. Das, S. K., Dickinson, C., Lafir, F., Brougham, D. F., & Marsili, E., (2012). Synthesis, characterization, and catalytic activity of gold nanoparticles biosynthesized with *Rhizopus oryzae* protein extract. *Green Chemistry, 14*, 1322–1334. doi: 10.1039/c2gc16676c.

20. Verma, A., Gautam, S., Bansal, K., Prabhakar, N., & Rosenholm, J., (2019). Green nanotechnology: Advancement in phytoformulation research. *Medicines, 6*, 39. doi: 10.3390/medicines6010039.

21. Jain, C., Khatana, S., & Vijayvergia, R., (2019). Bioactivity of secondary metabolites of various plants: A review. *International Journal of Pharmaceutical Sciences and Research, 10*(2), 494–504. doi: 10.13040/IJPSR.0975-8232.10(2).494-04.

22. Sajjad, S., Leghari, S. A. K., Ryma, N. U. A., & Farooqi, S. A., (2018). Green synthesis of metal-based nanoparticles and their applications. *Green Metal Nanoparticles*, 23–77. doi: 10.1002/9781119418900.ch2.

23. Ahmad, N. K. A., Fauzi, N. M., Buang, F., Mohd, S. Q. H., Husain, K., Jantan, I., & Jubri, Z., (2019). *Gynura procumbens* standardized extract reduces cholesterol levels and modulates oxidative status in postmenopausal rats fed with cholesterol diet enriched with repeatedly heated palm oil. *Evidence-Based Complementary and Alternative Medicine*, 1–15. doi: 10.1155/2019/7246756.

24. Khandel, P., Yadaw, R. K., Soni, D. K., Kanwar, L., & Shahi, S. K., (2018). Biogenesis of metal nanoparticles and their pharmacological applications: Present status and application prospects. *Journal of Nanostructure in Chemistry*. doi: 10.1007/s40097-018-0267-4.

25. Altemimi, A., Lakhssassi, N., Baharlouei, A., Watson, D., & Lightfoot, D., (2017). Phytochemicals: Extraction, isolation, and identification of bioactive compounds from plant extracts. *Plants, 6*, 42. doi: 10.3390/plants6040042.

26. Santos-Buelga, C., Gonzalez-Manzano, S., Dueñas, M., & Gonzalez-Paramas, A. M., (2012). Extraction and isolation of phenolic compounds. *Natural Products Isolation*, 427–464. doi: 10.1007/978-1-61779-624-1_17.

27. Sticher, O., (2008). Natural product isolation. *Natural Product Reports, 25*, 517–554. doi: 10.1039/b700306b.

28. Ong, E. S., (2004). Extraction methods and chemical standardization of botanicals and herbal preparations. *Journal of Chromatography B, 812*, 23–33. doi: 10.1016/j.jchromb.2004.07.041.

29. Sasidharan, S., Chen, D., Saravanan, K. M., Sundram, & Latha, Y. L., (2010). Extraction, isolation and characterization of bioactive compounds from plants 'extracts. *African Journal of Traditional and Complementary Alternative Medicine, 8*(1), 1–10. doi: 10.4314/ajtcam.v8i1.60483.

30. Rahman, M., (2018). Application of computational methods in isolation of plant secondary metabolites. *Computational Phytochemistry*, 107–139. doi: 10.1016/b9780-12-812364-5.00004-3.
31. Kavitha, A., Prabhakar, P., Narasimhulu, M., Vijayalakshmi, M., Venkateswarlu, Y., Venkateswara, R. K., & Balaraju, S. R. V., (2010). Isolation, characterization and biological evaluation of bioactive metabolites from nocardia Levis, MK-VL_113. *Microbiological Research, 165*(3), 199–210. doi: 10.1016/j.micres.2009.05.002.
32. Tistaert, C., Dejaegher, B., & Heyden, Y. V., (2011). Chromatographic separation techniques and data handling methods for herbal fingerprints: A review. *Analytica Chimica. Acta, 690*, 148–161. doi: 10.1016/j.aca.2011.02.023.
33. Romanik, G., Gilgenast, E., Przyjazny, A., & Kamiński, M., (2007). Techniques of preparing plant material for chromatographic separation and analysis. *Journal of Biochemical and Biophysical Methods, 70*, 253–261. doi: 10.1016/j.jbbm.2006.09.012.
34. Sarker, S. D., & Nahar, L., (2012). An introduction to natural products isolation. *Natural Products Isolation*, 1–25. doi: 10.1007/978-1-61779-624-1_1.
35. Zhao, Z., Dong, L., Wu, Y., & Lin, F., (2011). Preliminary separation and purification of rutin and quercetin from *Euonymus alatus* (Thunb.) Siebold extracts by macroporous resins. *Food and Bioproducts Processing, 89*(4), 266–272. doi: 10.1016/j.fbp.2010.11.001.
36. Lu, H., Yang, K., Zhan, L., Lu, T., Chen, X., Cai, X., & Chen, S., (2019). Optimization of flavonoid extraction in dendrobium officinale leaves and their inhibitory effects on tyrosinase activity. *International Journal of Analytical Chemistry*, 1–10. doi: 10.1155/2019/7849198.
37. Kwon, J. H., Oh, H. J., Lee, D. S., In, S. J., Seo, K. H., Jung, J. W., & Baek, N. I., (2019). Pharmacological activity and quantitative analysis of flavonoids isolated from the flowers of *Begonia semperflorens* link Et Otto. *Applied Biological Chemistry, 62*, 11. doi: 10.1186/s13765-019-0416-6.
38. Weber, P., Hamburger, M., Schafroth, N., & Potterat, O., (2011). Flash chromatography on cartridges for the separation of plant extracts: Rules for the selection of chromatographic conditions and comparison with medium pressure liquid chromatography. *Fitoterapia, 82*, 155–161. doi: 10.1016/j.fitote.2010.08.013.
39. Arora, S., & Itankar, P., (2018). Extraction, isolation, and identification of flavonoid from *Chenopodium* album aerial parts. *Journal of Traditional and Complementary Medicine*, 1–7. doi: 10.1016/j.jtcme.2017.10.002.
40. Mosad, A. G., Mohamed, R. H., Hanan, S. M., & Mohamed, S. A., (2018). Phytochemical analysis of *Eucalyptus camaldulensis* leaves extracts and testing its antimicrobial and schistosomicidal activities. *Bulletin of the National Research Centre, 42*, 16. doi: 10.1186/s42269-018-0017-2.
41. Silva, L., Alves, J., Da Silva, S. E., De Souza, N. M., Abreu, L., Tavares, J., & Zucolotto, S., (2018). Isolation and identification of the five novel flavonoids from *Genipa americana* leaves. *Molecules, 23*, 2521. doi: 10.3390/molecules23102521.
42. Shakthi, D. A., Sathish, K. T., Kumaresan, K., & Rapheal, V. S., (2014). Extraction process optimization of polyphenols from Indian citrus sinensis-as novel antiglycative agents in the management of diabetes mellitus. *Journal of Diabetes and Metabolic Disorders, 13*, 11. doi: 10.1186/2251-6581-13-11.

43. Birk, C. D., Provensi, G., Gosmann, G., Reginatto, F. H., & Schenkel, E. P., (2005). TLC Fingerprint of flavonoids and saponins from passiflora species. *Journal of Liquid Chromatography and Related Technologies, 28,* 2285–2291. doi: 10.1081/jlc-200064212.

44. Amor, S. E., Williams, W., Rautenbach, F., Le Roes-Hill, M., Mgwatyu, Y., Marnewick, J., & Hesse, U., (2019). Visualization of aspalathin in rooibos (*Aspalathus linearis*) plant and herbal tea extracts using thin-layer chromatography. *Molecules, 24,* 938. doi: 10.3390/molecules24050938.

45. West, C., Elfakir, C., & Lafosse, M., (2010). Porous graphitic carbon: A versatile stationary phase for liquid chromatography. *Journal of Chromatography A, 1217,* 3201–3216. doi: 10.1016/j.chroma.2009.09.052.

46. Claude, B., Morin, P., Lafosse, M., Belmont, A. S., & Haupt, K., (2008). Selective solid-phase extraction of a triterpene acid from a plant extract by molecularly imprinted polymer. *Talanta, 75,* 344–350. doi: 10.1016/j.talanta.2007.11.037.

47. Awouafack, M. D., Tane, P., & Morita, H., (2017). Isolation and structure characterization of flavonoids. *Flavonoids-From Biosynthesis to Human Health.* doi: 10.5772/67881.

48. Liang, Z., Li, B., Liang, Y., Su, Y., & Ito, Y., (2015). Separation and purification of two minor compounds from *Radix isatidis* by integrative MPLC and HSCCC with preparative HPLC. *Journal of Liquid Chromatography and Related Technologies, 38*(5), 647–653. doi: 10.1080/10826076.2014.936606.

49. Challal, S., Queiroz, E., Debrus, B., Kloeti, W., Guillarme, D., Gupta, M., & Wolfender, J. L., (2015). Rational and efficient preparative isolation of natural products by MPLC-UV-ELSD based on HPLC to MPLC gradient transfer. *Planta Medica, 81,* 1636–1643. doi: 10.1055/s-0035–1545912.

50. Crowley, T. E., (2020). High-performance liquid chromatography. *Purification and Characterization of Secondary Metabolites,* 49–58. doi: 10.1016/b978-0-12-813942-4.00005-x.

51. Latif, Z., (2006). Isolation by preparative high-performance liquid chromatography. *Natural Products Isolation,* 213–232. doi: 10.1385/1-59259-955-9:213.

52. Wang, S. P., & Huang, K. J., (2004). Determination of flavonoids by high-performance liquid chromatography and capillary electrophoresis. *Journal of Chromatography A, 1032,* 273–279. doi: 10.1016/j.chroma.2003.11.099.

53. Peasari, J. R., Motamarry, S. S., Varma, K. S., Anitha, P., & Potti, R. B., (2018). Chromatographic analysis of phytochemicals in *Costus igneus* and computational studies of flavonoids. *Informatics in Medicine Unlocked, 13,* 34–40. doi: 10.1016/j.imu.2018.10.004.

54. Zgórka, G., & Kawka, S., (2001). Application of conventional UV, photodiode array (PDA) and fluorescence (FL) detection to analysis of phenolic acids in plant material and pharmaceutical preparations. *Journal of Pharmaceutical and Biomedical Analysis, 24,* 1065–1072. doi: 10.1016/s0731-7085(00)00541-0.

55. Variyar, P. S., Chatterjee, S., & Sharma, A., (2011). Fundamentals and theory of HPTLC-based separation. In: Srivastava, M. M., (ed.), *High-Performance Thin-Layer Chromatography (HPTLC)* (pp. 27–39). doi: 10.1007/978-3-642-14025-9.

56. Patel, R. B., Patel, M. R., Bhatt, K. K., & Patel, B. G., (2011). Development and validation of HPTLC method for estimation of carbamazepine in formulations

and its *in vitro* release study. *Chromatography Research International,* 1–8. doi: 10.4061/2011/684369.

57. Thangaraj, P., (2015). Detection of phenolic and flavonoid compounds using high performance thin layer chromatography (HPTLC). *Pharmacological Assays of Plant-Based Natural Products,* 173–175. doi: 10.1007/978-3-319-26811-8_30.

58. Yilmaz, M. A., Ertas, A., Yener, I., Akdeniz, M., Cakir, O., Altun, M., & Temel, H., (2018). A comprehensive LC–MS/MS method validation for the quantitative investigation of 37 fingerprint phytochemicals in *Achillea* species: A detailed examination of *A. coarctata* and *A. monocephala. Journal of Pharmaceutical and Biomedical Analysis, 154,* 413–424. doi: 10.1016/j.jpba.2018.02.059.

59. Wang, Q., Kuang, Y., Song, W., Qian, Y., Qiao, X., Guo, D., & Ye, M., (2017). Permeability through the Caco-2 cell monolayer of 42 bioactive compounds in the TCM formula gegen-qinlian decoction by liquid chromatography tandem mass spectrometry analysis. *Journal of Pharmaceutical and Biomedical Analysis, 146,* 206–213. doi: 10.1016/j.jpba.2017.08.042.

60. De Rijke, E., Out, P., Niessen, W. M. A., Ariese, F., Gooijer, C., & Brinkman, U. A. T., (2006). Analytical separation and detection methods for flavonoids. *Journal of Chromatography A, 1112,* 31–63. doi: 10.1016/j.chroma.2006.01.019.

61. Dai, D., He, J., Sun, R., Zhang, R., Aisa, H. A., & Abliz, Z., (2009). Nuclear magnetic resonance and liquid chromatography-mass spectrometry combined with an incompleted separation strategy for identifying the natural products in crude extract. *Analytica Chimica Acta, 632,* 221–228. doi: 10.1016/j.aca.2008.11.002.

62. El Antri, A., Lachkar, N., El Hajjaji, H., Gaamoussi, F., Lyoussi, B., El Bali, B., & Lachkar, M., (2010). Structure elucidation and vasodilator activity of methoxy flavonols from *Calycotome villosa* subsp. intermedia. *Arabian Journal of Chemistry, 3,* 173–178. doi: 10.1016/j.arabjc.2010.04.006.

63. Keskes, H., Belhadj, S., Jlail, L., El Feki, A., Damak, M., Sayadi, S., & Allouche, N., (2016). LC-MS–MS and GC-MS analyses of biologically active extracts and fractions from Tunisian *Juniperus phoenice* leaves. *Pharmaceutical Biology, 55*(1), 88–95. doi: 10.1080/13880209.2016.1230139.

64. Wang, X. X., He, J. M., Wang, C. L., Zhang, R. P., He, W. Y., Guo, S. X., & Abliz, Z., (2011). Simultaneous structural identification of natural products in fractions of crude extract of the rare endangered plant *Anoectochilus roxburghii* using 1H NMR/RRLC-MS parallel dynamic spectroscopy. *International Journal of Molecular Sciences, 12,* 2556–2571. doi: 10.3390/ijms12042556.

65. Sharma, V., & Janmeda, P., (2017). Extraction, isolation, and identification of flavonoid from *Euphorbia neriifolia* leaves. *Arabian Journal of Chemistry, 10*(4), 509–514. doi: 10.1016/j.arabjc.2014.08.019.

66. Blunder, M., Orthaber, A., Bauer, R., Bucar, F., & Kunert, O., (2017). Efficient identification of flavones, flavanones and their glycosides in routine analysis via off-line combination of sensitive NMR and HPLC experiments. *Food Chemistry, 218,* 600–609. doi: 10.1016/j.foodchem.2016.09.077.

67. Francescato, L. N., Debenedetti, S. L., Schwanz, T. G., Bassani, V. L., & Henriques, A. T., (2013). Identification of phenolic compounds in *Equisetum giganteum* by LC–ESI-MS/MS and a new approach to total flavonoid quantification. *Talanta, 105,* 192–203. doi: 10.1016/j.talanta.2012.11.072.

68. Singh, A. P., Wilson, T., Luthria, D., Freeman, M. R., Scott, R. M., Bilenker, D., & Vorsa, N., (2011). LC-MS–MS characterization of curry leaf flavonols and antioxidant activity. *Food Chemistry, 127*, 80–85. doi: 10.1016/j.foodchem.2010.12.091.
69. Sekkoum, K., Belboukhari, N., & Cheriti, A., (2014). New flavonoids from bioactive extract of Algerian medicinal plant *Launeae arborescens. Asian Pacific Journal of Tropical Biomedicine, 4*(4), 267–271. doi: 10.12980/apjtb.4.2014c708.
70. Pereira, O. R., Silva, A. M. S., Domingues, M. R. M., & Cardoso, S. M., (2012). Identification of phenolic constituents of *Cytisus multiflorus. Food Chemistry, 131*, 652–659. doi: 10.1016/j.foodchem.2011.09.045.
71. Liu, G., Rajesh, N., Wang, X., Zhang, M., Wu, Q., Li, S., & Yao, S., (2011). Identification of flavonoids in the stems and leaves of *Scutellaria baicalensis* Georgi. *Journal of Chromatography B, 879*, 1023–1028. doi: 10.1016/j.jchromb.2011.02.050.
72. Sai, S. V., Saravanan, D., & Santhakumar, K., (2017). Isolation of quercetin from the methanolic extract of *Lagerstroemia speciosa* by HPLC technique, its cytotoxicity against MCF-7 cells and photocatalytic activity. *Journal of Photochemistry and Photobiology B: Biology, 171*, 20–26. doi: 10.1016/j.jphotobiol.2017.04.031.
73. Palit, S., & Hussain, C. M., (2018). Recent advances in green nanotechnology and the vision for the future. *Green Metal Nanoparticles: Synthesis, Characterization, and Their Applications, 1*–21. doi: 10.1002/9781119418900.ch1.
74. Koczkur, K. M., Mourdikoudis, S., Polavarapu, L., & Skrabalak, S. E., (2015). Polyvinylpyrrolidone (PVP) in nanoparticle synthesis. *Dalton Transactions, 44*, 17883–17905, RSC. doi: 10.1039/c5dt02964c.
75. Mourdikoudis, S., Pallares, R. M., & Thanh, N. T. K., (2018). Characterization techniques for nanoparticles: Comparison and complementarity upon studying nanoparticle properties. *Nanoscale, 10*(27), 12871–12934. doi: 10.1039/c8nr02278j.
76. Chauhan, N., Tyagi, A. K., Kumar, P., & Malik, A., (2016). Antibacterial potential of *Jatropha curcas* synthesized silver nanoparticles against food borne pathogens. *Frontiers in Microbiology, 7*, 1748. doi: 10.3389/fmicb.2016.01748.
77. Nasrollahzadeh, M., Mahmoudi-Gom Y. S., Motahharifar, N., & Ghafori, G. M., (2019). Recent developments in the plant-mediated green synthesis of Ag–based nanoparticles for environmental and catalytic applications. *The Chemical Record, 19*, 1–45. doi: 10.1002/tcr.201800202.
78. Singh, J., Dutta, T., Kim, K. H., Rawat, M., Samddar, P., & Kumar, P., (2018). "Green" synthesis of metals and their oxide nanoparticles: Applications for environmental remediation. *Journal of Nanobiotechnology, 16*(1). doi: 10.1186/s12951-018-0408-4.
79. Boroumand, M. A., Namvar, F., Moniri, M., Md. Tahir, P., Azizi, S., & Mohamad, R., (2015). Nanoparticles biosynthesized by fungi and yeast: A review of their preparation, properties, and medical applications. *Molecules, 20*, 16540–16565. doi: 10.3390/molecules200916540.
80. Das, R. K., Pachapur, V. L., Lonappan, L., Naghdi, M., Pulicharla, R., Maiti, S., & Brar, S. K., (2017). Biological synthesis of metallic nanoparticles: Plants, animals and microbial aspects. *Nanotechnology for Environmental Engineering, 2*, 18. doi: 10.1007/s41204-017-0029-4.
81. Sharma, D., Kanchi, S., & Bisetty, K., (2015). Biogenic synthesis of nanoparticles: A review. *Arabian Journal of Chemistry*. doi: 10.1016/j.arabjc.2015.11.002.

82. Zheng, M., Zhang, S., Ma, G., & Wang, P., (2011). Effect of molecular mobility on coupled enzymatic reactions involving cofactor regeneration using nanoparticle-attached enzymes. *Journal of Biotechnology, 154*, 274–280. doi: 10.1016/j.jbiotec.2011.04.013.

83. Saravanan, S., Sameera, D. K., Moorthi, A., & Selvamurugan, N., (2013). Chitosan scaffolds containing chicken feather keratin nanoparticles for bone tissue engineering. *International Journal of Biological Macromolecules, 62*, 481–486. doi: 10.1016/j.ijbiomac.2013.09.034.

84. Mousavi-Khattat, M., Keyhanfar, M., & Razmjou, A., (2018). A comparative study of stability, antioxidant, DNA cleavage and antibacterial activities of green and chemically synthesized silver nanoparticles. *Artificial Cells, Nanomedicine, and Biotechnology*. doi: 10.1080/21691401.2018.1527346.

85. Buazar, F., (2019). Impact of biocompatible nanosilica on green stabilization of subgrade soil. *Scientific Reports, 9*, 15147. doi: 10.1038/s41598-019-51663-2.

86. Seabra, A. B., Haddad, P., & Duran, N., (2013). Biogenic synthesis of nanostructured iron compounds: Applications and perspectives. *IET Nanobiotechnology, 7*(3), 90–99. doi: 10.1049/iet-nbt.2012.0047.

87. Yu, J., Zhao, H., Wang, D., Song, X., Zhao, L., & Wang, X., (2017). Extraction and purification of five terpenoids from olibanum by ultrahigh pressure technique and high-speed counter current chromatography. *Journal of Separation Sciences, 40*(13), 2732–2740. doi: 10.1002/jssc.201700215.

88. Wink, M., (2015). Modes of action of herbal medicines and plant secondary metabolites. *Medicines, 2*, 251–286. doi: 10.3390/medicines2030251.

89. Almadiy, A. A., & Nenaah, G. E., (2018). Ecofriendly synthesis of silver nanoparticles using potato steroidal alkaloids and their activity against phytopathogenic fungi. *The Brazilian Archives of Biology and Technology, 61*, e18180013. doi: 10.1590/1678-4324-2018180013.

90. Vukics, V., & Guttman, A., (2010). Structural characterization of flavonoid glycosides by multi-stage mass spectrometry. *Mass Spectrometry Reviews, 29*, 1–16. doi: 10.1002/mas.20212.

91. Chernavskii, P. A., Peskov, N. V., Mugtasimov, A. V., & Lunin, V. V., (2007). Oxidation of metal nanoparticles: Experiment and model. *Russian Journal of Physical Chemistry B, 1*(4), 394–411. doi: 10.1134/s1990793107040082.

92. Verwey, E. J., & Overbeek, J. T. G., (1947). Theory of the stability of lyophobic colloids. Elsevier, Amsterdam. *Journal of Physical Chemistry, 51*(3), 631–636. https://doi.org/10.1021/j150453a001.

93. Njagi, E. C., Huang, H., Stafford, L., Genuino, H., Galindo, H. M., & Collins, J. B., (2011). Biosynthesis of iron and silver nanoparticles at room temperature using aqueous sorghum bran extracts. *Langmuir, 27*(1), 264–271. doi: 10.1021/la103190n.

94. Yang, L., Cao, Z., Sajja, H. K., Mao, H., Wang, L., & Geng, H., (2008). Development of receptor targeted magnetic iron oxide nanoparticles for efficient drug delivery and tumor imaging. *Journal of Biomedical Nanotechnology, 4*(4), 439–449. doi: 10.1166/jbn.2008.007.

95. Mystrioti, C., Xanthopoulou, T., Tsakiridis, P., Papassiopi, N., & Xenidis, A., (2016). Comparative evaluation of five plant extracts and juices for nanoiron synthesis and

application for hexavalent chromium reduction. *Science of the Total Environment, 539*, 105–113. doi: 10.1016/j.scitotenv.2015.08.091.

96. Machado, S., Pinto, S. L., Grosso, J. P., Nouws, H. P., Albergaria, J. T., & Delerue-Matos, C., (2013). Green production of zerovalent iron nanoparticles using tree leaf extracts. *Science of the Total Environment, 15*(445, 446), 1–8. doi: 10.1016/j.scitotenv.2012.12.033.

97. Harshiny, M., Iswarya, C. N., & Matheswaran, M., (2015). Biogenic synthesis of iron nanoparticles using *Amaranthus dubius* leaf extract as a reducing agent. *Powder Technology, 286*, 744–749. doi: 10.1016/j.powtec.2015.09.021.

98. Wang, T., Jin, X., Chen, Z., Megharaj, M., & Naidu, R., (2014). Green synthesis of Fe nanoparticles using eucalyptus leaf extracts for treatment of eutrophic wastewater. *Science of the Total Environment, 1*(466/ 467), 210–213. doi: 10.1016/j.scitotenv.2013.07.022.

99. Karimian, H., & Babaluo, A. A., (2007). Halos mechanism in stabilizing of colloidal suspensions: Nanoparticle weight fraction and pH effects. *Journal of the European Ceramic Society, 27*(1), 19–25. doi: 10.1016/j.jeurceramsoc.2006.05.109.

100. Armendariz, V., Herrera, I., Jose-yacaman, M., Troiani, H., Santiago, P., & Gardea-Torresdey, J. L., (2004). Size controlled gold nanoparticle formation by *Avena sativa* biomass: Use of plants in nanobiotechnology. *Journal of Nanoparticle Research, 6*(4), 377–382. doi: 10.1007/s11051–004–0741–4.

101. Shim, J. Y., & Gupta, V. K., (2007). Reversible aggregation of gold nanoparticles induced by pH dependent conformational transitions of a self-assembled polypeptide. *Journal of Colloid and Interface Science, 316*(2), 977–983. doi: 10.1016/j.jcis.2007.08.021.

102. Jeevanandam, J., Chan, Y. S., & Danquah, M. K., (2017). Biosynthesis and characterization of MgO nanoparticles from plant extracts via induced molecular nucleation. *New Journal of Chemistry, 41*(7), 2800–2814. doi: 10.1039/c6nj03176e.

103. Izadiyan, Z., Shameli, K., Miyake, M., Hara, H., Mohamad, S. E. B., Kalantari, K., & Rasouli, E., (2018). Cytotoxicity assay of plant-mediated synthesized iron oxide nanoparticles using Juglans regia green husk extract. *Arabian Journal of Chemistry*. doi: 10.1016/j.arabjc.2018.02.019.

104. Prasad, P. R., Kanchi, S., & Naidoo, E. B., (2016). *In-vitro* evaluation of copper nanoparticles cytotoxicity on prostate cancer cell lines and their antioxidant, sensing and catalytic activity: One-pot green approach. *Journal of Photochemistry and Photobiology B: Biology, 161*, 375–382. doi: 10.1016/j.jphotobiol.2016.06.008.

105. Sathishkumar, M., Sneha, K., & Yun, Y. S., (2010). Immobilization of silver nanoparticles synthesized using Curcuma longa tuber powder and extract on cotton cloth for bactericidal activity. *Bioresource Technology, 101*(20), 7958–7965. doi: 10.1016/j.biortech.2010.05.051.

106. Dubey, S. P., Lahtinen, M., & Sillanpää, M., (2010). Tansy fruit mediated greener synthesis of silver and gold nanoparticles. *Process Biochemistry, 45*(7), 1065–71. doi: 10.1016/j.procbio.2010.03.024.

107. Basnet, P., InakhunbiChanu, T., Samanta, D., & Chatterjee, S., (2018). A review on bio-synthesized zinc oxide nanoparticles using plant extracts as reductants and stabilizing agents. *Journal of Photochemistry and Photobiology B: Biology, 183*, 201–221. doi: 10.1016/j.jphotobiol.2018.04.036.

108. Iravani, S., & Zolfaghari, B., (2013). Green Synthesis of silver nanoparticles using *Pinus* eldarica bark extract. *BioMed Research International*, 1–5. doi: 10.1155/2013/639725.

109. Dwivedi, A. D., & Gopal, K., (2010). Biosynthesis of silver and gold nanoparticles using Chenopodium album leaf extract. *Colloids Surf. A Physicochemical and Engineering, 369*(1–3), 27–33. doi: 10.1016/j.colsurfa.2010.07.020.

110. Martínez-Cabanas, M., López-García, M., Barriada, J. L., Herrero, R., & De Vicente, M. E. S., (2016). Green synthesis of iron oxide nanoparticles. Development of magnetic hybrid materials for efficient As (V) removal. *Chemical Engineering Journal, 301*, 83–91. doi: 10.1016/j.cej.2016.04.149.

111. Kuang, Y., Wang, Q., Chen, Z., Megharaj, M., & Naidu, R., (2013). Heterogeneous Fenton-like oxidation of monochlorobenzene using green synthesis of iron nanoparticles. *Journal of Colloid and Interface Science, 410*, 67–73. doi: 10.1016/j.jcis.2013.08.020.

112. Narayanan, K. B., & Sakthivel, N., (2011). Extracellular synthesis of silver nanoparticles using the leaf extract of *Coleus amboinicus Lour. Materials Research Bulletin, 46*(10), 1708–171. doi: 10.1016/j.materresbull.2011.05.041.

113. Balavijayalakshmi, J., & Ramalakshmi, V., (2017). Carica papaya peel mediated synthesis of silver nanoparticles and its antibacterial activity against human pathogens. *Journal of Applied Research and Technology, 15*(5), 413–422. doi: 10.1016/j.jart.2017.03.010.

114. Yallappa, S., Manjanna, J., Sindhe, M. A., Satyanarayan, N. D., Pramod, S. N., & Nagaraja, K., (2013). Microwave assisted rapid synthesis and biological evaluation of stable copper nanoparticles using *T. arjuna* bark extract. *Spectrochimica Acta Part A: Molecular and Biomolecular Spectroscopy, 110*, 108–115. doi: 10.1016/j.saa.2013.03.005.

115. Li, S., Shen, Y., Xie, A., Yu, X., Qiu, L., Zhang, L., & Zhang, Q., (2007). Green synthesis of silver nanoparticles using *Capsicum annuum* L. extract. *Green Chemistry, 9*(8), 852–858. doi: 10.1039/b615357g.

116. Jinu, U., Gomathi, M., Saiqa, I., Geetha, N., Benelli, G., & Venkatachalam, P., (2017). Green engineered biomolecule-capped silver and copper nanohybrids using *Prosopis cineraria* leaf extract: Enhanced antibacterial activity against microbial pathogens of public health relevance and cytotoxicity on human breast cancer cells (MCF-7). *Microbial Pathogenesis, 105*, 86–95. doi: 10.1016/j.micpath.2017.02.019.

117. Rauwel, P., Küünal, S., Ferdov, S., & Rauwel, E., (2015). A review on the green synthesis of silver nanoparticles and their morphologies studied via TEM. *Advances in Materials Science and Engineering.* doi: 10.1155/2015/682749.

118. Hulkoti, N. I., & Taranath, T. C., (2014). Biosynthesis of nanoparticles using microbes: A review. *Colloids and Surfaces B: Biointerfaces, 121*, 474–483. doi: 10.1016/j.colsurfb.2014.05.027.

119. Vitta, Y., Figueroa, M., Calderon, M., & Ciangherotti, C., (2019). Synthesis of Iron Nanoparticles from aqueous extract of *Eucalyptus robusta* Sm. and evaluation of antioxidant and antimicrobial activity. *Materials Science for Energy Technologies.* doi: 10.1016/j.mset.2019.10.014.

120. Sravanthi, K., Ayodhya, D., & Yadgiri, S. P., (2018). Green synthesis, characterization of biomaterial-supported zero-valent iron nanoparticles for contaminated water

treatment. *Journal of Analytical Science and Technology, 9,* 3. doi: 10.1186/s40543-017-0134-9.

121. Wang, Z., Fang, C., & Megharaj, M., (2014). Characterization of iron-polyphenol nanoparticles synthesized by three plant extracts and their Fenton oxidation of azo dye. *ACS Sustainable Chemistry and Engineering, 2*(4), 1022–1025. doi: 10.1021/sc500021n.

122. Kanagasubbulakshmi, S., & Kadirvelu, K., (2017). Green synthesis of iron oxide nanoparticles using *Lagenaria siceraria* and evaluation of its antimicrobial activity. *Defense Life Science Journal, 2*(4), 422–427. doi: 10.14429/dlsj.2.12277.

123. Soliemanzadeh, A., Fekri, M., Bakhtiary, S., & Mehrizi, M. H., (2016). Biosynthesis of iron nanoparticles and their application in removing phosphorus from aqueous solutions. *Chemical Ecology, 32*(3), 286–300. doi: 10.1080/02757540.2016.1139091.

124. Singh, A., Singh, N. B., Hussain, I., & Singh, H., (2017). Effect of biologically synthesized copper oxide nanoparticles on metabolism and antioxidant activity to the crop plants *Solanum lycopersicum* and *Brassica oleracea* var. botrytis. *Journal of Biotechnology, 262,* 11–27. doi: 10.1016/j.jbiotec.2017.09.016.

125. Hassanien, R., Husein, D. Z., & Al-Hakkani, M. F., (2018). Biosynthesis of copper nanoparticles using aqueous *Tilia* extract: Antimicrobial and anticancer activities. *Heliyon, 4*(12), e01077. doi: 10.1016/j.heliyon.2018.e01077.

126. Chung, I., Abdul, R. A., Marimuthu, S., Vishnu, K. A., Anbarasan, K., Padmini, P., & Rajakumar, G., (2017). Green synthesis of copper nanoparticles using *Ecliptica prostrata* leaves extract and their antioxidant and cytotoxic activities. *Experimental and Therapeutic Medicine, 14,* 18–24. doi: 10.3892/etm.2017.4466.

127. Sivaraj, R., Rahman, P. K. S. M., Rajiv, P., Salam, H. A., & Venckatesh, R., (2014). Biogenic copper oxide nanoparticles synthesis using *Tabernaemontana* divaricate leaf extract and its antibacterial activity against urinary tract pathogen. *Spectrochimica Acta Part A: Molecular and Biomolecular Spectroscopy, 133,* 178–181. doi: 10.1016/j.saa.2014.05.048.

128. Khani, R., Roostaei, B., Bagherzade, G., & Moudi, M., (2018). Green synthesis of copper nanoparticles by fruit extract of *Ziziphus spina-christi* (L.) Willd.: Application for adsorption of triphenylmethane dye and antibacterial assay. *Journal of Molecular Liquids, 255,* 541–549. doi: 10.1016/j.molliq.2018.02.010.

129. Nazar, N., Bibi, I., Kamal, S., Iqbal, M., Nouren, S., Jilani, K., & Ata, S., (2018). Cu nanoparticles synthesis using biological molecule of P. granatum seeds extract as reducing and capping agent: Growth mechanism and photo-catalytic activity. *International Journal of Biological Macromolecules, 106,* 1203–1210. doi: 10.1016/j.ijbiomac.2017.08.126.

130. Rehana, D., Mahendiran, D., Kumar, R. S., & Rahiman, A. K., (2017). Evaluation of antioxidant and anticancer activity of copper oxide nanoparticles synthesized using medicinally important plant extracts. *Biomedicine and Pharmacotherapy, 89,* 1067–1077. doi: 10.1016/j.biopha.2017.02.101.

131. Aritonang, H. F., Koleangan, H., & Wuntu, A. D., (2019). Synthesis of silver nanoparticles using aqueous extract of medicinal plants' (*Impatiens balsamina* and *Lantana camara*) fresh leaves and analysis of antimicrobial activity. *International Journal of Microbiology,* 1–8. doi: 10.1155/2019/8642303.

132. Singh, C., Kumar, J., Kumar, P., Chauhan, B. S., Tiwari, K. N., Mishra, S. K., & Singh, J., (2019). Green synthesis of silver nanoparticles using aqueous leaf extract of *Premna integrifolia* (L.) rich in polyphenols and evaluation of their antioxidant, antibacterial and cytotoxic activity. *Biotechnology and Biotechnological Equipment*, 1–13. doi: 10.1080/13102818.2019.1577699.

133. Jain, S., & Mehata, M. S., (2017). Medicinal plant leaf extract and pure flavonoid mediated green synthesis of silver nanoparticles and their enhanced antibacterial property. *Sci. Rep., 7*, 15867. doi: 10.1038/s41598-017-15724-8.

134. Ambika, S., & Sundrarajan, M., (2015). Antibacterial behavior of Vitex negundo extract assisted ZnO nanoparticles against pathogenic bacteria. *Journal of Photochemistry and Photobiology B: Biology, 146*, 52–57. doi: 10.1016/j.jphotobiol.2015.02.020.

135. Bhuyan, T., Mishra, K., Khanuja, M., Prasad, R., & Varma, A., (2015). Biosynthesis of zinc oxide nanoparticles from *Azadirachta indica* for antibacterial and photocatalytic applications. *Materials Science in Semiconductor Processing, 32*, 55–61. doi: 10.1016/j.mssp.2014.12.053.

136. Sadeghi, B., & Gholamhoseinpoor, F., (2015). A study on the stability and green synthesis of silver nanoparticles using *Ziziphora tenuior* (Zt) extract at room temperature. *Spectrochimica Acta Part A: Molecular and Biomolecular Spectroscopy, 134*, 310–315. doi: 10.1016/j.saa.2014.06.046.

137. Morel, A. L., Giraud, S., Bialecki, A., Moustaoui, H., De La Chapelle, M. L., & Spadavecchia, J., (2017). Green extraction of endemic plants to synthesize gold nanoparticles for theranostic applications. *Frontiers in Laboratory Medicine, 1*, 158–171. doi: 10.1016/j.flm.2017.10.003.

138. Nasrollahzadeh, M., & Sajadi, S. M., (2015). Preparation of Au nanoparticles by anthemis xylopoda flowers aqueous extract and their application for alkyne/aldehyde/amine A3-type coupling reactions. *RSC Advances, 5*, 46240–46246. doi: 10.1039/c5ra08927a.

139. Nasrollahzadeh, M., Maham, M., Rostami-Vartooni, A., Bagherzadeh, M., & Sajadi, S. M., (2015). Barberry fruit extract assisted in situ green synthesis of Cu nanoparticles supported on a reduced graphene oxide: $Fe_3O_4$ nanocomposite as a magnetically separable and reusable catalyst for the O-arylation of phenols with aryl halides under ligand-free conditions. *RSC Advances, 5*, 64769–64780. doi: 10.1039/c5ra10037b.

140. Nasrollahzadeh, M., Momeni, S. S., & Sajadi, S. M., (2017). Green synthesis of copper nanoparticles using *Plantago asiatica* leaf extract and their application for the cyanation of aldehydes using $K_4Fe(CN)_6$. *Journal of Colloid and Interface Science, 506*, 471–477. doi: 10.1016/j.jcis.2017.07.072.

141. Nasrollahzadeh, M., Atarod, M., & Sajadi, S. M., (2017). Biosynthesis, characterization and catalytic activity of $Cu/RGO/Fe_3O_4$ for direct cyanation of aldehydes with $K_4[Fe(CN)_6]$. *Journal of Colloid and Interface Science, 486*, 153–162. doi: 10.1016/j.jcis.2016.09.053.

142. Nava, O. J., Luque, P. A., Gómez-Gutiérrez, C. M., Vilchis-Nestor, A. R., Castro-Beltrán, A., Mota-González, M. L., & Olivas, A., (2017). Influence of Camellia sinensis extract on zinc oxide nanoparticle green synthesis. *Journal of Molecular Structure, 1134*, 121–125. doi: 10.1016/j.molstruc.2016.12.069.

143. Luo, F., Yang, D., Chen, Z., Megharaj, M., & Naidu, R., (2015). The mechanism for degrading Orange II based on adsorption and reduction by ion-based nanoparticles synthesized by grape leaf extract. *Journal of Hazardous Materials, 296*, 37–45. doi: 10.1016/j.jhazmat.2015.04.027.

144. Yugandhar, P., Vasavi, T., & Jayavardhana, R. Y., (2018). Cost effective, green synthesis of copper oxide nanoparticles using fruit extract of *Syzygium alternifolium* (Wt.) Walp., characterization and evaluation of antiviral activity, *Journal of Cluster Science, 29*, 743–755. doi: 10.1007/s10876-018-1395-1.

145. Kumar, P. P. N. V., Shameem, U., Kollu, P., Kalyani, R. L., & Pammi, S. V. N., (2015). Green synthesis of copper oxide nanoparticles using aloe vera leaf extract and its antibacterial activity against fish bacterial pathogens. *Bio. Nano Science, 5*, 135–139. doi: 10.1007/s12668015–0171-z.

146. Sharma, P., Pant, S., Dave, V., Tak, K., Sadhu, V., & Reddy, K. R., (2019). Green synthesis and characterization of copper nanoparticles by *Tinospora cardifolia* to produce nature-friendly copper nano-coated fabric and their antimicrobial evaluation. *Journal of Microbiological Methods, 160*, 107–116. doi: 10.1016/j.mimet.2019.03.007.

147. Gondwal, M., & Joshi, N. P. G., (2018). Synthesis and catalytic and biological activities of silver and copper nanoparticles using cassia occidentalis. *International Journal of Biomaterials*, 1–10. doi: 10.1155/2018/6735426.

148. Umaralikhan, L., & Jamal, M. J. M., (2016). Green synthesis of MgO nanoparticles and it antibacterial activity. *Iranian Journal of Science and Technology, Transactions A: Science, 42*(2), 477–485. doi: 10.1007/s40995-016-0041-8.

149. Ramesh, M., Anbuvannan, M., & Viruthagiri, G., (2014). Green synthesis of ZnO nanoparticles using Solanum nigrum leaf extract and their antibacterial activity. *Spectrochimica Acta Part A: Molecular and Biomolecular Spectroscopy, 136*, 864–870. doi: 10.1016/j.saa.2014.09.105.

150. Chaudhuri, S. K., & Malodia, L., (2017). Biosynthesis of zinc oxide nanoparticles using leaf extract of *Calotropis gigantea*: Characterization and its evaluation on tree seedling growth in nursery stage. *Applied Nanoscience, 7*, 501–512. doi: 10.1007/ s13204-017-0586-7.

151. Nagajyothi, P. C., Cha, S. J., Yang, I. J., Sreekanth, T. V. M., Kim, K. J., & Shin, H. M., (2015). Antioxidant and anti-inflammatory activities of zinc oxide nanoparticles synthesized using *Polygala tenuifolia* root extract. *Journal of Photochemistry and Photobiology B: Biology, 146*, 10–17. doi: 10.1016/j.jphotobiol.2015.02.008.

152. Murali, M., Mahendra, C., Nagabhushan, Rajashekar, N., Sudarshana, M. S., Raveesha, K. A., & Amruthesh, K. N., (2017). Antibacterial and antioxidant properties of biosynthesized zinc oxide nanoparticles from *Ceropegia candelabrum* L.: An endemic species. *Spectrochimica Acta Part A: Molecular and Biomolecular Spectroscopy, 179*, 104–109. doi: 10.1016/j.saa.2017.02.027.

153. Santhoshkumar, J., Kumar, S. V., & Rajeshkumar, S., (2017). Synthesis of zinc oxide nanoparticles using plant leaf extract against urinary tract infection pathogen. *Resource-Efficient Technologies, 3/4*, 459–465. doi: 10.1016/j.reffit.2017.05.001.

154. Mohan, K. K., Mandal, B. K., Siva, K. K., Sreedhara, R., P., & Sreedhar, B., (2013). Biobased green method to synthesize palladium and iron nanoparticles using

*Terminalia chebula* aqueous extract. *Spectrochimica Acta Part A: Molecular and Biomolecular Spectroscopy, 102,* 128–133. doi: 10.1016/j.saa.2012.10.015.

155. Devatha, C. P. Jagadeesh, K., & Patil, M., (2018). Effect of green synthesized iron nanoparticles by *Azardirachta indica* in different proportions on antibacterial activity. *Environmental Nanotechnology, Monitoring, and Management, 9,* 85–94. doi: 10.1016/j.enmm.2017.11.007.

156. Saranya, S., Vijayarani, K., & Pavithra, S., (2017). Green synthesis of iron nanoparticles using aqueous extract of *Musa ornata* flower sheath against pathogenic bacteria. *Indian Journal of Pharmaceutical Sciences, 79*(5), 688–694. www.ijpsonline.com (accessed on 10 November 2020).

157. Radini, I. A., Hasan, N., Malik, M. A., & Khan, Z., (2018). Biosynthesis of iron nanoparticles using *Trigonella foenum-graecum* seed extracts for photocatalytic methyl orange dye degradation and antibacterial applications. *Journal of Photochemistry and Photobiology B: Biology, 183,* 154–163. doi: 10.1016/j.jphotobiol.2018.04.014.

158. Da'na, E., Taha, A., & Afkar, E., (2018). Green synthesis of iron nanoparticles by *Acacia* nilotica pods extract and its catalytic, adsorption, and antibacterial activities. *Applied Sciences, 8,* 1922. doi: 10.3390/app8101922.

159. Samrot, A. V., Senthilkumar, P., Rashmitha, S., Veera, P., & Sahithya, C. S., (2018). *Azadirachta indica* influenced biosynthesis of super-paramagnetic iron-oxide nanoparticles and their applications in tannery water treatment and x-ray imaging. *Journal of Nanostructure in Chemistry, 8,* 343–351. doi: 10.1007/s40097-018-0279-0.

160. Jagathesan, G., & Rajiv, P., (2018). Biosynthesis and characterization of iron oxide nanoparticles using *Eichhornia crassipes* leaf extract and assessing their antibacterial activity. *Biocatalysis and Agricultural Biotechnology, 13,* 90–94. doi: 10.1016/j.bcab.2017.11.014.

# Index

## N

For Product Safety Concerns and Information please contact our EU
representative GPSR@taylorandfrancis.com
Taylor & Francis Verlag GmbH, Kaufingerstraße 24, 80331 München, Germany